NUTRITIONAL NEEDS IN HOT ENVIRONMENTS

Applications for Military Personnel in Field Operations

Committee on Military Nutrition Research

Food and Nutrition Board
Institute of Medicine

Bernadette M. Marriott, Editor

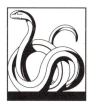

NATIONAL ACADEMY PRESS
Washington, D.C.   1993

NATIONAL ACADEMY PRESS • 2101 Constitution Avenue, N.W. • Washington, D.C. 20418

NOTICE: The project that is the subject of this report was approved by the Governing Board of the National Research Council, whose members are drawn from the councils of the National Academy of Sciences, the National Academy of Engineering, and the Institute of Medicine. The members of the committee responsible for the report were chosen for their special competencies and with regard for appropriate balance. Part I of this report has been reviewed by a group other than the authors according to procedures approved by a Report Review Committee consisting of members of the National Academy of Sciences, the National Academy of Engineering, and the Institute of Medicine.

The Institute of Medicine was established in 1970 by the National Academy of Sciences to enlist distinguished members of the appropriate professions in the examination of policy matters pertaining to the health of the public. In this, the Institute acts under both the Academy's 1863 congressional charter responsibility to be an adviser to the federal government and its own initiative in identifying issues of medical care, research, and education. Dr. Kenneth R. Shine is president of the Institute of Medicine.

This report was produced under grants DAMD17-86-G-6036/R and DAMD17-92-J-2003 between the National Academy of Sciences and the U.S. Army Medical Research and Development Command. The views, opinions, and/or findings contained in chapters in Parts II and III that are authored by U.S. Army personnel are those of the authors and should not be construed as official Department of the Army positions, policies, or decisions, unless so designated by other official documentation. Human subjects who participated in studies described in those chapters gave their free and informed voluntary consent. Investigators adhered to U.S. Army regulation 70-25 and United States Army Medical Research and Development Command regulation 70-25 on use of volunteers in research. Citations of commercial organizations and trade names in this report do not constitute an official Department of the Army endorsement or approval of the products or services of these organizations. The chapters are approved for public release; distribution is unlimited.

The serpent has been a symbol of long life, healing, and knowledge among almost all cultures and religions since the beginning of recorded history. The image adopted as a logotype by the Institute of Medicine is based on a relief carving from ancient Greece, now held by the Staatlichemuseen in Berlin.

COMMITTEE ON MILITARY NUTRITION RESEARCH

FOOD AND NUTRITION BOARD

Staff

CATHERINE E. WOTEKI, Director
MARCIA S. LEWIS, Administrative Assistant
SUSAN M. WYATT, Financial Associate

Preface

This publication, *Nutritional Needs in Hot Environments*, is another in a series of reports based on workshops sponsored by the Committee on Military Nutrition Research (CMNR) of the Food and Nutrition Board (FNB), Institute of Medicine, National Academy of Sciences. Other workshops or mini-symposia have included such topics as body composition and physical performance, nutrition and physical performance, cognitive testing methodology, and fluid replacement and heat stress. These workshops form a part of the response that the CMNR provides to the Assistant Surgeon General of the Army regarding issues brought to the committee through the Military Nutrition Division of the U.S. Army Institute of Environmental Medicine (USARIEM) at Natick, Massachusetts.

FOCUS OF THE REPORT

The timing of the request in the late fall of 1990 from the Nutrition Division of the U.S. Army Institute of Environmental Medicine (USARIEM) to examine the topic of nutritional needs in hot environments was undoubtedly influenced by the initiation of Operation Desert Shield (later Desert Storm) and the deployment of military personnel in the harsh desert environment of the Middle East. The ability of troops to perform under these extreme conditions was naturally a matter of concern to military commanders.

The past 50 years have produced only a limited number of studies focused on the influence of heat on nutrient requirements and work performance that can be directly applied to military nutrition issues (see the selected bibliography in Appendix B). Recent military-based research has been concerned with nutrient and caloric requirements for work in cold environments (cf. Edwards et al., 1990a,b; Morgan et al., 1988). In 1990, the CMNR produced the report of a workshop, *Fluid Replacement and Heat Stress* (Marriott and Rosement, 1991), which presented a general review of fluid intake and replacement and also specifically addressed concerns related to military combat activities in both temperate and warm conditions. This report and the previous work of military researchers at the USARIEM formed the basis for the nutritional advice contained in the pocket guide prepared by USARIEM staff for personnel involved in Operation Desert Storm (Glenn et al., 1990).

The present report builds further on *Fluid Replacement and Heat Stress* and summarizes the current state of knowledge about the influence of high temperatures on nutrient requirements—other than water—for work in hot environments. It also identifies specific areas for additional study. The report discusses as well some of the important issues in delivering nutrients to military personnel through combat field feeding systems. During Operation Desert Storm, Army food scientists prepared an initial review of hot weather feeding and provided recommendations related to feeding and food management issues (Norman and Gaither, 1991).

HISTORY OF THE COMMITTEE

The Committee on Military Nutrition Research (CMNR) was established in October 1982 following a request by the Assistant Surgeon General of the Army that the Food and Nutrition Board of the National Academy of Sciences set up a committee to advise the U.S. Department of Defense on the need for and conduct of nutrition research and on related issues. The committee's tasks are to identify nutritional factors that may critically influence the physical and mental performance of military personnel under all environmental extremes; to identify deficiencies in the existing data base; to recommend research that would remedy these deficiencies and approaches for studying the relationship of diet to physical and mental performance; and to review and advise on standards for military feeding systems. Within this context the CMNR was asked to focus on nutrient requirements for performance during combat missions rather than requirements for military personnel in garrison. (The latter were judged as not significantly different from those of the civilian population.)

Although the membership of the committee has changed periodically, the disciplines represented have consistently included human nutrition, nutritional biochemistry, performance physiology, food science, and psychology. For issues that require broader expertise than exists within the committee, the CMNR has convened workshops. These workshops provide additional state-of-the-art scientific information and informed opinion for the consideration of the committee in its evaluation of the issues at hand.

COMMITTEE TASK AND PROCEDURES

In late 1990, personnel from the USARIEM requested that the CMNR examine the current state of knowledge concerning the influence of a hot environment on nutrient requirements of military personnel. The nutritional needs of the thousands of troops deployed to the desert environment of Saudi Arabia and other areas of the Middle East for Operation Desert Storm made this an especially urgent issue. A parallel concern was to ensure that performance would not decline as a result of inadequate nutrition.

The committee was aware of the limited studies conducted on this topic for or by the military since World War II. It decided that the best way to review the state of knowledge in this diverse area was through a small workshop at which knowledgeable researchers could review published research and provide an update on current knowledge. Such a workshop would enable the CMNR to review the adequacy of the current nutrient specifications for military operational rations and to identify gaps in the knowledge base that might be filled by future research.

A subgroup of the committee met in December 1990, determined the key topics for review, identified speakers with expertise in these topics, and planned the workshop for April 1991. Invited speakers were asked to prepare a review paper on their assigned topic for presentation and publication and to identify gaps in the data base. The CMNR also believed that it would be beneficial to obtain actual observations from a military field research team to aid in evaluating the performance of current field feeding systems used in Operation Desert Storm. The stress on logistical systems during the operation did not permit fielding a research group specifically for this purpose; however, the committee identified two speakers who were in the operation theater on other assignments and who presented informal commentary at the workshop on troop feeding during Operation Desert Storm. In addition, four scientists who had conducted a controlled research project at the USARIEM on dietary sodium levels during heat acclimation presented their results.

At the workshop, each speaker gave a formal presentation, which was followed by questions and a brief discussion period. The proceedings were tape-recorded and professionally transcribed. At the end of the presentations, a general discussion of the overall topic was held. The next day, the CMNR met in executive session to review the issues, draw some tentative conclusions, and assign the preparation of draft reviews and summaries of specific topics to individual committee members. Committee members subsequently met in a series of working sessions and worked separately and together using the authored papers and additional reference material to draft the summary and recommendations. The final report was reviewed and approved by the entire group. These working sessions included Andre Bensadoun, Bill Evans, Joel Grinker, Richard Jansen, Gil Levielle, John Milner, and Allison Yates. At the request of the committee chairman, Allison Yates developed a summary paper for the committee to stimulate discussion and raise important questions primarily related to heat, food intake, and appetite. This discussion paper is included in Chapter 15 in Part IV.

The summary and recommendations of the Committee on Military Nutrition Research constitute Part I of this volume, and the papers presented at the workshop make up Parts II and III. Part I has been reviewed anonymously by an outside group with expertise in the topic area and experience in military issues. The authored papers in Parts II, III, and IV have undergone limited editorial change, have not been reviewed by the outside group, and represent the views of the individual authors. Selected questions directed toward the speakers and their responses are provided at the end of each chapter to give an indication of the discussion after each presentation. The invited speakers were also requested to submit a brief list of selected background papers prior to the workshop. These recommended readings, as well as relevant citations obtained through a computerized literature search, and the citations from each chapter are included in the Selected Bibliography (Appendix B).

ACKNOWLEDGMENTS

It is my pleasure as chairman of the CMNR to acknowledge the contributions of the FNB staff, particularly the excellent technical and organizational skills of Bernadette Marriott, Ph.D., the FNB program director for the CMNR. Her assistance in organizing the workshop, and in bringing the proceedings to the point of publication, is greatly appreciated. I wish to acknowledge as well the fine contributions by the workshop speakers and their commitment to participate and prepare detailed review papers on relatively short notice. The CMNR appreciates the assistance of COL E. Wayne Askew and others from the USARIEM for their assistance in identifying issues of concern to the military and obtaining the involvement of the military personnel who participated in the workshop. COL David Schnakenberg's scientific expertise and his historical knowledge of relevant military studies contributed significantly, as in the past, to the success of this workshop. An earlier summary of the history of the Military Recommended Dietary Allowances, prepared by COL Schnakenberg, was invaluable in developing this report. The critiques of the anonymous reviewers and Food and Nutrition Board liaison member, Johanna Dwyer, in addition to comments by

FNB director Catherine Woteki, provided helpful insight in the development of this final document. The editorial efforts of Judy Grumstrup-Scott and Leah Mazade are gratefully acknowledged. The assistance of Valerie Breen, CMNR project assistant, and Connie Rosemont, FNB research assistant, in word processing, editing, and proofreading this report is greatly appreciated.

Finally, I am grateful to the members of the committee who participated significantly in the discussions at the workshop and in the preparation of the summaries of the proceedings. In particular, I want to thank former committee members Andre Bensadoun and Bill Evans who wrote substantive portions of the initial drafts of Chapter 1. The commitment of the members of this committee, who serve without compensation, to provide sound, timely recommendations for consideration by the military, is commendable. I am personally inspired by my work with this group of dedicated professionals.

ROBERT O. NESHEIM, *Chairman*
Committee on Military Nutrition Research

REFERENCES

Edwards, J.S.A., D.R. Roberts, J. Edinberg, and T.E. Morgan
1990a   The Meal, Ready-to-Eat Consumed in a Cold Environment. Report No. T9-90. United States Army Research Institute of Environmental Medicine. Natick, Mass.
Edwards, J.S.A., D.C. Roberts, S.H. Mutter, and R.J. Moore
1990b   A Comparison of the Meal, Ready-to-Eat VIII with Supplemental Pack and the Ration, Cold Weather Consumed in an Arctic Environment. Report No. T21-90. United States Army Research Institute of Environmental Medicine. Natick, Mass.
Glenn, J.R.,R.E. Burr, R.W. Hubbard, M.Z. Mays, R.J. Moore, B.H. Jones, and G.P. Krueger, eds.
1990   Sustaining Health and Performance in the Desert: A Pocket Guide to Environmental Medicine for Operations in Southwest Asia. Technical Note 91-2. United States Army Research Institute of Environmental Medicine. Natick, Mass.
Marriott, B.M., and C. Rosemont, eds.
1991   Fluid Replacement and Heat Stress: Proceedings of a Workshop. Second printing. Washington, D.C.: National Academy Press.
Morgan, T.E., L.A. Hodgess, D. Schilling, R.W. Hoyt, E.J. Iwanyk, G. McAninch, T.C. Wells, and E.W. Askew
1988   A Comparison of the Meal, Ready-to-Eat, Ration, Cold Weather, and Ration, Lightweight Nutrient Intakes During Moderate Altitude Cold Weather Field Training Operations. Report No. T5-89. United States Army Research Institute of Environmental Medicine. Natick, Mass.
Norman, E.J., and R.M. Gaither
1991   Review of Army Food Related Operations in Hot Desert Environments. Technical Report Natick/TR-91/008. United States Army Natick Research, Development and Engineering Center. Natick, Mass.

Contents

PART I

Committee Summary
and Recommendations

OVERVIEW

PART I CONSISTS OF TWO CHAPTERS. Chapter 1 provides the background for the report. It describes the task presented to the Committee on Military Nutrition Research (CMNR) by the Military Nutrition Division, U.S. Army Institute for Environmental Medicine (USARIEM), U.S. Army Medical Research and Development Command; summarizes the relevant background material; and presents the committee's findings. The Army posed 11 questions to the committee; these questions are also listed in Chapter 1. In addition, this chapter presents an overview of the relevant areas of concern, a review of current military dietary standards, and a summary of the committee's interpretation of the current scientific knowledge in these areas. Chapter 2 presents the committee's answers to the questions posed by the Army and its conclusions. Chapter 2 also includes specific and general recommendations developed by the CMNR.

1

Introduction and Background

THE COMMITTEE'S TASK

The Committee on Military Nutrition Research (CMNR) of the Food and Nutrition Board (FNB), Institute of Medicine (IOM), National Academy of Sciences (NAS), was asked by the Division of Military Nutrition, U.S. Army Institute of Environmental Medicine (USARIEM), U.S. Army Medical Research and Development Command (USARMRDC), to review current research pertaining to nutrient requirements for working in hot environments and to comment on how this information might be applied to military nutrient standards and military rations. The committee was thus tasked with providing a thorough review of the literature in this area and with interpreting these diverse data in terms of military applications. In addition to a focus on specific nutrient needs in hot climates, the committee was asked to consider factors that might change food intake patterns and therefore overall calories. The CMNR was presented with this problem as a direct result of the movement of the Armed Forces into Saudi Arabia in Operation Desert Shield in the autumn of 1990; the committee was organizing the workshop that resulted in this report while the American Armed Forces were actively engaged in Operation Desert Storm in early 1991. Although concern for adequate nutrition for U.S. soldiers in Saudi Arabia prompted the initiation of this project, its scope was defined as including the nutrient needs of individuals who may be actively working in both hot-dry and hot-moist climates.

The CMNR was asked to address the following questions:

1. What is the evidence that there are any significant changes in nutrient requirements for work in a hot environment?

2. If such evidence exists, do the current Military Recommended Dietary Allowances provide for these changes?

3. Should changes be made in military rations that may be used in hot environments to meet the nutrient requirements of soldiers with sustained activity in such climates?

4. Specifically, are the meals, ready-to-eat (MREs) good hot-weather rations? Should the fat content be lower? Should the carbohydrate content be higher?

5. What factors may influence food intake in hot environments?

6. To what extent does fluid intake influence food intake?

7. Is there any scientific evidence that food preferences change in hot climates?

8. Are there special nutritional concerns in desert environments in which the daily temperature may change dramatically?

9. Is there an increased need for specific vitamins or minerals in the heat?

10. Does working in a hot climate change an individual's absorptive or digestive capability?

11. Does work at a moderate to heavy rate increase energy requirements in a hot environment to a greater extent than similar work in a temperate environment?

To assist the CMNR in responding to these questions, a workshop was convened on April 11-12, 1991, that included presentations from individuals familiar with or having expertise in digestive physiology, energetics, macronutrients, vitamins, minerals, appetite, psychology, sociology, and olfaction. The invited speakers discussed their presentations with committee members at the workshop and submitted the content of their verbal presentations as written reports. The committee met after the workshop to discuss the issues raised and the information provided. The CMNR later reviewed the workshop presentations and drew on its collective expertise and the scientific literature to develop the following summary, conclusions, and recommendations.

MILITARY RECOMMENDED DIETARY ALLOWANCES

History

The history of the Military Recommended Dietary Allowances (MRDAs) is related to the history of both the Recommended Dietary Allowances (RDAs) and the Food and Nutrition Board of the National Academy of Sciences. The Food and Nutrition Division, Office of the Surgeon General, U.S. Army, was established in 1917 to (1) safeguard the nutritional interests of the Army; (2) inspect food supplied to the Army to ensure the proper amount and distribution of nutrients; and (3) obtain data on which to base intelligent alterations of military rations. During World War I, the Food and Nutrition Division of the Army conducted nutrition surveys at Army training camps to determine food consumption and wastage. Based on these early surveys, the first recommended nutrient requirements for the training of soldiers were developed in 1919. They were listed as follows: protein, 12.5 percent kcal; fat, 25 percent kcal; and carbohydrate, 62.5 percent kcal (Murlin and Miller, 1919).

During World War II the responsibilities for nutrition of the Office of the Surgeon General were expanded to provide more direct nutrition guidance. In 1940 the Food and Nutrition Board (FNB) of the National Academy of Sciences was organized in conjunction with the defense program to help the Army establish a satisfactory standard for operational rations. From 1943 until 1947 the Surgeon General's Office accepted diets as nutritionally adequate if they met the recommended allowances of the FNB. Beginning with Army Regulation (AR) 40-250 Nutrition (October 28, 1947), the Office of the Surgeon General initiated the first use of a specified "Minimum Nutrient Intake" for military personnel. These standards incorporated an adjusted caloric standard for the extreme cold.

The military nutrient standards were patterned after the current FNB Recommended Dietary Allowances (RDAs) with modifications to meet the needs of Army personnel beginning with AR 4-564 (February 9, 1956). The first Tri-Service regulation (AR 40-25, 1968) based on the RDAs with modifications was issued on July 2, 1968. The military nutrition standards were first termed "Military Recommended Dietary Allowances" with the May 15, 1985, revision of AR 40-25. The CMNR provided commentary to the Army during the revision process. This regulation also designated the Army Surgeon General as the Department of Defense (DOD) Executive Agent for Nutrition for the military. The 1985 MRDAs are adapted from the ninth edition of the RDAs (NRC, 1980) and are the current standard for all branches of the military.

Current MRDAs

The MRDA regulation (AR 40-25, 1985) is presently under revision.[1] The revised standards will reflect changes in the nutrition knowledge base,

---

[1] At the request of the Army Medical Research and Development Command representative, the Committee on Military Nutrition Research held a meeting on November 27, 1990, at the

changes in the RDAs based on the tenth edition (NRC, 1989b), and military nutrition initiatives for the twenty-first century. AR 40-25 (1985) not only lists the nutrient standards but includes definitions of terminology, guidelines for healthful diets, and clarification of the use of the MRDAs for menu planning, dietary evaluations, nutrition education, and food research and development in the military. A separate table provides nutritional standards for operational and restricted rations. AR 40-25 is included in full in Appendix A.

One purpose of the present study was to comment on the applicability of the current MRDAs for work in hot environments. Table 1-1 is a comparison of the nutrient recommendations in the latest edition of the RDAs (NRC, 1989b) and those in AR 40-25 (1985). Table 1-2 compares the estimated safe and adequate ranges for selected vitamins and minerals from the same two sources. These tables provide a reference for the physiological and nutrient-by-nutrient discussion that follows.

PHYSIOLOGICAL CHANGES ARISING FROM EXERCISE AND HEAT

For the most part, reported studies in the areas of physiology and gastrointestinal function have examined the effect on physiological function of an increased core temperature, whether as a result of exercise or increased ambient temperature. In only a few cases are the effects of exercise on body core temperature compared with the effects of a hot environment alone, whether in exercising or resting people. A few studies are described in the historical perspective in Chapter 6. Important physiological considerations related to performance are reviewed below.

Exercise

Muscular exercise can increase metabolism by up to 15 times the basal rate (see discussion in Chapter 3). Most of the heat resulting from this level of energy expenditure needs to be removed to maintain thermostasis. Heat loss occurs through both insensible (evaporative) and sensible (radiative and convective) mechanisms. These are controlled by a thermoregulatory center in the hypothalamus; this center, through the autonomic nervous system, controls heat transfer from the body core to the skin primarily via

---

National Academy of Sciences in Washington, D.C., to discuss the status and the direction of the revision of the MRDAs. Dietitians and representatives from the Army, Navy, Air Force, Marines, and Coast Guard attended and discussed specific service-based concerns regarding MRDA revisions and issues related to military nutrition initiatives for the future. They also covered garrison menu planning and general implementation of the MRDAs in various non-garrison military settings.

blood circulation. The increased blood flow to the surface raises the temperature of the skin and allows sensible heat loss by radiative and convective mechanisms. Evaporative heat loss occurs through sweating (see Chapters 3, 4, and 5).

Heavy exercise at increased ambient temperatures decreases the skin-to-ambient-temperature gradient, thus substantially decreasing sensible heat loss. Under these conditions, most heat loss by the body will occur through evaporative cooling (i.e., sweating). As is well known, heat loss by this mechanism can be greatly decreased under conditions of high humidity. The resulting dehydration from excess sweating can reduce blood volume and cardiac filling. If compensatory circulatory and cardiac changes are insufficient, skin and muscle blood flow will be impaired, thus reducing sensible heat loss and physical performance. A state of adequate hydration is therefore important in maintaining the effectiveness of the physiological mechanisms involved in heat dissipation.

Heat Stress

Thermoregulation can be defined as the summation of the mechanisms by which the body adapts to a heat stress in order to maintain thermoneutrality. Body core and skin temperatures have been used as indices of the ability of the body to thermoregulate, along with cardiovascular changes in heart rate, blood volume (see Harrison, 1985, for a comprehensive review) and blood pressure, with sweat rate as a visible mechanism of adaptation. Acclimatization is the process of adapting to prolonged exposure to a new environment, so that the mechanisms that result in initial responses are modified to allow increased endurance with less strain on body functions.

The ability to defend one's body temperature against heat stress is influenced by level of activity, acclimatization state, aerobic fitness, and hydration level. In heat-acclimatized[2] individuals, the thermoregulatory mechanisms involved in dissipating heat become fully operative. Although some investigators report that to perform a given submaximal exercise task the metabolic rate is greater in a hot compared to a temperate environment (Consolazio et al., 1961, 1963; Dimri et al., 1980, Fink et al., 1975), other investigators report lower metabolic rates in the heat (Brouha et al., 1960; Petersen and Vejby-Christensen, 1973; Williams et al., 1962; Young et al., 1985). A person's state of heat acclimatization does not account for whether individuals demonstrate an increased or decreased metabolic rate during submaximal exercise in the heat; other mechanisms explain this discrep-

---

[2]The term heat acclimatization is used here to refer to the adaptive changes that occur due to exposure to a hot natural environment; heat acclimation will be used to refer to adaptive changes to a hot environment under controlled conditions, such as in an environmental chamber.

TABLE 1-1 Comparison of the Current Military Recommended Dietary Allowances (MRDAs) (AR 25-40, 1985) That Are Based in Part on the Ninth Edition of the Recommended Dietary Allowances (RDAs) (NRC, 1980) with the Most Recent RDAs (NRC, 1989b)

Nutrient	Unit	MRDAs[a]		RDAs[b]			
		Men (17-50 y)	Women (17-50 y)	Men (19-24 y)	Men (25-50 y)	Women (19-24 y)	Women (25-50 y)
Energy	Kcal	3200 (2800-3600)[c,d]	2400 (2000-2800)[c,d]	2900[e]	2900[e]	2200[e]	2200[e]
	MJ	13.4 (11.7-15.1)	10.0 (8.4-11.7)				
Protein	g	100[f]	80[f]	58	63	46	50
Vitamin A[g]	μg RE	1000	800	1000	1000	800	800
Vitamin D[h]	μg	5-10[i]	5-10[i]	10	5	10	5
Vitamin E[j]	mg TE	10	8	10	10	8	8
Ascorbic Acid	mg	60	60	60	60	60	60
Thiamin (B$_1$)	mg	1.6	1.2	1.5	1.5	1.1	1.1
Riboflavin (B$_2$)	mg	1.9	1.4	1.7	1.7	1.3	1.3
Niacin[k]	mg NE	21	16	19	19	15	15
Vitamin B$_6$	mg	2.2	2.0	2.0	2.0	1.6	1.6
Folacin	μg	400	400	200	200	180	180
Vitamin B$_{12}$	μg	3.0	3.0	2.0	2.0	2.0	2.0
Calcium	mg	800-1200[i]	800-1200[i]	1200	800	1200	800
Phosphorus	mg	800-1200[i]	800-1200[i]	1200	800	1200	800
Magnesium	mg	350-400[i]	300[i]	350	350	280	280
Iron	mg	10-18[i]	18[i]	10	10	15	15
Zinc	mg	15	15	15	15	15	15
Iodine	μg	150	150	150	150	150	150
Sodium	mg	See note[l]	See note[l]	500[m]	500[m]	500[m]	500[m]

[a]MRDA for moderately active military personnel, ages 17 to 50 years, are based in part on the *Recommended Dietary Allowances*, ninth revised edition, 1980. The MRDAs are currently under revision.

[b]For the RDAs, the allowances, expressed as average daily intakes over time, are intended to provide for individual variations among most normal persons as they live in the United States under usual environmental stresses. Diets should be based on a variety of common foods in order to provide other nutrients for which human requirements have been less well defined. See text for detailed discussion of allowances and of nutrients not tabulated. Values are taken from the RDAs, tenth edition (NRC, 1989b).

[c]Energy allowance ranges are estimated to reflect the requirements of 70 percent of the moderately active military population. One megajoule (MJ) equals 239 kcal.

[d]Dietary fat calories should not contribute more than 35 percent of total energy intake.

[e]From Table 3-5 from the RDAs, tenth edition (NRC, 1989b) by using the assumption of light to moderate activity for each age and gender group. These figures were calculated using the World Health Organization (WHO, 1985) equations for resting energy expenditure multiplied by an activity factor as described in the text (NRC, 1989b) pp. 25-33.

[f]Protein allowance is based on an estimated protein requirement of 0.8 g per kilogram (kg) desirable body weight. By using the reference body weight ranges for males of 60 to 79 kilograms and for females of 46 to 63 kilograms, the protein requirement is approximately 48 to 64 grams for males and 37 to 51 grams for females. These amounts have been approximately doubled to reflect the usual protein consumption levels of Americans and to enhance diet acceptability.

[g]One microgram of retinol equivalent (µg RE) equals 1 microgram of retinol, or 6 micrograms beta-carotene, or 5 international units (IU).

[h]As cholecalciferol, 10 micrograms of cholecalciferol equals 400 IU of vitamin D.

[i]High values reflect greater vitamin D, calcium, phosphorus, magnesium, and iron requirements for 17- to 18-year olds than for older ages.

[j]One milligram of alpha-tocopherol equivalent (mg TE) equals 1 milligram d-alpha-tocopherol.

[k]One milligram of niacin equivalent (mg NE) equals 1 milligram niacin or 60 milligram dietary tryptophan.

[l]The safe and adequate levels for dietary sodium intake of 1100 to 3300 mg published in the RDAs (NRC, 1980) are currently impractical and unattainable within military food service systems. However, an average of 1700 milligrams of sodium per 1000 kilocalories of food served is the target for military food service systems. This level equates to a daily sodium intake of approximately 5500 milligrams for males and 4100 milligrams for females. [Note: This comment is based on the ninth edition of the RDAs (NRC, 1980). The MRDAs are currently under revision in light of the 1989 publication of the tenth edition of the RDAs (NRC, 1989b).]

[m]Estimated minimum requirements for healthy persons. No allowance has been included for large, prolonged losses from skin through sweat. There is no evidence that higher intakes confer any health benefit.

SOURCE: Adapted from Table 2-1, MRDA for selected nutrients, p. 2-4 (AR 25-40, 1985) and National Research Council *Recommended Dietary Allowances* (1989b), p. 284, and Tables 3-4, 3-5, and 11-1; pp. 29, 33, and 253.

TABLE 1-2   Comparison of the Estimated Safe and Adequate Daily Dietary Intake Ranges of Selected Vitamins and Minerals from the Military Recommended Dietary Allowances (AR 25-40, 1985) That Are Based in Part on the Ninth Edition of the Recommended Dietary Allowances (RDAs) (NRC, 1980) with the Values from the Tenth Edition of the RDAs (NRC, 1989b)

Nutrient	Unit	From MRDAs[a]	From RDAs[b]
Vitamins			
Vitamin K	μg	70-140	65, 80[c]
Biotin	μg	100-200	30-100
Pantothenic Acid	mg	4-7	4-7
Trace Elements[d]			
Fluoride	mg	1.5-4.0	1.5-4.0
Selenium	μg	50-200	55, 70[c]
Molybdenum	mg	0.15-0.50	0.075-0.250
Copper	mg	2-3	1.5-3.0
Manganese	mg	2.5-5.0	2.0-5.0
Chromium	μg	50-200	50-200
Electrolytes			
Potassium	mg	1875-5625	2000
Chloride	mg	1700-5100	750

[a]MRDAs = Military Recommended Dietary Allowances. Data in this portion of the table are based in part on the *Recommended Dietary Allowances*, ninth edition, 1980, Table 10, "Estimated Safe and Adequate Daily Dietary Intakes of Selected Vitamins and Minerals." Estimated ranges are provided for these nutrients because sufficient information upon which to set a recommended allowance is not available. Values reflect a range of recommended intake over an extended period of time.

[b]RDAs = Recommended Dietary Allowances. Because there is less information on which to base allowances, these figures were not given in the main table of RDA and were provided in the form of ranges of recommended intakes.

[c]First number is the RDA for women aged 19-50; the second number is the RDA for men of the same age range. With the publication of the tenth edition of the RDAs, vitamin K and selenium were moved into the summary chart for recommended, age and gender-based dietary allowances.

[d]Since the toxic levels for many trace elements may be only several times usual intakes, the upper levels for the trace elements given in this table should not be habitually exceeded.

SOURCE: MRDA values adapted from Table 2-2, p. 2-5 (AR 40-25, 1985); RDA values adapted from Table 11-1, p. 253; Summary Table: Estimated Safe and Adequate Daily Dietary Intakes of Selected Vitamins and Minerals, p. 284, and the Recommended Dietary Allowances, tenth edition, 1989, Summary Table, p. 285 (NRC, 1989b).

ancy. Most investigators have only calculated the aerobic metabolic rate during submaximal exercise, ignoring the contribution of anaerobic metabolism to total metabolic rate. Although both increases and decreases have been observed in metabolic rate in the heat, it does not appear that the presence or absence of heat acclimatization has an effect on metabolic rate (see Chapters 3 and 6 for further discussion).

Muscular activity produces an enormous amount of heat, with the amount of heat production directly related to the intensity of exercise (Nadel et al., 1977). The amount of heat production generated by the increased energy metabolism of skeletal muscle during exercise may be as much as 100 times that of inactive muscle. The mechanisms for dissipating this heat are generally well regulated. Although heat loss occurs through evaporation of sweat and by conduction, convection, and radiation, evaporation of sweat is clearly the most effective avenue of heat loss during exercise. The sweat glands are capable of secreting up to 30 grams of sweat per minute, removing approximately 18 kcal of heat in the process. Sweat rate is directly associated with exercise intensity (Maughan, 1985; Nadel et al., 1977).

Gastrointestinal Functioning

It has been reported (see Chapter 4) that gastric emptying and intestinal motility decrease as core temperature increases during exercise and in hypohydration. Some, but not all, investigators have also observed reductions in intestinal absorption of nutrients under these conditions.

Most of the studies on the effects of exercise and heat on gastrointestinal function have been carried out in endurance athletes such as marathon runners. Gastrointestinal symptoms under these conditions are often severe, although transient. They include cramps, belching, gastrointestinal reflux, flatulence, bloody stools, vomiting, diarrhea, and nausea. Mechanisms for these effects are discussed in Chapter 4. The relevance of these findings to the range of physical activity in the military is not at all clear, and the findings appear transient when associated with extreme physical activity. Instances of levels of physical activity in the military approaching those of highly competitive endurance athletes would appear to be the exception rather than the rule.

CHANGES IN NUTRIENT REQUIREMENTS FOR HOT ENVIRONMENTS

Fluid and Dehydration

The requirement for water in a hot environment depends on the amount of fluid loss, which in turn depends on such factors as exercise intensity, exercise duration, environmental conditions (dry heat versus humid heat), state of training and heat acclimatization, sex, and age (see Chapter 5). The increased heat production of exercise, an increased sweat rate, and inadequate hydration predispose soldiers in hot environments to dehydration.

Along with exercise intensity, sweat rate is related to environmental conditions, clothing, and acclimatization state (Shapiro et al., 1982). In hot, dry conditions, water loss from the skin and respiratory surfaces can be as much as 2 to 3 liters per hour (Wenger, 1988). In hot, moist (humid) conditions, sweat losses are measurably less than in hot, dry conditions. In a study that measured physiologic changes and sweat losses in healthy young men during hyperthermia induced by humid heat in an environmental chamber, total sweat losses averaged 7 liters per 24 hours (Beisel et al., 1968). However, humidity per se does not appear to affect core (rectal) temperature (Morimoto, 1967). In terms of military apparel, the nuclear-biological-chemical (NBC) protective clothing worn by many military personnel prevents the normal dissipation of body heat because of the cloth's lack of moisture permeability and its insulating properties. As a result, body temperature may rise excessively, producing high levels of sweat (1 to 2 liters per hour) that cannot evaporate effectively because air turnover is reduced, and caution must be taken (Muza et al., 1988; Pimental et al., 1987).

If the fluid involved in excessive sweat loss is not replaced, total body water, along with the total blood volume, will be decreased. A water loss as small as 1 percent of body weight will induce changes such as increased heart rate during rest and exercise, and decreased performance. However, a 1 percent loss is difficult to discern relative to what might be regarded as initial water balance. Thus, it is hard to attribute physiological changes to a 1 percent loss, but such changes can be readily observed at losses of 2.0 to 2.5 percent. A 10 percent loss of body weight through dehydration[3] is life-threatening (Adolf, 1947). Water loss from the blood leads to a decrease in sweat rates and skin blood flow (Sawka and Pandolph, 1990; Wyndham, 1977), which results in less evaporative cooling and a risk of heat stroke (Wyndham, 1977). The normal compensatory response to exercise and heat stress is increased peripheral blood flow to maximize heat dissipation and prevent hyperthermia. However, in dehydrated individuals with greatly diminished blood volume, skin blood flow is reduced to maintain cardiac output and blood pressure.

Reductions in blood volume can result in a reduced flow of blood to organs during exercise and reduced venous flow in return. This reduced venous return to the heart decreases stroke volume and causes a compensatory increase in the heart rate to maintain cardiac output and blood pressure.

---

[3] The term *dehydration* is used here to refer to the process of losing body water, while the term *hypohydration* will be used to denote the result of the dehydration process.

This reflex increase in heart rate, however, is not sufficient to compensate for the decrease in stroke volume (Rowell et al., 1966); consequently, maximal cardiac output is reduced.

Several studies have shown that cardiovascular performance is compromised following thermal or exercise-induced hypohydration (≤2 percent body weight loss) (Armstrong et al., 1985; Costill et al., 1976; Pitts et al., 1944; Saltin, 1964). Cardiac output is reduced by almost 2 liters per minute with decreased blood volume (Fortney et al., 1983; Nadel et al., 1980). This reduction in cardiac output can almost entirely account for decreases in $V_{O_2 max}$ as a result of hypohydration (Rowell et al., 1966; Saltin, 1964). Significant reductions in physical work capacity have been seen in wrestlers after hypohydration-caused weight loss (Herbert and Ribisl, 1972), as well as in runners after diuretic-induced weight loss (Armstrong et al., 1986).

The acute heat stress in hot climates that causes and is caused by dehydration has been associated with several factors. It can be precipitated by an increase in resting and submaximal exercise metabolic rates (Consolazio et al., 1961, 1963; Dimri et al., 1980; Fink et al., 1975), increases in plasma or muscle lactate levels (Dill et al., 1930; Dimri et al., 1980; Fink et al., 1975; Nadel, 1983; Robinson et al., 1941; Young et al., 1985), and glycogenolysis during submaximal exercise.

Effect of Gender

Early studies that investigated dehydration and exercise in heat and humidity found differences in sweat rate and endurance, with women sweating less than men for a given thermal stress (Fox et al., 1969; Wyndham, 1965). These studies were initially interpreted as evidence that women were not as capable as men in coping with heat stress. More recent studies comparing the effects of exercising in heat and humidity in men and women continue to find differences in sweat rate. Gender differences in response to thermal stress (body core temperature, acclimatization, etc.) however, appear to result from differences in aerobic power, due to disparities in body weight-to-mass ratio or level of physical fitness (Armstrong et al., 1990; Avellini et al., 1980; Dill et al., 1977; Grucza et al., 1985; Havenith and van Middendorp, 1990; O'Toole, 1989; Paolone et al., 1978; White et al., 1992; Chapter 5, this volume).

Avellini et al. (1980) compared acclimation to work in humid heat in an environmental chamber in men and women with similar aerobic capacities and surface-area-to-mass ratios. The women were tested both pre- and post-ovulation. Prior to acclimation, the women sweated less than the men, their endurance was greater, and their rectal temperature and heart rate did not increase to the level seen in men. After acclimation, rectal temperature and heart rates were similar, although there was an increased difference in sweat rates between the two groups. Women had the greatest tolerance to the exercise and lowest rectal temperature prior to acclimation if they were in the pre-ovulatory phase, whereas post-ovulation, rectal temperature was similar to men while sweat rate and heart rate continued to be significantly lower. In women there was also a lag period before sweating began in the post-ovulatory phase, resulting in core temperatures rising above those seen in the pre-ovulatory phase. The differences seen in sweat rate pre- and post-ovulation in women, however, were not of the same magnitude as those seen when they were compared to men (Avellini et al., 1980).

Studies comparing men to women in hot environments have shown that women acclimated to the same work load as men demonstrate decreased sweat rates, but similar core (rectal) temperatures (Avellini et al., 1980; Wyndam, 1965). Other studies comparing men and women exercising in hot environments (Dill et al., 1977; Morimoto et al., 1967; Weinman et al., 1967) have consistently demonstrated less elevation of total body sweat rates (in milliliters per meter squared per hour) among women. Although heat and dehydration affect thermoregulatory responses such as sweating in men more severely than in women (Grucza et al., 1987), it is not gender but an individual's surface area, fitness or aerobic capacity, and acclimatization status that determine the relative heat strain in a given environment (Havenith and van Middendorp, 1990).

Overall, therefore, women do not seem to have less heat tolerance than men when they are exercising at equivalent intensities in relation to their aerobic capacities. Whereas women sweat less, they rely on circulatory cooling to a greater extent for heat dissipation. Therefore well-trained, heat acclimatized women show similar responses to hot-humid and hot-dry environments as do men.

Effect of Age

Apparent heat intolerance among the aged has been attributed to a reduction in sweating capacity and a decline in aerobic fitness (see Kenney and Gisolfi, 1986, for a review). It appears that the development of the decline in heat tolerance normally associated with men and women beginning around age 50 to 60 can be attributed to reduced cardiovascular fitness and a lack of prior heat exposure that would allow for heat acclimatization. One study (Robinson, et al., 1986) cited by Gisolfi (Chapter 5) demonstrated decreased sweating capacity in four men age 44 to 60 compared with measurements made 21 years earlier. However, this decline did not affect the ability of the older men to become acclimated to a hot-dry environment (as defined by a decreased body core temperature after 6 to 8 days) and to work at the same level and intensity as they had previously worked.

In contrast, a study done with five older men (aged 61 to 67), in which they were compared to six younger men (aged 21 to 29) who were matched for height, weight, and body surface area, but not percent body fat, demonstrated that the older men were less able to respond to a single 3-hour period of thermal dehydration than the younger men (Miescher and Fortney, 1989). Rectal temperatures in the older men increased more rapidly while sweat rates were not significantly different. In addition, plasma volume decreased and plasma osmolality increased to a larger extent in the older men. Within 30 minutes of rehydration, plasma volume and osmolality had returned to normal in the young men, while the older men took 60 minutes to restore plasma osmolality, and 90 minutes to restore plasma volume. Since these older subjects were not considered "extremely" fit, did not have similar ratios of body fat compared to the younger subjects, and since the protocol did not call for work or exercise during the 3 hour period, it is possible that the differences noted were due to these factors and not age per se.

Military researchers have measured thermoregulatory responses and acclimation in two groups of nine men who were matched for body weight, surface area, percent body fat, and maximal aerobic power, but with average ages of 21 and 46 (Pandolf et al, 1988). Initially, the older group demonstrated increased performance time with decreased rectal and skin temperatures and increased body sweat loss. After acclimation (measured after 10 days), no differences were seen between the two groups in thermoregulatory responses, including sweating rate, or performance time. The authors also noted that those in the older group who engaged in regular weekly aerobic activity were better able to initially respond to the thermal stress, although such differences were not evident after heat acclimation.

An additional study, compared a group of eight sedentary men, average age 34, with six "moderately active" older men, average age 57 (Smolander et al., 1990). The men in both groups walked on a treadmill at 30 percent $V_{O_2 max}$ for up to 3.5 hours in thermoneutral, warm-humid, and hot-dry environments. There was little difference in the ability of the older men to tolerate the protocol when compared with the younger men. The authors concluded that the ability to exercise in hot environments may not necessarily be associated with calendar age but more importantly with factors such as physical activity habits and aerobic capacity.

Based on these studies, it appears that for the age group of the active military, it is important to take into consideration the level of fitness of military troops regardless of age, particularly when going into a hot environment in which significant work is initially expected.

Effect on Electrolyte Balance

Although electrolytes are lost with sweat, these losses, except in some extreme cases, are usually not large enough to affect performance capacity

(Costill et al., 1976; Koslowski and Saltin, 1964). (Plasma concentrations may even rise as a result of the relatively larger fluid losses.) Renal retention of electrolytes during exercise can compensate for some of these electrolyte losses; following exercise, normal dietary intake can replenish these losses. In extreme cases in which sweat loss is great enough to result in a significant electrolyte deficit, the dehydration itself may cause debilitating conditions.

Summary

Increased physical activity in hot environments can result in severe hypohydration. This is particularly true when fluids are in short supply or not very palatable. Hypohydration can cause large decrements in performance and can greatly increase the risk of heat casualties. The risk of hypohydration is reduced in individuals who have been acclimatized to the heat and who are physically fit. The papers presented in this volume (see, in particular, Chapters 3-5 and 12-14) provide the scientific information necessary for understanding both acute and long-term adaptations to heat stress, particularly when combined with exercise. The physiological mechanisms that lead to increased water loss during heat exposure and the adaptability of such mechanisms to chronic heat exposure must be well understood to begin to make nutritional recommendations for soldiers subjected to these conditions for long periods. As Gisolfi (Chapter 5) concludes, sweat rates, proportional to metabolic rates, can reach as much as 10 liters per day. Training and heat acclimatization can increase the rate of sweating (and therefore the ability to work in a hot environment) by 10 to 20 percent or 200 to 300 milliliters per hour. Although men sweat more than women and require more water, well-trained, heat-acclimatized women can adapt to heat as effectively as men. Within the age range of the active-duty military force, there is no predicted decrement in sweating with increasing age; therefore, the water requirement during exercise in the heat is unchanged.

Sodium Levels for Work in the Heat

During the past several years there has been an emphasis on reducing the sodium content of foods and the sodium intake of the U.S. population. *The Surgeon General's Report on Nutrition and Health* (U.S. Department of Health and Human Services, 1988) recommended a reduction in sodium intakes, the latest version of the Recommended Dietary Allowances (RDAs) (NRC, 1989b) lowered the estimated minimum sodium requirements for healthy adults to 500 milligrams (mg) per day, and the Food and Nutrition Board's *Diet and Health* (NRC, 1989a) also recommended significant reductions in sodium in all diets. The 1989 RDAs contain a footnoted caution, however, that "no allowance has been included for large, prolonged losses from the skin through sweat."

The military has endeavored to reduce the sodium intake of its personnel through modifications of garrison and operational ration guidelines. Dietary surveys conducted at various military facilities have documented changes in the dietary intakes of several nutrients, but the sodium intake of personnel eating in military dining halls has remained relatively stable at 1500 to 1850 mg of sodium per 1000 kcal of diet (IOM, 1991). The MRDAs set forth a goal of 1700 mg of sodium per 1000 kcal of diet for foods served in military dining halls. This level is estimated to equal a daily sodium intake of approximately 5500 mg for men and 4100 mg for women. For operational rations[4] the MRDAs specify a range of 5000 to 7000 mg of sodium per day, excluding the additional salt packets that are packed with the rations. Restricted rations[5] have sodium levels, as established by the MRDAs, of 2500 to 3500 mg of sodium per day.

In an earlier report (IOM, 1991), the CMNR evaluated the sodium content of military rations. The committee urged caution in arbitrarily reducing sodium intake drastically from current levels and noted that studies were needed to evaluate the impact of reductions on personnel who might not be heat acclimatized and who were routinely consuming diets that provided sodium in the range of 1700 to 1850 mg per 1000 kcal of diet. The committee recommended that the "total daily intake of salt should be limited to 10 grams or less (4000 mg sodium) except under conditions in which salt requirements exceed values due to large salt losses such as those associated with heavy physical work in hot environments."

Chapters 12 through 14 in Part III summarize the details of studies by researchers from the USARIEM who investigated the impact of reducing intake from 8 grams to 4 grams of sodium chloride per day (3200 to 1600 mg sodium) for individuals working in a hot environment. The primary concern of the CMNR in including this study as part of this report was a consideration of the possible detrimental effects on troops of being suddenly deployed from a temperate environment to a desert or a jungle without an opportunity for acclimatizing to the heat. A mobilization of this kind would also result in soldiers' consuming combat rations that would provide significantly lower levels of sodium than they had been consuming prior to deployment. The committee's concern centers on the ability of troops to

---

[4] Operational rations typically are composed of nonperishable items that are designed for use under actual or simulated combat conditions.

[5] Restricted rations are designed for use under more specific operational scenarios such as long-range patrol, assault, and reconnaissance when troops are required to subsist for short periods (up to 10 days) on an energy-restricted ration. These rations require no further preparation; because they are intended for short-range patrols, they provide suboptimal levels of energy and nutrients.

perform immediately in a combat situation without a period of heat accli-matization. Furthermore, it should be noted that most of the sodium con-sumed by troops is derived from the consumption of food. Therefore a reduction in food, which is frequently observed during deployment, will likely result in a significant drop in sodium intake.

The data presented in Chapters 12 to 14 show that soldiers acclimated fairly rapidly to the hot environment and adapted to the lowered salt intake over the 10-day study period. However, there were increased symptoms of heat exhaustion during the first two days, which could be a significant problem for troops involved in military operations. These symptoms might have been even more severe had the subjects not been following a careful fluid intake schedule to maintain hydration during the study. It is also pos-sible that the tendency toward heat illness would have been greater if these subjects had not been adapted to 8 grams per day of sodium chloride rather than the levels found in garrison dietary surveys (approximately 12 to 13 grams per day). Therefore, although the CMNR supports the goals of reduc-ing the sodium intake of the U.S. population as well as military personnel, the committee does not recommend a reduction in the sodium content of operational rations at this time. As stated in the committee's report *Military Nutrition Initiatives* (IOM, 1991), it is not reasonable to expect the dietary sodium intake of military personnel in garrison to be different from that of the civilian population, which for adults is estimated to range from 1800 to 5000 mg per day in some reports (NRC, 1989a,b), and at a slightly higher level of 4000 to 6000 mg of sodium per day in other reports (U.S. Depart-ment of Health and Human Services, 1988). In addition, reducing sodium levels in operational rations must follow the efforts to reduce sodium intake in the general population to minimize the potential for compromising sol-dier performance in the days following deployment to hot environments.

Macronutrients

Chapter 6 provides a review of the influence of heat on macronutrient needs and soldier performance. A summary of this information is provided below.

Protein

Various authors over the past 40 years have reviewed the protein re-quirements for individuals working in the heat. Mitchell and Edman (1951) stated that "considering all evidence, it may be concluded that protein re-quirements may be slightly increased in the tropics by some 5-10 grams daily." They postulated that the slight increase in requirements may be due to a stimulation of tissue catabolism if pyrexia occurs and to compensation for sweat losses of nitrogen by diminished losses in the urine. Consolazio and Shapiro (1964) found that protein intakes of men exercising in a hot climate exceeded the *then* National Research Council (NRC) recommended allowances of 100 grams per day. They felt that the increased protein intake in the heat was not due to an innate desire for protein but to the relatively greater caloric intake that the men were consuming. Paul (1989) has suggested that because protein and amino acids contribute 5 to 15 percent of the energy for prolonged exercise, with the higher value perhaps associated with glycogen depletion, adequate protein intake is important when exercising in the heat. In Chapter 6, Buskirk concludes nevertheless, that there appears to be no evidence that protein intakes in excess of 1 to 1.5 grams per kilogram (kg) of body weight offer any advantage to the mature military person. Indeed, higher protein intakes may be a disadvantage, given the obligatory urine volume required to excrete the products of protein breakdown. The generous protein level of the MRDAs would suggest that somewhat lower levels might reduce body heat production while maintaining nutritional adequacy under conditions of high ambient temperatures. It should also be kept in mind that the matter of the relative proportions of protein, carbohydrate, and fat in hot environments is not yet entirely resolved.

Energy

Caloric requirements of troops are largely determined by the physical activities in which troops are engaged. The higher caloric intakes recommended for cold environments are largely due to the need to maintain thermal balance. It is interesting that studies of troops who operated in cold, moderate, and hot environments doing moderate work had essentially the same caloric requirements when calculated on the basis of body weight plus clothing and equipment being manually transported. In addition, a study that examined the performance of well-fed troops who were actively exercising in a hot environment with a group who experienced moderate energy restriction over a 12-day period found no difference in task performance between the groups, with both groups exhibiting weight loss (Crowdy et al., 1982). Buskirk (Chapter 6) concludes that for troops working in a hot environment, the submaximal exercise they perform has a far greater impact on their physiological functioning than if they performed the same tasks in a more comfortable environment. He also concludes that acclimatization plays a valuable role in physiological adaptation but that the process has only a minor part in modifying energy turnover and caloric requirements.

A major factor in meeting macronutrient requirements is the tendency for appetites to be adversely affected when unacclimatized personnel are suddenly exposed to a hot environment. Therefore, careful attention should be paid to those factors that will encourage adequate ration consumption to minimize the potential for reduced nutrient intake over time.

It is also fitting to consider the quote from Dill (1985) cited by Buskirk:

> In the hot desert even a well trained human can sprint only about half the distance one would guess before collapsing. One should respect the incredible intensity of the desert, protect oneself with shade, spare water, slow movement, equally-minded partners, then enjoy and relish its beauty.

Buskirk continues:

> Unfortunately, military personnel engaged in combat or under the threat of combat may not have the luxury of contemplating beauty, but they nevertheless must deal with the "incredible intensity of the desert."

Vitamins

There has been considerable research dealing with the effects of temperature and exercise on vitamin requirements, particularly requirements for the B vitamins and vitamin C. A review of this published literature was presented at the workshop by Priscilla M. Clarkson (Chapter 8).

B Vitamins

Although there is limited evidence of small increases in the loss of some B vitamins in sweat during work in hot environments, these losses are not sufficient to increase the requirements beyond the intakes recommended in the current MRDAs. Because the vitamins thiamin, riboflavin, niacin, and vitamin B_6 are important in energy metabolism, their intake should be related to energy intake. As noted earlier, the MRDAs are based on the RDAs and are revised periodically to reflect the regular revision of the RDAs. For these vitamins, the current MRDAs (see Table 1-1) are based directly on the amounts given in the ninth edition of the RDAs (NRC, 1980) (vitamin B_6) or are based on the amounts given in the ninth edition of the RDAs with a higher assumed caloric intake (thiamin, riboflavin, and niacin). The MRDAs are currently undergoing revision to reflect the changes in the tenth edition of the RDAs (NRC, 1989b), current scientific knowledge, and the demands of military tasks. Thus, the recommendations contained in the present MRDAs for these B vitamins appear sufficient to satisfy requirements for hot environments as long as the rations are consumed in adequate amounts. Furthermore, consideration can be given to decreasing the MRDAs for these nutrients in the revised edition of this regulation, in keeping with the recommendations of the tenth edition of the RDAs and on the basis of caloric intake.

There is no evidence that the levels of folic acid and B_{12} required for work in the heat are increased beyond the levels recommended in the 1989 RDAs. The folate allowance was lowered in the tenth edition of the RDAs because it was recognized that diets containing approximately half the RDA listed in the ninth edition maintained both an adequate folate status and ample liver stores (NRC, 1989b). Similarly, the RDA for vitamin B_{12} in the tenth edition was reduced by one-third for the adult age groups. The committee that wrote the RDAs commented that this was a conservative approach, which left the recommendation at approximately twice the level deemed safe by the Food and Agricultural Organization of the United Nations (FAO, 1988). The MRDAs (see Table 1-1) directly reflect the values of the ninth edition and presumably can be revised downward in a similar fashion without undue concern about the levels needed for work in hot environments.

Vitamin C

There is some evidence that increased intake of vitamin C may help to reduce heat stress during acclimatization, particularly in those individuals who may have low intakes that are nevertheless considered to be in the adequate range. There is some limited evidence that excess vitamin C may adversely affect the absorption of vitamin B_{12}. The recommended dietary allowance for vitamin C remained at 60 mg per day in the tenth edition of the RDAs (NRC, 1989b). Vitamin C levels in the MRDAs directly reflect the RDAs for this nutrient (see Table 1-1). More research is needed before any conclusions can be drawn.

Fat-Soluble Vitamins

At present there is no evidence that requirements for fat-soluble vitamins increase for people working in hot environments. Vitamin D levels appear adequate for work in hot environments, and the exposure to sunlight in these climates would likely be adequate to meet any increased need that might exist.

Vitamins A and E, as well as vitamin C, function as antioxidants and may be useful in the reduction of lipid peroxidation induced by exercise stress. However, there are no studies that have adequately examined this issue. Intakes of vitamins A, D, and E, as recommended in the 1989 RDAs, appear adequate to meet the requirements for military personnel performing their duties in hot environments. The MRDAs are based directly on the 1980 RDAs; the 1989 revision of the RDAs for these vitamins did not change appreciably (see Table 1-1). Further studies on whether these vitamins will be important as antioxidants for those living and working in a hot environment are warranted.

Summary

It appears that the intake of vitamins at levels recommended in the 1989 RDAs and in the current MRDAs is adequate for military personnel working in hot environments. Operational rations are the primary source of nutrients during the early stages of military deployment and may be used for extended periods, as apparently was the case in Operations Desert Storm and Desert Shield. It is important therefore that operational rations be formulated in accordance with the MRDAs and that the acceptance of all ration components—particularly those that may be the principal carrier of vitamin fortification—be such that these intakes are achieved over extended periods of use.

Minerals

Chapter 7 presents a review of the effects of exercise and heat on mineral metabolism and requirements. Current data are not adequate to determine under what conditions strenuous exercise or heat, or both, increase mineral requirements beyond the levels set by the MRDAs. A major difficulty is that past research on this topic has focused on sweat losses, plasma changes, and mineral balances rather than on biochemical indicators of nutritional status and functional indicators such as performance, immunity, antioxidant defense, resistance to injury, and recovery from illness or trauma.

There is no doubt that during profuse sweating (>5 liters per day), mineral losses can be substantial. In some experiments, the concentrations of minerals in plasma increased with intense exercise, whereas in other cases plasma mineral levels decreased, accompanied by substantial tissue redistribution (see Chapter 7). The significance of plasma changes is not clear. Likewise, reduced urinary excretion, which has also been observed following profuse sweating, can reflect tissue conservation or reduced tissue stores, or both. In most of the studies carried out to date, the effect of exercise has not been separated from the effects of increased ambient temperature. Moreover, there are few data that demonstrate beneficial effects from mineral supplements on either biochemical or functional indicators.

Sodium, Potassium, and Chloride

As discussed extensively in a previous report of the CMNR, *Fluid Replacement and Heat Stress* (Marriott and Rosemont, 1991), sweat losses of sodium, potassium, and chloride can be substantial under conditions of profuse sweating. For sodium, the problem is particularly acute for people who are not heat acclimatized (see section: Sodium Levels for Work in the Heat in this chapter). The committee previously concluded that there are circumstances in which the performance of military personnel would be improved by the use of electrolyte-carbohydrate beverages (see Marriott and Rosemont, 1991). In these cases, such beverages should provide approximately 20 to 30 milliequivalents (mEq) of sodium and 2 to 5 mEq of potassium per liter, with chloride as the only anion.

Iodide, Chromium, and Selenium

Sweat losses of iodide, chromium, and selenium are appreciable with intense exercise or in a hot environment. In the case of iodide, the losses that occur during profuse sweating make the use of iodized salt highly desirable. With intense exercise, plasma chromium increases, urinary chromium decreases, and plasma selenium decreases. As discussed above, the significance of these changes for the mineral status of an individual is not clear.

Iron

Iron deficiency can reduce physical performance; it has also been reported to result in a defect in thermoregulation. Losses of iron during heavy sweating can be considerable. Although anemia (i.e., "sports anemia") may occur during training, it is transitory and due in part to plasma volume expansion. Iron deficiency anemia is not commonly seen with chronic intense exercise, although low serum ferritin levels have been observed. Low serum ferritin levels are an indication that iron stores are not high and that an acute loss of iron or a decrease in intake will almost certainly result in anemia. However, caution must be employed when using iron supplements because of their reported adverse effect on zinc absorption and the potential for creating iron overload in some individuals if used for a prolonged period.

Zinc

Sweat losses of zinc can present a significant problem for military personnel in a hot environment, whether they are exercising or not. Intense exercise has been observed in some instances to increase, and in others to decrease, plasma zinc concentrations. The low plasma zinc values could also result from an acute metallothionein-induced sequestration of zinc within hepatic cells. Such interleukin-1 (IL-1) generated zinc redistribution occurs during many stress situations, and does not cause loss of zinc from the body. The frequent observation of lowered plasma zinc levels during chronic and prolonged exercise, when considered together with the high sweat losses that have been observed, suggests the appropriateness of zinc supplements under these conditions. However, no clear evidence indicates whether zinc in excess of the MRDAs should be recommended. Once again, caution is required in considering supplementation: zinc supplements reportedly lower the absorption of copper, a nutrient that already may be marginal in many diets (NRC, 1989b).

Magnesium and Copper

Sweat losses of magnesium and copper, like those of other trace elements, can be appreciable. Negative nitrogen, potassium, and magnesium balances were produced in young men by diminished dietary intake, increased urinary excretion, and sweat losses during hyperthermia induced by humid heat in an experimental chamber (Beisel et al., 1968). In some studies involving intense exercise the plasma levels of these elements have increased and in other studies they decreased. It should be noted however, that plasma levels of both elements are not a useful measure of body stores.

Calcium and Phosphorus

Calcium and phosphorus were not addressed specifically at the workshop. Based on current knowledge, the existing MRDAs for these nutrients appear to be sufficient for nutritional needs even during profuse sweating in a hot environment.

Summary

It is unclear whether mineral losses resulting from chronic heat exposure or exercise, or both, result in compromised health and performance (endurance capacity, immune defense, antioxidant defense, or recovery from illness or trauma). This information is essential before the applicability of the MRDAs can be fully assessed for military personnel working in hot environments.

FACTORS THAT MAY INFLUENCE EATING PATTERNS, FOOD PREFERENCES, AND FOOD INTAKE IN HOT ENVIRONMENTS

Olfaction and Taste

Chapter 9 reviews flavor effects (taste-gustation, smell-olfaction) and trigeminal sensation including touch, temperature, and pain, as well as color and psychological factors that affect sensory aspects of food consumption. Subject variables (age, gender, ethnic group, disease state, etc.) were not explored.

The effects of changes in temperature on sensory perception and preferences have been examined by using several different approaches. On the one hand, the perceived intensity of sucrose solutions has been reported as greater (sweeter) at higher temperatures (Bartoshuk et al., 1982); alternatively, taste thresholds for salt at cold (0°C) and hot (55°C) temperatures did not differ markedly (Pangborn et al., 1970). The effects of increased temperature on suprathreshold intensity estimates are unclear. The threshold for detecting the four basic tastes reportedly varies in a U-shaped function with the minimum at 20° to 30°C. Thus, when food or beverages of low or threshold concentrations are heated to 30°C (86°F) or above, taste thresholds become more difficult to detect.

Cooling the tongue reduced the perceived intensity of the sweetness of sucrose and the bitterness of caffeine test solutions (Green and Frankmann, 1987). However, the perceived saltiness of sodium chloride (NaCl) and the sourness of citric acid were not affected. The temperature of the tongue reportedly was the critical factor in decreasing the sweetness and bitterness. Again, the measured responses for the four basic tastes after changes in tongue temperature were not the same.

Warming a familiar food reportedly "enhances" flavor and aroma, which suggests that for certain foods, warm temperatures can enhance immediate consumption (Trant and Pangborn, 1983). However, studies examining the effects of warming on subsequent intake have not been conclusive. Further studies with other types of foods and drinks are desirable to clarify relationships among environmental temperature and mode of presentation, familiar and novel foods, hot or cold temperatures, and immediate or delayed effects.

Most experiments have primarily employed model chemosensory stimuli rather than real foods and have manipulated stimulus temperature alone rather than stimulus temperature plus environmental temperature. In addition, other aspects of sensory responsiveness, such as the physical properties of smoothness, creaminess, and thickness, need to be examined in the context of stimulus and oral (tongue) temperature differences. Capsaicin and other chemical irritants appear to increase the sensory impact of foods (Rozin et al., 1982). It is worth noting that these foods tend to be consumed predominately in hot environments.

It is unclear whether a dry-hot versus a humid-hot environment produces differential sensory responses or food consumption. The degree to which subject differences (for example, weight or fatness, age, and gender) affect responses is unknown. Under experimental conditions, decreased sweating responses have been demonstrated in older individuals at 50 percent relative humidity (Robinson et al., 1986; see previous discussion in this chapter). A question relevant to this report therefore is, How do these subject variables affect sensory responses?

When discussing preferences for sweet and fat tastes, it should be emphasized that although a preference for sweet foods may be universal, a preference for fat appears to be specific to the individual and therefore a learned response. Some preferences for combinations of fat and carbohydrate foods have been examined (typically dessert type foods), but preferences for foods high in protein and fat have not been examined in detail. Gender differences in preferences for different macronutrients also have not been well studied. In addition, the intake of specific foods during different seasons, such as fresh corn during the summer months, appears to be primarily a function of availability and learning. (See additional discussion of seasonality of food intake below).

Hotter-temperature foods generally are rated as having greater intensity of taste and smell. Further studies with various types of drinks and foods are necessary to clarify whether temperature or mode of presentation can, in fact, influence satiety. Largely unexamined is the degree to which variations in the temperature of foods (rather than preloads) or variations in ambient temperature influence the intake of specific meals or the intake of subsequent meals.

Appetite

It is important to distinguish among appetite, hunger, and intake. "Appetite" will be used here to refer to the subjective desire to eat, whereas "hunger" usually refers to a more objective deprivation state. In humans, it is possible to distinguish between what a person wants (appetite) or needs (hunger) and what a person eats (intake). These distinctions are useful because large-scale or clinical human studies often involve combinations of measures, including choice or preference ratings, in discussions of food intake. These clearly are not always the same. For example, preference ratings do not accurately predict food intake.

Thermoregulation

One of the body's major physiological concerns is thermoregulation, the maintenance of body thermoneutrality. Eating appears to be a major contributor to maintaining body heat. The "thermostatic" hypothesis of feeding is that the body experiences a temperature-dependent variation in energy needs that should be reflected in appetite. If normal food intake continues under conditions of heat stress, the additional heat that must be dissipated as a result of the amounts ingested may lead to a breakdown in the body's heat mechanisms (see Chapter 15).

In a series of studies by Hamilton (1963a), rats exposed to a temperature of 35°C ate only 2 grams of food during the first 24 hours, compared with a previous intake of more than 20 grams at 24°C; mild (32°C) and severe (35°C) heat stress over 21 days resulted in a continued lower level of food intake. At 40°C, rats stop eating altogether; if force-fed by intubation, they suffer heat stress and occasionally die (Hamilton, 1967). Studies in a number of experimental animals demonstrate cessation of eating at high temperatures, with the possibility that continued eating would probably lead to hyperthermia. The marked decrease in food intake is followed by a decrease in body weight and fat (Jakubczak, 1976). Reduced intake in the heat would thus seem to be adaptive. Keys and coworkers (1950) found that their semistarved volunteers complained of the cold even in warm summer weather. This indicates that a reduction in food intake may actually be a mechanism to cope with hot environments. There is thus significant research in various models to support the observation that food intake drops as the environmental temperature increases from normal to hot ambient temperatures, followed by a decrease in body weight.

Heating the preoptic and anterior hypothalamic regions in animals appears to act in much the same fashion as external cues to inhibit eating (Andersson and Larsson, 1961). Opposite results, however, were obtained by Spector and colleagues (1968). Heating of the preoptic medialis region caused increased eating when the temperature of the area was raised to 43°C; decreased eating occurred when the ambient temperature was raised to 35°C. Local temperature in the anterior hypothalamic area reportedly drops at the onset of eating in the monkey, which is the opposite of what would be expected (Hamilton, 1963b). It appears that the effect of brain temperature on eating may be more a result of external ambient temperature than of localized temperature changes. In addition, it may be due to the rate of heat flow from the body's core to the periphery or vice versa, as no single temperature uniquely governs the level of food intake (Spector et al., 1968).

Thermogenic Effect of Food

Studies of the theory that animals stop eating to prevent hyperthermia have noted differences in the resulting thermic effect of the food ingested (dietary induced thermogenesis, or specific dynamic action) as a possible triggering mechanism (Chapter 15). The caloric intake of rats that were fed special diets during mild heat stress was inversely related to the thermogenic effect of the diet selected (Hamilton, 1963a). It appears that fats may be the preferred energy source in heat stress (Salganik, 1956) and that in conditions of severe heat, rats avoid protein because of the comparatively high amount of heat it creates (Hamilton, 1963a). Under this theory, body temperature should be highly correlated with hunger and satiety, yet there appears to be no consistently observed relationship between them. LeBlanc and Cabanac (1989) recently demonstrated that the postprandial thermogenic effect of food intake has both a cephalic and a gastrointestinal phase. The cephalic effect (which was evident in subjects who did not even swallow the food but merely chewed and spit it out) was stronger than the subsequent gastrointestinal effect following consumption. Some researchers (Penicaud et al., 1986) argue that temperature control has primacy over food intake control.

Dehydration

Osmotic factors have also been shown to affect food intake (see discussion in Chapter 15). Ingestion or intubation of hypertonic solutions results in decreased food intake in rats (Ehman et al., 1972; Kozub, 1972). This reduction in intake is a protective mechanism that is demonstrated under conditions of total water deprivation, which drastically reduces eating in most species (Thompson, 1980). It appears that, to a large extent, decreased food intake in unacclimatized subjects in tropical climates may be mediated by hypertonicity associated with initial dehydration and may improve as acclimatization occurs (Bass et al., 1955).

Influence of Physique

Chapter 10 provides a discussion of the evolutionary aspects of survival in hot environments. For example, a bulkier shape minimizes heat loss, because the bulkier animal has a relatively smaller ratio of skin surface to metabolically active bulk and skin surface determines heat dissipation (Beller, 1977). Physical anthropologists (see Beller, 1977, for a review) have long noted a correspondence between physique and climate. The fact that linear physiques generally do better in the heat may be seen as an evolutionary selection principle. The endomorphy of a population, however, is not correlated with mean annual temperature so much as with mean January temperature (in northern latitudes) (Beller, 1977). It is quite possible that adaptation to one sort of challenge may prove to be contra-adaptive in some other sense. Animals and people who maintain a body weight below the set-point show aberrant eating patterns, hyperemotionality (including irritability), distractibility, and a reduced sex drive (Nisbett, 1972).

Heat as a Stressor

Body temperature increases under acute stress, which may elevate the thermoregulatory set-point—or simply add metabolic heat. Normal eaters in both laboratory and field settings respond to stress by decreasing their food intake. Not only does the stress of a hot environment involve the need for thermoregulation and maintenance hydration, but it encompasses psychological stress as well. It is difficult to ascertain the difference between appetite and hunger in animals; in humans, however, for whom other factors, such as situational stress, may affect hunger and appetite differently, it may be important to differentiate the two. Both, singly or in combination, will affect food intake. Given the stress expected with military excursions into hot and tropical environments and the rapid deployment that troops often experience, any evaluation of food intake and habits in hot environments should include all possible stressors to determine the potential combined effects of these factors.

Food Preferences in Hot Environments

In studies to determine the preferred types of foods for consumption in hot environments, palatability per se has not been measured in hot versus cold environments. In temperate environments, studies show that humans have an expressed preference for fats and sweets (Drewnowski et al., 1989). There is currently a dearth of solid experimental research on human food consumption in response to variations in heat. In terms of the proportions of various macronutrients in the diet, protein as a percentage of energy remained constant in military nutrition studies conducted during different seasons over the course of World War II (Edholm et al., 1964; Johnson and Kark, 1947). These data were supported by animal studies (Donhoffer and Vonotsky, 1947). Rolls and others (1990), however, found almost no relation between how hungry or satiated people claimed to be and how much they subsequently ate.

One classic study in food intake changes among military personnel was conducted by Edholm and Goldsmith (1966). Two similar groups of military men were followed in carefully controlled conditions. One group had spent a year in Bahrain prior to the experiment; the second group was first studied for 12 days in the United Kingdom and then flown to Bahrain, where it joined the first group. Both groups of subjects spent the first 4 days engaged in hard work, the next 4 days engaged in lighter work, and the final 4 days engaged in hard work in tents and outside. Both groups then returned to the United Kingdom for a repeat of the 12-day protocol.

In Bahrain the daytime temperature rarely went below 30°C (86°F), with a relative humidity of 40 to 90 percent. The mean food intake in Bahrain was approximately 25 percent less than that in the United Kingdom; however, the percentages of calories from fat and carbohydrate were similar, as was the percentage of calories from protein. While in Bahrain, the unacclimatized group lost an average body weight of 2.5 kg over 12 days, and the acclimatized group lost 1.1 kg. The lost weight was not quickly recovered upon the groups' return to the United Kingdom. This result led researchers to believe that the caloric deficit, rather than the state of hydration, was responsible for the majority of the weight lost in the hot environment.

A number of military studies conducted by the U.S. Department of Defense have looked at garrison feeding, food choices, and food waste; they have also conducted tests of the rations that have been developed. In each case these studies have been conducted during only one season, usually fall or spring; thus comparative information regarding summer food choices is not available.

A few studies have investigated the relationship between seasonal changes in body composition and seasonal changes in caloric intake and body weight. Some of these studies have also evaluated nutrient intake in adults by season of the year in hot environments. Decreased intake of several nutrients, such as vitamins A and C (Aldashev et al., 1986) and protein, vitamin C, and total energy (Mommadov and Grafova, 1983), has been reported. However, these studies did not evaluate changes in food preferences or appetite.

Empirical data, based on observations and practices in food service in both the military and the commercial sector, indicate a change in food preferences during seasons associated with elevated mean environmental temperatures. Few basic studies have attempted to specifically address food patterns that change according to season in self-selected diets. In a study of seasonal variations in self-selected lunches in a large employee cafeteria in Maryland, Zifferblatt and colleagues (1980) found a decreased selection of starches and cooked vegetables with increased purchases of fruits, salads, yogurt, and cottage cheese as the noontime temperature rose. As the temperature increased, average caloric purchases also tended to decrease. The workplace cafeteria, along with the work areas of most of the employees, was kept at 72°F; and thus, the environmental temperature of the location at which the food was ingested may have only moderately influenced workers' appetites.

National surveys have investigated the food consumption patterns of Americans, but they have not gathered recent data on the same individuals or on individuals in similar geographic areas at different times of the year. Such data would help determine whether changes of season, and thus changes in environmental temperatures, affect appetite (resulting in changes in food intake) or food selection patterns. The 1977-1978 Nationwide Food Consumption Survey reported three-day food intake information for about 36,100 individuals from a sample of households in 48 states that included four seasonal samples. The seasonal differences in average intakes of 10 major food groups were low—11 percent or less. For the major food groups, average intakes were typically higher in one season than in the three others with intakes of vegetables, fruits, and beverages increasing in the summer. Intake of legumes, sugars and sweets, meats, and eggs was at a seasonal low in the summer. Data on the intake of food subgroups appear to mirror the seasonal availability. With the subgroups of fruits, for example, more noncitrus fruit was eaten in the summer than in other seasons, the intake of citrus fruits and juices was highest in the winter months, while apple intake was highest in the fall with a drop progressively from winter through summer. In contrast, the average intake of bananas was the same in all four seasons. Intake of fats and oils varied little across the seasons with a slight drop in reported intake of table fats in the summer but this corresponded with a slight increase in the use of salad dressings in spring and summer months. Thus, people do alter their eating behavior during the year, but to some extent these alterations are based on availability and prices of food items. Whether changes also occur in appetite (considered to be the desire to eat) is unknown from these data.

There was no discussion at the workshop or in the literature surveyed by the committee of the interaction of ethnic food preferences with appetite and intake or related variables in hot environments. This topic is undoubtedly one that should be considered for future research in light of the changing ethnic composition of the military services.

Summary

Herman's presentation in Chapter 10 raises several questions about appetite and provides a philosophical base from which to study the problem of changes in appetite in the heat. The studies cited suggest that the thermoregulatory value of decreased food intake in hot environments should be stressed. The percentage of body weight lost and the nutritional adequacy of the diet are thus major concerns. Studies that have documented voluntary decreased food intake in individuals in hot environments and animal studies that have supported the concept that decreased food intake is an adaptive mechanism to ameliorate the increased need for thermoregulation, make it clear that optimal nutrition is compromised if intake decreases to the extent of consuming inadequate levels of key nutrients.

SOCIAL AND PSYCHOLOGICAL INFLUENCES ON FOOD INTAKE DURING MILITARY OPERATIONS

Situational Influences on Food Intake

A common observation is that food consumption is reduced in battle situations. In attempting to address this issue, the Army is confronted by a set of complex interacting variables (the lack of palatable or familiar foods, environmental stress, time of meals, fatigue, etc.) that could lead to reduced food intake. Another difficulty is the problem encountered trying to simulate combat conditions in the laboratory. In Chapter 11, Hirsch and Kramer ask, What are the limiting factors that lead to this drop in food intake? These authors report that the meals, ready-to-eat rations (MREs) are not actively disliked by troops and thus conclude that unpalatability must be only one limiting factor. Their data suggest that when normal volunteers are fed a consistent diet of MREs, food intake, which initially is no different from that of controls, drops by the sixth week. Lack of convenience, difficulty of preparation, poor palatability, and lack of menu variety are all factors that could contribute to this decreased intake. Situational influences—for example, meal location (eating in the field versus in dining facilities)—appear to have primary importance in determining the amount of food eaten.

Research indicates that the environmental factors impinging on food intake are often confounded with social factors. Social influences, time of day (breakfast versus dinner), and ease of preparation or accessibility of the food (see Chapter 11) also appear to be important influences on the amount of food consumed. Field troops in Operations Desert Shield and Desert Storm reportedly ate more food when they were served hot meals from the kitchen than when they ate self-prepared meals or MREs. Laboratory studies suggest that food intake can be increased when new foods are offered after satiation with familiar ones, when variety is increased, and when individuals eat together in small groups. The stimulation afforded by the sounds associated with eating in social settings also leads to increased meal size (de Castro and de Castro, 1989; Klesges et al., 1984).

Animal data (Collier 1989) and human data (Levitz, 1975; Meyer and Puddel, 1977; Meyers et al., 1980) support the contention that even relatively minor changes in accessibility and the effort required to obtain food can lead to significant changes in food consumption. Other studies suggest that greater amounts of food are consumed when presented in a smorgasbord fashion (i.e., self-selection), compared with a more typical restaurant presentation (Stunkard and Kaplan, 1977; Stunkard and Mayer, 1978). Eating in small groups facilitates both increased food consumption and increased meal duration. In addition, individual group members can, by statement or example, influence the amount consumed by others (Engell et al., 1990; Polivy et al., 1979), which suggests that food acceptance can be increased by explicit examples.

In summary, evaluation of the suitability of the MREs as a hot-weather ration requires careful consideration not only of their nutrient content but of the social influences on eating. Modification of troop feeding practices based on the results of ration field trials can potentially increase the intake of MREs through the enhancement of effective social stimuli.

Field Observations of Food Intake

During the workshop, military personnel indicated that the environment in which food is provided, the soldier's understanding of the ration's nutrient content, and the form of the ration are as important to the soldier's dietary intake as the ration's actual nutrient composition. These comments were primarily based on anecdotal information provided by two short-term observers during Operation Desert Storm and should be considered in the context of other information that has been provided from other sources who were also present during the deployment.

Environmental Concerns

In a hot, dry environment, sand became an unwelcome but constant additive to all food items wherever food handling was involved. Protection from tents that had been set up decreased the amount of sand to some extent, but did not eliminate it entirely. As a result, some of the steps required for food preparation of field rations, such as heating and rehydration, may not be possible in a desert setting because of the introduction of sand as a contaminant.

It also appears that during the extremely hot part of the day, soldiers would not eat, although they would drink. When field kitchens became available, the time of meal service was adjusted as much as possible to coincide with cooler environmental temperatures. Even when they were hungry during the hotter periods of the day, soldiers often did not want to eat the kinds of food provided, but they did have ideas of what they would have liked to eat.

Dehydration and Constipation

A significant concern to soldiers during Desert Storm and Desert Shield was constipation; many held the belief that consuming the ration would result in constipation. In the recent Gulf War, constipation apparently was prevented by strict adherence to the water discipline regimen that had been established to prevent significant dehydration. However, the distant placement of sheltered latrines in the field resulted in decreased fluid consumption after dark to prevent having to get dressed, put on gear, and go through the dark to the latrine. Female soldiers in particular restricted their fluid intake; male soldiers could urinate in more convenient unsheltered latrines. In addition, some soldiers voluntarily restricted fluid intake prior to operations (i.e., when they were going on convoys, flying a mission, etc.). This practice resulted in the potential for fluid restriction both at night and dur-

ing the day for the same individual. Some soldiers also reported self-medi-
cation to prevent defecation while on 3- to 4-day missions.

Food Preferences

As might be expected, foods that were commercially labeled—even
though they were not as heat stable and in certain cases showed evidence of
some deterioration—were preferred to the field ration (MRE). Apparently,
soldiers had greater confidence—in terms of meeting their appetite and
nutritional needs—in foods that seemed to be the same (including packaging) as those they had consumed at home. This was particularly true for
flavored beverage powder. A significant concern of soldiers was the com-
patibility of foods in each MRE. For example, an MRE that contained a
slice of ham as an entree did not come with cheese, which would have been
preferable for making a sandwich. It instead was packaged with peanut
butter. Likewise, peanut butter and jelly were not packed together in any
MRE pouch because they were both considered "spreads." To overcome
this problem, soldiers would "rob" one MRE pouch to obtain the other
spread and then discard the remaining contents.

Because the Desert Shield operation lasted from summer to winter, it
was necessary to provide foods appropriate to the prevailing climatic conditions. In the summer, the amount of beverage bases provided in each MRE
pouch was not adequate to flavor all the water that was consumed. (Soldiers
deemed it necessary to flavor the water because of its unpalatability.) Individuals were drinking from 8 to 9 bottles per day; thus, three beverage
bases were needed to flavor 1½ liters of water per bottle. Likewise, during
the colder season, the soldiers all wanted cocoa, which had been discarded
during the summer. Because cocoa was not included in every MRE pouch,
often a hot drink choice was not available with each meal. Concomitantly,
in order to have a hot drink, soldiers in the field who did not have access to
kerosene heaters needed hot tabs.[6] This had a direct effect on the acceptability of the rations. In 130°F weather, soldiers did not want a hot meal but
rather the MRE entrees that were intended to be eaten without heating. In
essence, they would have preferred entrees that were cool or cold.

Social/Psychological Aspects of Eating

The use of individual MREs decreased socialization because there was
no need for a field kitchen and a common mess. To soldiers with little
access to information about what was going on in the war, this practice

---

[6] Hot tabs are small portable elements for warming ration components. They are included
only with rations that require heating.

decreased morale, because the opportunity for bringing the unit together on at least a daily basis was not available. Thus, the use of MREs, in decreasing social interaction, acted as a psychological stressor.

Caffeine consumption changed dramatically depending on the situation of the troops, and the use of smokeless tobacco increased as a result of light (fire) discipline and the fire hazards associated with smoking. It was reported by the two observers that these changes affected eating patterns but no quantitative information was available. In addition, the use of meal shifts changed normal times of meals and the types of food associated with certain meals, as well as the desire, among some soldiers, to have a meal.

Nutrition Understanding

The observations presented concerning Desert Shield and Desert Storm reinforced the committee's belief that a broad program of educating soldiers with regard to the ration and its contents, and how it would influence their desire to maintain or change body weight, was needed on the unit level. Many soldiers apparently read the packaging labels on their foods; this could be a vehicle for additional information and education. It may be appropriate to determine the need, if any, for a general policy regarding vitamin and mineral supplementation. Many soldiers reported their consumption of supplements from personal supplies or packages that were requested from home. The CMNR recommended in an earlier review of the MREs and T rations (NRC, 1986) that the distribution of vitamin and mineral supplements was unnecessary and ill-advised if the rations were well fortified by meeting the MRDAs and if the soldiers ate the rations in sufficient quantities to meet their caloric needs.

Summary

The following recommendations, gleaned from anecdotal comments of soldiers in the field during Operations Desert Shield and Storm, were discussed informally at the workshop: (1) pouch bread should be available at every meal, if at all possible; (2) more eat-on-the-go-type foods are necessary, such as cookie bars or snack items that could be saved and eaten later; (3) food items within the individual MREs should be packaged together so that they form complementary alternative foods, such as sandwich ingredients; (4) although salt packets are rarely used, other condiment packets such as pepper or mustard should be provided to add variety to the meal; (5) MREs should be unitized, along with sundry packs, supplement packs, and other such items, so that each pallet has a variety when it is moved forward to the field of operation. Although, it must be recognized that the decision to fortify certain foods within the MRE places the onus on the soldier to eat that specific item in order to meet the MRDA, practice in the field indicates that this was not always achieved.

CONCLUSION

The magnitude of the stress imposed by exercise in hot environments depends on an individual's nutritional status and his or her ability to regulate metabolic events and dissipate heat. Increased heat production, increased sweat losses, and inadequate hydration predispose soldiers in hot environments to dehydration. It is of paramount importance that hydration be preserved to maintain performance. Although it is generally recognized that some losses of minerals and vitamins occur during intense exercise in hot environments, available information suggests that the present MRDAs are adequate for achieving optimal work performance and preventing overt clinical deficiencies. The absence of sensitive, reliable indicators of many nutritional inadequacies limits the detection of subtle changes in dietary practices on health and performance. The interrelationships of exercise in hot environments and nutrient requirements, as influenced by eating behavior, age, gender, and body composition, are unclear. These factors clearly deserve additional investigation. There is substantial evidence that food intake decreases markedly as the environmental temperature increases, which probably reflects the need to control thermogenesis. It thus becomes prudent to provide palatable, nutrient-rich foods that reduce the monotony of eating during extremely hot conditions. Quoting E. R. Buskirk (Chapter 6): "Finally, as the nutritional situation during the recent operations of Desert Shield and Desert Storm is reviewed, a comment by R. M. Kark (1954) comes to mind:

> 'Field studies have shown that physical deterioration in soldiers may be due to inadequate nutrition, but perhaps what is more important, they have shown that loss of military efficiency through inadequate nutrition is most often due to inadequate planning, catering or supply, and to inadequate training or indoctrination. . . . Maintaining good nutrition is like maintaining freedom of speech or democracy. You need eternal vigilance to make it work.'"

REFERENCES

Adolph, E.I.
   1947   Physiology of Man in the Desert. New York, N.Y.: Interscience.
Aldashev, A.A., B.I. Kim, O.A. Kolesova, V.L. Reznik, and V.V. Subach
   1986   Indices of the nutritional status of workers in the oil and gas production industry
           adapting to the extreme conditions of an arid zone. (in Russian) Vopr. Pitan. May-
           June (3):25-28.
Andersson, B., and B. Larsson
   1961   Influence of local temperature changes in the preoptic area and rostral hypothala-
           mus on the regulation of food and water intake. Acta Physiol. Scand. 52:75-89.

Armstrong, L.E., D.L. Costill, and W.J. Fink
  1985   Influence of dehydration on competitive running performance. Med. Sci. Sports Exerc. 17:456-461.
Armstrong, L.E., R.W. Hubbard, B.H. Jones, and J.T. Daniels
  1986   Preparing Alberto Salazar for the heat of the 1984 Olympic Marathon. Physician Sportsmed. 14:73-81.
Armstrong, L.E., J.P. DeLuca, E.L. Christensen, and R.W. Hubbard
  1990   Mass-to-surface area index in a large cohort. Am. J. Phys. Anthropol. 83:321-329.
AR 40-25
  1968   *See* U.S. Departments of the Army, the Navy, and the Air Force. 1968.
  1985   *See* U.S. Departments of the Army, the Navy, and the Air Force. 1985.
Avellini, B.A., E. Kamon, and J.T. Krajewski
  1980   Physiological responses of physically fit men and women to acclimation to humid heat. J. Appl. Physiol.: Respirat. Environ. Exercise Physiol. 49:254-261.
Bartoshuk, L.M., K. Rennert, H. Rodin, and J.C. Stevens
  1982   Effects of temperature on the perceived sweetness of sucrose. Physiol. Behavior 28:905-910.
Bass, D.E., C.R. Kleeman, M. Quinn, A. Henschel, and A.H. Hegnauer
  1955   Mechanisms of acclimatization to heat in man. Med. Anal. Rev. 34:323-380.
Beisel, W.R., R.F. Goldman, and R.J.T. Joy
  1968   Metabolic balance studies during induced hyperthermia in man. J. Appl. Physiol. 24:1-10.
Beller, A.S.
  1977   Fat and Thin: A Natural History of Obesity. New York, N.Y.: Farrar, Straus, and Giroux.
Brouha, L., P.E. Smith, Jr., R. De Lanne, and M.E. Maxfield
  1960   Physiological reactions of men and women during muscular activity and recovery in various environments. J. Appl. Physiol. 16:133-140.
Collier, G.
  1989   The economics of hunger, thirst, satiety and regulation. Ann. N.Y. Acad. Sci. 575:136-154.
Consolazio, C.R., and R. Shapiro
  1964   Energy requirements of men in extreme heat. Pp. 121-124 in Environmental Physiology and Psychology in Arid Conditions: Proceedings of the Lucknow Symposium. Liège, Belgium: United Nations Educational, Scientific, and Cultural Organization.
Consolazio, C.F., R. Shapiro, J.E. Masterson, and P.S.L. McKinzie
  1961   Energy requirements of men in extreme heat. J. Nutr. 73:126-134.
Consolazio, C.F., L.O. Matoush, R.A. Nelson, J.A. Torres, and G.J. Isaac
  1963   Environmental temperature and energy expenditures. J. Appl. Physiol. 18:65-68.
Costill, D.L., R. Cote, and W. Fink
  1976   Muscle water and electrolytes following varied levels of dehydration in man. J. Appl. Physiol. 40:6-11.
Crowdy, J.P., C.F. Consolazio, A.L. Forbes, M.F. Haisman, and D.E. Worsley
  1982   Nutrition in adverse environments, 3: The metabolic effects of a restricted food intake on men working in a tropical environment. Hum. Nutri. Appl. Nutr. 36A:325-344.
de Castro, J.M., and E.S. de Castro
  1989   Spontaneous meal patterns of humans: Influence of the presence of other people. Am. J. Clin. Nutr. 50:237-247.
DHHS
  1988   *See* U.S. Department of Health and Human Services, 1988.

Dill, D.B.
    1985   The Hot Life of Man and Beast. P. 185. Springfield, Ill.: Charles C. Thomas.
Dill, D.B., H.T. Edwards, P.S. Bauer, and E.J. Levenson
    1930   Physical performance in relation to external temperature. Arbeitsphysiologie 3:508-
              518.
Dill, D.B., L.F. Soholt, D.C. McLean, T.F. Drost, Jr., M.T. Loughran
    1977   Capacity of young males and females for running in desert heat. Med. Sci. Sports
              9:137-142.
Dimri, G.P., M.S. Malhortra, J. Sen Gupta, T.S. Kumar, and B.S. Aora
    1980   Alterations in aerobic-anaerobic proportions of metabolism during work in heat. J.
              Appl. Physiol. 45:43-50.
Drewnowski, A., E.E. Shrager, C. Lipsky, E. Stellar, and M.R.C. Greenwood
    1989   Sugar and fat: Sensory and hedonic evaluation of liquid and solid foods. Physiol.
              Behav. 45:177-184.
Donhoffer, S., and J. Vonotsky
    1947   The effect of environmental temperature on food selection. Am. J. Physiol. 150:329-
              333.
Edholm, O.G, and R. Goldsmith
    1966   Food intakes and weight changes in climatic extremes. Proc. Nutr. Soc. 25:113-
              119.
Edholm, O.G., R.H. Fox, R. Goldsmith, I.F.G. Hampton, C.R. Underwood, E.J. Ward,
          H.S. Wolf, J.M. Adam, and J.R. Allan
    1964   Report to the Medical Research Council, London: Army Personnel Research Committee,
              No. APRC64/65. 240 pp.
Ehman, G.K., D.J. Albert, and J.L. Jamieson
    1972   Injections into the duodenum and the induction of satiety in the rat. Can. J. Psychol.
              25:147-166.
Engell, D., F.M. Kramer, S. Luther, and S.O. Adams
    1990   The effect of social influences on food intake. Unpublished manuscript presented
              at the Society for Nutrition Education 1990 Annual Meeting, Anaheim, Calif.
Fink, W.J., D.L. Costill, and W.J. Van Handel
    1975   Leg muscle metabolism during exercise in the heat and cold. Eur. J. Appl. Physiol.
              34:183-190.
FAO (Food and Agriculture Organization)
    1988   Requirements of Vitamin A, Iron, Folate and Vitamin B12. Report of a Joint FAO/
              WHO Expert Consultation. FAO Food and Nutrition Series no. 23. Rome: Food
              and Agriculture Organization.
Fortney, S.M., C.B. Wenger, J.R. Bove, and E.R. Nadel
    1983   Effect of blood volume on forearm venous and cardiac stroke volumes during
              exercise. J. Appl. Physiol. 55:884-890.
Fox, R.H., B.E. Lofstedt. P.M. Woodward, E. Eriksson, and B. Werkstrom
    1969   Comparison of thermoregulatory function in men and women. J. Appl. Physiol.
              26:444-453.
Green, B.G., and S.P. Frankmann
    1987   The effect of cooling the tongue on the perceived intensity of taste. Chem. Sens.
              12:609-619.
Grucza, R., J.L. Lecroart, J.J. Hauser, and Y. Houdas
    1985   Dynamics of sweating in men and women during passive heating. Eur. J. Appl.
              Physiol. 54:309-314.
Grucza, R., J.L. Lecroart, G. Carette, J.J. Hauser, and Y. Houdas
    1987   Effect of voluntary dehydration on thermoregulatory responses to heat in men and
              women, Eur. J. Appl. Physiol. 56:317-322.

Hamilton, C.L.
 1963a   Interactions of food intake and temperature regulation in the rat. J. Comp. Physiol. Psychol. 56:476-488.
 1963b   Hypothalamic temperature records of a monkey. Proc. Soc. Exp. Biol. Med.112:55-57.
 1967   Food and temperature. Pp. 303-317 in Handbook of Physiology: section 6, Volume 1, C.F. Code, ed. Washington, D.C.: American Physiological Society

Harrison, M.H.
 1985   Effects of thermal stress and exercise on blood volume in humans. Physiol. Rev. 65:149-209.

Havenith, G., and H. van Middendorp
 1990   The relative influence of physical fitness, acclimatization or state, anthropometric measures and gender on individual reactions to heat stress. Eur. J. Appl. Physiol. 61:419-427.

Herbert, W.E., and P.M. Ribisl
 1972   Effects of dehydration upon physical working capacity of wrestlers under competitive conditions. Res. Q. Am. Assoc. Health Phys. Educ. 43:416-421.

IOM (Institute of Medicine)
 1991   Military Nutrition Initiatives. A Brief Report Submitted by the Committee on Military Nutrition Research. Washington, D.C.: Food and Nutrition Board.

Jakubczak, L.F.
 1976   Food and water intakes of rats as a function of strain, age, temperature, and body weight. Physiol. Behav. 17:251-258.

Johnson, R.E., and R.M. Kark
 1947   Environment and food intake in man. Science 105:378-379.

Kark, R.M.
 1954   Studies on troops in the field. Pp. 193-195 in Nutrition Under Climatic Stress, H. Spector and M.S. Peterson, eds. Washington, D.C.: National Academy of Sciences/National Research Council.

Kenney, M.J., and C.V. Gisolfi
 1986   Thermal regulation: effects of exercise and age, Pp. 133-134 in Sports Medicine for the Mature Athlete. J.R. Sutton and R.M. Brock, eds. Indianapolis, Ind.: Benchmark Press.

Keys, A., J. Brozek, A. Henschel, O. Mickelson, and L.L. Taylor
 1950   The Biology of Starvation. Minneapolis, Minn.: University of Minnesota Press.

Klesges, R.C., D. Barsch, J.D. Norwood, D. Kautzman, and D. Haugrud
 1984   The effects of selected social and environmental variables on the eating behavior of adults in the natural environment. Int. J. Eating Dis. 3:35-41.

Koslowski, S., and B. Saltin
 1964   Effect of sweat loss on body fluids. J. Appl. Physiol. 19:1119-1124.

Kozub, F.J.
 1972   Male-female differences in response to stomach loads of hypertonic NaCl in rats. Psychon. Sci. 28:149-151.

LeBlanc, J., and Cabanac, M.
 1989   Cephalic postprandial thermogenesis in human subjects. Physiol. Behav. 46:479-482.

Levitz, L.S.
 1975   The susceptibility of human feeding behavior to external control. Pp. 53-61 in Obesity in Perspective, G. A. Bray, ed. DHEW Publication No. NIH75-708. Washington, D.C.: U.S. Government Printing Office.

Marriott, B.M., and C. Rosemont
 1991   Fluid Replacement and Heat Stress: Proceedings of a Workshop. 2nd printing. Washington, D.C.: National Academy Press.

Maughan, R.J.
1985 Thermoregulation and fluid balance in marathon competition at low ambient temperature. Int. J. Sports Med. 6:15-19.

Meyer, J.E., and Puddel, V.E.
1977 Experimental feeding in man: A behavioral approach. Psychosom. Med. 39:153-157.

Meyers, A.W., A.J. Stunkard, and M. Coll
1980 Food accessibility and food choice. Arch. Gen. Psychiat. 37:1133-1135.

Miescher, E., and S.M. Fortney
1989 Responses to dehydration and rehydration during heat exposure in young and older men. Am. J. Physiol. 257 (Regulatory Integrative Comp. Physiol. 26): R1050-R1056.

Mitchell, H.H., and M. Edman
1951 Nutrition and Climatic Stress with Particular Reference to Man. Springfield, Ill.: Charles C. Thomas.

Mommadov, I.M., and V.A. Grafova
1983 Daily diet and ascorbic acid intake in man during work in the Arid zone. Human Physiol. 9(4):224-228.

Morimoto, T., Z. Slabochova, R.K. Naman, and F. Sargent II
1967 Sex differences in physiological reactions to thermal stress. J. Appl. Physiol. 22:526-532.

Murlin, J.R., and Miller, C.W.
1919 Preliminary results of nutritional surveys in United States Army camps. Am. J. Publ. Health 9(6):401-413.

Muza, S.R., N.A. Pimental, H.M. Cosimini, and M.N. Sawka
1988 Portable ambient air microclimate cooling simulated desert and tropic conditions. Aviat. Space Environ. Med. 59:553-558.

Nadel, E.R.
1983 Effects of temperature on muscle metabolism. Pp. 134-143 in Biochemistry of Exercise, H. G. Knuttgen, J.A. Vogel, and J.Poortmans, eds. Champaign, Ill.: Human Kinetics Publishers.

Nadel, E.R., C.B. Wenger, M.F. Roberts, J.A.J. Stolwijk, and E. Cafarelli
1977 Physiological defenses against hyperthermia of exercise. Ann. N.Y. Acad. Sci. 301:98-109.

Nadel, E.R., S.M. Fortney, and C.B. Wenger
1980 Effect of hydration state on circulatory and thermal regulations. J. Appl. Physiol. 49:715-721.

NRC (National Research Council)
1980 Recommended Dietary Allowances, Ninth Edition. Washington, D.C.: National Academy Press.
1986 Military Nutrition Research, Report of Committee Activities, August 1, 1985-July 31, 1986. Washington, D.C.: National Academy Press.
1989a Diet and Health: Implications for Reducing Chronic Disease Risk. Washington, D.C.: National Academy Press.
1989b Recommended Dietary Allowances, Tenth Edition. Washington, D.C.: National Academy Press.

Nisbett, R.E.
1972 Hunger, obesity, and the ventromedial hypothalamus. Psychol. Rev. 79:433-453.

O'Toole, M.L.
1989 Gender differences in the cardiovascular response to exercise [a review]. Cardiovasc. Clin. 19:17-33.

Pandolf, K.B., B.S. Cadarette, M.J. Sawka, A.J. Young, R.P. Francesconi, and R.R. Gonzalez
    1988   Thermoregulatory responses of middle-aged and young men during dry-heat accli-
            mation. J. Appl. Physiol. 65:65-71.
Pangborn, R.M., R.B. Chrisp, and L.L. Bertolero
    1970   Gustatory, salivary, and oral thermal responses to solutions of sodium chloride at
            four temperatures. Percept. and Psychophys. 8:69-75.
Paolone, A.M., C.L. Wells, and G.T. Kelly
    1978   Sexual variations in thermoregulation during heat stress. Aviat. Space Environ.
            Med. 49:715-719.
Paul, G.L.
    1989   Dietary protein requirements of physically active individuals. Sports Med. 8:154-
            176.
Penicaud, L., D.A. Thompson, and J. Le Magnen
    1986   Effects of 2-deoxy-*d*-glucose on food and water intake and body temperature in
            rats. Physiol. Behav. 36:431-435.
Petersen, E.S., and H. Vejby-Christensen
    1973   Effect of body temperature on steady-state ventilation and metabolism in exercise.
            Acta Physiol. Scand. 89:342-351.
Pimental, N.A., H.M. Cosimini, M.N. Sawka, and C.B. Wenger
    1987   Effectiveness of an air-cooled vest using selected air temperature and humidity
            combinations. Aviat. Space Environ. Med. 58:119-124.
Pitts, G.C., R.E. Johnson, and C.F. Consolazio
    1944   Work in the heat as affected by intake of water, salt, and glucose. Am. J. Physiol.
            142:253-259.
Polivy, J., C.P. Herman, J.C. Younger, and B. Erskine
    1979   Effects of a model on eating behaviour: The induction of a restrained eating style.
            J. of Pers. 47:100-117.
Robinson, S., D.B. Dill, J.W. Wilson, and M. Nielson
    1941   Adaptations of white men and negroes to prolonged work in humid heat. Am. J.
            Trop. Med. 21:261-287.
Robinson, S., H.S. Belding, F.C. Consolazio, S.M. Horvath, and E.S. Turrell
    1986   Acclimatization of older men to work in heat. J. Appl. Physiol. 20(4):583-586.
Rolls, B.J., I.C. Federoff, J.F. Guthrie, and L.J. Laster
    1990   Effects of temperature and mode of presentation of juice on hunger, thirst and
            food intake in humans. Appetite 15:199-208.
Rowell, L.B., H.J. Marx, R.A. Bruce, R.D. Conn, and F. Kusumi
    1966   Reductions in cardiac output, central blood volume and stroke volume with ther-
            mal stress in normal men during exercise. J. Clin. Invest. 45:1801-1816.
Rozin, P., L. Ebert, and J. Schull
    1982   Some like it hot: A temporal analysis of hedonic responses to chili pepper. Appe-
            tite 3:13-22.
Salganik, R.I.
    1956   Nutrition in high environmental temperatures. (in Russian) Vopr. Pitan. 33:3-11.
Saltin, B.
    1964   Aerobic and anaerobic work capacity after dehydration. J. Appl. Physiol. 19:1114-
            1118.
Sawka, M.N., and K.B. Pandolph
    1990   Effects of body water loss on exercise performance and physiological functions.
            Pp. 1-8 in Perspectives in Exercise Science and Sports Medicine, Vol. 3, Fluid
            Homeostasis During Exercise, C.V. Gisolfi and D.R. Lamb, eds. Indianapolis,
            Ind.: Benchmark Press.

Shapiro, Y., K.B. Pandolf, and R.F. Goldman
   1982   Predicting sweat loss response to exercise, environment and clothing. Eur. J. Appl. Physiol. 48:83-96.
Smolander, J., O. Korhonen, and R. Ilmarinen
   1990   Responses of young and older men during prolonged exercise in dry and humid heat. Eur. J. Appl. Physiol. 61:413-418.
Spector, N.H., J.R. Brobeck, and C.L. Hamilton
   1968   Feeding and core temperature in albino rats: Changes induced by preoptic heating and cooling. Science 161:286-288.
Stunkard, A., and B. Kaplan
   1977   Eating in public places. Int. J. Obesity 1: 89-91.
Stunkard, A., and A.J. Mayer
   1978   Smorgasbord and obesity. Psychosom. Med. 40: 173-176.
Thompson, C.I.
   1980   Controls of Eating. New York, N.Y.: Spectrum Publications.
Trant, A.S., and F.M. Pangborn
   1983   Discrimination, intensity, and hedonic responses to color, aroma, viscosity, and sweetness of beverages. Lebensmittel Wissenschaff und Technologie 16:147-152.
USDA (U.S. Department of Agriculture)
   1983   Food Intakes: Individuals in 48 States, Year 1977-78. Consumer Nutrition Division, Human Nutrition Information Service, Report No. I-1. August. Hyattsville, Maryland: U.S. Department of Agriculture.
U.S. Department of Health and Human Services
   1988   Summary and recommendations. Pp. 1-21 in The Surgeon General's Report on Nutrition and Health. Washington, D.C.: U.S. Government Printing Office.
U.S. Departments of the Army, the Navy, and the Air Force
   1968   Army Regulation 40-25, BUMED Instruction No. 10110.3, Air Force Regulation No. 160-95. "Nutritional Standards." July 2. Washington, D.C.
   1985   Army Regulation 40-25/Naval Command Medical Instruction 10110.1/Air Force Regulation 160-95. "Nutrition Allowances, Standards, and Education." May 15. Washington, D.C.
Weinman, K.P., Z. Slabochova, E.M. Bernauer, T. Morimoto, and F. Sargent II
   1967   Reactions of men and women to repeated exposure to humid heat. J. Appl. Physiol. 22:533-538.
Wenger, C.B.
   1988   Human heat acclimatization. Pp. 153-197 in Human Performance Physiology and Environmental Medicine at Terrestrial Extremes, K.B. Pandolf, M.N. Sawka, and R.R. Gonzalez, eds. Indianapolis, Ind.: Benchmark Press.
White, M.D., W.D. Ross, and I.B. Mekjavic
   1992   Relationship between physique and rectal temperature cooling rate. Undersea Biomed. Res. 19:121-130.
Williams, C.G., G.A.G. Bredell, C.H. Wyndham, N.B. Strydom, J.F. Morrison, J. Peter, P.W. Fleming, and J.S. Ward
   1962   Circulatory and metabolic reactions to work in heat. J. Appl. Physiol. 17:625-638.
WHO (World Health Organization)
   1985   Energy and Protein Requirements. Report of a Joint FAO/WHO/UNU Expert Consultation. Technical Report Series 724. World Health Organization, Geneva. 206 pp.
Wyndham, C.H.
   1977   Heatstroke and hyperthermia in marathon runners. Pp. 129-138 in The Marathon:

Physiological, Medical, Epidemiological and Psychological Studies, P. Milvy, ed. New York, N.Y.: New York Academy of Science.

Wyndham, C.H., J.F. Morrison, and C.G. Williams
1965   Heat reactions of male and female Caucasians. J. Appl. Physiol. 20:357-364.

Young, A.J., M.N. Sawka, L. Levine, B.S. Cadarette, and K.B. Pandolf
1985   Skeletal muscle metabolism during exercise is influenced by heat acclimation. J. Appl. Physiol. 59:1929-1935.

Zifferblatt, S.M., C.S. Wilbur, and J.L. Pinsky
1980   Influence of ecologic events on cafeteria food selections; Understanding food habits. J. Am. Dietet. Assoc. 76:9-14.

2

Conclusions and Recommendations

CONCLUSIONS

As stated in Chapter 1, the Committee on Military Nutrition Research (CMNR) was asked to respond to 11 specific questions dealing with nutrient requirements for work in hot environments. The committee's responses to these questions appear below:

1. What is the evidence that there are any significant changes in nutrient requirements for work in a hot environment?

Sensible and insensible water losses are increased markedly by work in a hot environment, resulting in an increased need for water. In general, energy requirements decline somewhat in a hot environment, primarily because of the tendency to reduce activity. However, other factors, including the degree of acclimatization, may modify the body's energy requirement in the heat. In addition, there is considerable individual variation. Recent evidence suggests that slight increases in protein may be required for work in hot environments; however, the Military Recommended Dietary Allowance (MRDA) for protein already includes an amount sufficient to meet this increased level given adequate consumption of kilocalories. Significant losses of several minerals occur with profuse sweating; however, current methodology does not provide data that indicate the need for measurable increases in requirements. Based on losses in sweat and the potential for dehydration, people working in hot environments may require additional sodium and other electrolytes. Vitamin requirements do not appear to increase with exposure to a hot environment; however, few studies have examined this issue. In particular, the role of antioxidant vitamins (A, C, and E) in reducing lipid peroxidation induced by exercise in a hot environment should be examined.

2. If such evidence exists, do the current Military Recommended Dietary Allowances (MRDAs) provide for these changes?

The variations in nutrient requirements, including sodium, that may occur as a result of working—and sweating—in a hot environment are reasonably covered by the nutrient content of the MRDAs, because the MRDAs provide generous allowances over most nutrient requirements. If military rations are consumed in amounts that approximate energy expenditures, it is likely that the nutrient requirements of soldiers will be met.

3. Should changes be made in military rations that may be used in hot environments to meet the nutrient requirements of soldiers with sustained activity in such climates?

Based on the evidence available at this time, the nutrient content of military rations does not need to be changed. Nevertheless, because appetite is depressed and food preferences and eating patterns are changed in response to short-term and long-term exposure to heat, changes should be made in ration components to enhance intake. Military feeding in hot environments needs to take into account what is known about these changes in food preferences and meal schedules. The components of the rations and field feeding environments should be adjusted to encourage consumption of military rations. Convenience, taste, and acceptability become all important.

4. Specifically, are the meals, ready-to-eat (MREs) good hot weather rations? Should the fat content be lower? Should the carbohydrate content be higher?

The nutritional composition of MRE rations is appropriate for use in a hot environment. There are no consistent data that suggest that the relative proportions of protein, carbohydrate, and fat should be altered. It is clear, however, that the experience gained during Operation Desert Storm regarding the acceptability of the various MRE rations and ration components needs to be evaluated.

Significant components, including the entrees, in the MREs available in 1991 required heating to provide the most palatable meal. As noted in anecdotes from those conducting observations in the Persian Gulf area during hot weather, the shift in soldiers' food preferences to a desire for cooler items (salads, sandwiches, etc.) confirms that the MREs were not designed specifically for long-term consumption in hot climates. Data from animal studies show an increase in fat consumption in the heat, with a decrease in protein consumption. As a result of the organoleptic changes in fat within foods in conditions of extreme heat, however, food products that contain significant amounts of fat may be deemed unacceptable by soldiers and thus may not be consumed.

The requirement for sustained physical activity in hot environments might result in the need for a modified ration that would encourage food consumption, for example, one lower in fat and higher in carbohydrate that could be consumed with little preparation. Heat-stable food products that are similar to those available in the private sector appear to be preferred by soldiers in terms of appetite. In designing MRE rations for use in hot environments, information from the experience gained during Operations Desert Shield and Desert Storm should be combined with what is known about how food preferences change in the heat. Moreover, factors other than ration composition that may influence food intake need to be considered. These include the availability of potable liquids in generous supply, the eating situation of troops (i.e., alone or in groups), the time of day when food may be offered, and the convenience of consuming the rations. Nonnutritional factors such as these can have a significant influence on ration intake.

5. What factors may influence food intake in hot environments?

The major factors that appear to influence food intake in hot environments are the need to maintain body temperature (through decreased intake to reduce the thermic effect of food) and the apparent relationship between decreased body weight and decreased body temperature. With the hydration regimens in place in the military, which appear to encourage adequate fluid intake, and the awareness among military personnel of potential heat stroke, the observation in laboratory animals of markedly decreased food intake to prevent hyperthermia is probably not a significant concern within the military population.

Other factors such as psychological stress may further depress food intake. In addition, the lack of a desire in hot environments to eat hot foods (even though their palatability may be greater than that of cold foods) and the concomitant increased desire to consume cold foods are documented somewhat subjectively in nationwide surveys of food intake of individuals from households in the U.S. general population during various seasons. The intake of food by humans in a hot environment may be further influenced by the availability of cool potable water, the time of day, the psychosocial environment, and ration components.

6. To what extent does fluid intake influence food intake?

Animal studies demonstrate that dehydration markedly decreases voluntary food intake and that forcing foods during dehydration results in increased mortality. Although there have been a few human studies of this question, it appears that rehydration is necessary in humans before depressed food intake returns to normal. To maximize the energy intake of military personnel in hot environments in which significant physical activity is required, maintenance of adequate hydration status should be a primary objective of all policies related to soldier readiness. Maintenance of states of proper hydration was also identified as the most critical issue facing soldiers in desert environments in an Army report on food management issues written during Operation Desert Storm (Norman and Gaither, 1991). The recent CMNR report *Fluid Replacement and Heat Stress* (Marriott and Rosemont, 1991) thoroughly addressed this issue.

7. Is there any scientific evidence that food preferences change in hot climates?

Several animal studies document changes in food preferences in hot environments. There are also a limited number of studies that show decreased caloric intake in humans when working in a hot environment. Most of these studies did not allow for acclimatization of subjects to the hot climate. In the one major study that did, food intake decreased less markedly in the acclimatized individuals, with no change in percent distribution of kilocalories from fat, carbohydrate, or protein. In the summer season food choices do change, but whether this is due to environmental temperature or other factors such as price and availability has not been well established. Thus, to date, most information on changes in food preferences in humans is limited to anecdotal observations or studies that were not balanced with respect to temporal adaptation to climatic change.

8. Are there special nutritional concerns in desert environments in which the daily temperature may change dramatically?

If rations are consumed in adequate amounts, no specific nutrient concerns need be addressed as a result of the dramatic changes in temperature that frequently occur in the desert. Adequate intake of fluid to avoid dehydration and help maintain food intake is obviously important. The levels of nutrients specified by the MRDAs appear to be adequate to meet the nutrient needs of soldiers if rations are consumed in appropriate amounts.

9. Is there an increased need for specific vitamins or minerals in the heat?

Although small increases may occur in the losses of B vitamins in sweat during work in hot environments, these losses do not appear to be great enough to justify increasing the requirement over that established in the MRDAs. There is limited evidence that vitamin C may have an effect in reducing heat stress during periods of acclimatization, particularly if the individual has had a low vitamin C intake prior to exposure to the heat.

However, there is insufficient evidence at this time to recommend an increase in vitamin C beyond that currently supplied by the MRDA.

Prolonged moderate- to high-intensity activity in hot environments will result in a significant loss of electrolytes (sodium, potassium, magnesium), particularly among troops who are not adapted to hot environments. However, if fluid intake is maintained to prevent dehydration and consumption of military rations is at or near energy requirements, sufficient intake of electrolytes should occur.

10. Does working in a hot climate change an individual's absorptive or digestive capability?

There is evidence that gastric emptying may be reduced during heat stress. Although the mechanisms responsible for this observation are unclear, they may be associated with dehydration, which frequently occurs when working in the heat, and with reduced splanchnic blood flow. Studies have also demonstrated that elevations in core body temperature can reduce stomach and intestinal motility. It is apparent that maintaining adequate fluid intake is important as an aid in reducing heat stress from working in a hot environment.

Limited evidence suggests that net calcium absorption may be reduced as a result of increased fecal losses during profuse sweating while working in hot environments. Some investigators have reported reduced intestinal absorption during exercise. However, other studies, by using more direct techniques of segmental perfusion, have shown no effect of either exercise intensity or duration on fluid absorption. In short, individuals who are well trained, acclimatized to heat, and accustomed to endurance exercise seem to experience fewer symptoms of gastrointestinal stress than less well conditioned and acclimatized individuals.

11. Does work at a moderate to heavy rate increase energy requirements in a hot environment to a greater extent than similar work in a temperate environment?

Uncertainty exists about the influence on energy requirements of working in the heat (see Chapter 6). Submaximal exercise in a hot environment does not appear to have an impact greater than that occurring in a more comfortable environment. Maintaining adequate food intake in the temperature extremes of hot environments to meet caloric needs is a higher priority than concern over small differences in energy requirements.

RECOMMENDATIONS

On the basis of the papers presented by the invited speakers, discussion at the workshop, and subsequent committee deliberations, the Committee on

Military Nutrition Research finds that the nutritional requirements for work in hot environments are not significantly different from those needed in more moderate conditions. The nutrient content of the military's operational rations is adequate to provide for any variation that may occur as a result of work in the heat. There are, however, significant concerns about inadequate intakes of soldiers engaged in field operations, exercises, or combat in that the nutrients actually consumed may be less than the amounts specified in the MRDAs. Special attention should be given to ensuring that the intake of rations by soldiers is adequate to meet caloric needs, thereby ensuring that each individual's nutrient requirements are met. Of primary consideration is maintaining adequate fluid intake to avoid dehydration and consequent decreased food intake. This topic has been addressed in a previous CMNR report, *Fluid Replacement and Heat Stress* (Marriott and Rosemont, 1991). The committee wishes to reiterate that water is the most important nutrient for maintaining the performance of the soldier.

The committee offers the following recommendations regarding nutrient requirements for work in hot environments.

1. The maintenance of adequate hydration should be the major objective of efforts to maintain the sustained performance of troops in hot environments. As recognized by current Army doctrine, water is an essential nutrient.

2. Maintaining an adequate intake of operational rations should also be an important objective, particularly in hot environments, to ensure that troops will meet their nutritional needs over the course of extended military operations.

3. Based on observations of the decreased food intake in hot environments, changes should be made in rations and their components to enhance appetite and food intake. These changes should include ensuring the delivery of a variety of ration options to avoid menu fatigue.

4. Delivery systems and feeding situations should be designed to enhance intake and take into account the environmental factors, including psychosocial factors, that influence food consumption. The following should be considered:

- availability of cool, flavored, potable water,
- a cooling environment such as shade,
- time of day for meal service,
- the social situation during meals,
- ration preparation requirements,
- use of familiar commercial food products, and
- ethnic food preferences.

5. Variations in ration components for different environments (hot-dry, hot-humid, moderate, and cold) should be evaluated.

AREAS FOR FUTURE RESEARCH

The Committee on Military Nutrition Research suggests a number of areas for future research within the military related to nutrition for soldiers working in hot environments. The CMNR believes that the military services, through their pool of volunteer personnel, offer an excellent and often unique opportunity to generate research data and statistics on the nutrition, health, and well-being of service personnel. These findings can be directly applied to improve both the health of military personnel and that of the general U.S. population.

Future Research Needs

• The observed decreases in food intake in hot environments and the previous lack of research emphasis on this subject urge the investigation of factors that affect food intake in a hot ambient environment. Such factors include but are not limited to the following:

— environmental conditions in the dining situation such as meal setting, menu item variability, food item temperature, social setting, and meal timing and frequency;

— ethnic and gender differences in food preferences;

— the relationship of food preferences to climate, with a focus on carefully controlled studies of the same individuals in temperate and hot environments (both dry and humid);

— chemosensory perception of foods and menus in relation to climate; and

— composition of the ration, that is, proportion of fat, carbohydrates, etc.

• In addition to the application of current biochemical indicators, an important area of research is the development and validation of appropriate functional indicators of nutritional status, with an emphasis on vitamins and minerals for which sweat losses are significant. These functional indicators should relate to endurance, immunity, antioxidants, nutrient deficiencies, and recovery from illness/trauma. A particular concern would be the iron status of military women under conditions that produced significant sweating.

• The potential role in stress responses of higher dietary intakes of zinc, vitamin C, and other antioxidants could be explored further with emphasis on heat stress.

• Studies that focus on gastrointestinal function in the heat are important, in particular, the effects of various levels of militarily relevant physical activity and the interaction of physical activity with psychological stress and gastrointestinal function.

• More research is needed to evaluate the impact of adequate mineral intake on physical performance in a hot environment. Such research would allow the development of more specific recommendations concerning circumstances in which mineral supplements or food fortification is indicated. In particular, studies are needed that separate the effects of exercise from the effects of an elevated ambient temperature, and studies that evaluate the effects of higher levels of mineral intake on functional indicators.

• Does heat enhance satiety or impair hunger? These questions could be addressed through research that more specifically addresses whether the effect of heat on appetite suppression is expressed in terms of smaller meals—presumptive satiety effects—or less frequent meals—presumptive hunger effects.

• In light of animal studies of hypoxia, additional research appears warranted to evaluate whether the decreased human food intake in hot environments serves a protective metabolic effect.

• The committee has noted in a number of research projects presented for its review, that there is a decrease in food intake of military personnel under operational conditions regardless of environmental climate. Based on these results it is recommended that a study be conducted to determine why soldiers don't consume adequate amounts of food to maintain body weight under operational conditions, and to evaluate steps that may be taken to achieve adequate ration intake.

The Committee on Military Nutrition Research is pleased to participate with the Division of Nutrition, U.S. Army Research Institute of Environmental Medicine, U.S. Army Medical Research and Development Command, in programs related to the nutrition and health of American military personnel. The CMNR hopes that this information will be useful and helpful to the Department of Defense in developing programs that continue to improve the lifetime health and well-being of service personnel.

REFERENCES

Marriott, B.M., and C. Rosemont, eds.
  1991   Fluid Replacement and Heat Stress: Proceeding of a Workshop, 2nd printing. Washington, D.C.: National Academy Press.
Norman, E.J., and R.M. Gaither
  1991   Review of Army Food Related Operations in Hot Desert Environments. Technical Report Natick/TR-91/008. United States Army Natick Research, Development and Engineering Center. Natick, Mass.

PART II

Invited Presentations

OVERVIEW

IN PART II THE EXPERT PAPERS that formed the basis for the development of the basic science summary and recommendations in Part I are included here in the order they were presented at the workshop. A sub-committee of the CMNR worked with the Army Grant Officer Representative, COL E. Wayne Askew to define the focus for the workshop and the report. Speakers were selected who were active senior investigators and well known for their research in the specific area. Each speaker was asked to carefully review the literature in his or her field of expertise as it related to the eleven questions posed to the Committee, and provide copies of scientific articles as background papers to the CMNR prior to the workshop. In their presentation and in their chapter, the invited experts were requested to make critical comments on the relevant research and conclude with their personal recommendations. There was a recorded question and answer period at the end of each presentation. Selected questions directed toward the speakers and their responses that were recorded during the workshop are included at the end of each chapter. After the workshop, authors were given the opportunity to revise or add to their papers based on committee questions. The final papers were used by the committee in the development of Part I.

A computerized literature search was conducted as part of the planning for this workshop. Selected citations from Part I, the following chapters, and the literature search have been compiled into the Selected Bibliography on Nutritional Needs in Hot Environments in Appendix B. Although the conclusions of the following chapters focused on the impact of a hot environment on work in a military setting, these chapters provide a state-of-the-art review of effect of heat on any type of outdoor activity whether heavy work, sports, or recreation.

3

Physiological Responses to Exercise in the Heat

Michael N. Sawka,[1] C. Bruce Wenger, Andrew J. Young, and Kent B. Pandolf

INTRODUCTION

Humans often exercise strenuously in hot environments for reasons of recreation, vocation, and survival. The magnitude of physiological strain imposed by exercise-environmental stress depends on the individual's metabolic rate and capacity for heat exchange with the environment. Muscular exercise increases metabolism by 5 to 15 times the resting rate to provide energy for skeletal muscle contraction. Depending on the type of exercise, 70 to 100 percent of the metabolism is released as heat and needs to be dissipated in order to maintain body heat balance. The effectiveness of the thermoregulatory system in defending body temperature is influenced by the individual's acclimatization state (Wenger, 1988), aerobic fitness (Armstrong and Pandolf, 1988), and hydration level (Sawka and Pandolf, 1990). Aerobically fit persons who are heat acclimatized and fully hydrated have less body heat storage and perform optimally during exercise-heat stress. To regulate body temperature, heat gain and loss are controlled by the autonomic nervous system's alteration of (a) heat flow from the core to the skin via the blood and (b) sweating. Thermoreceptors in the skin and body core provide input into the hypothalamic thermoregulatory center where this information is processed, via a proportional control system, with a resultant

---

[1] Michael N. Sawka, Ph.D., Thermal Physiology and Medicine Division, U.S. Research Institute of Environmental Medicine, Kansas Street, Natick, MA 01760-5007

signal for heat loss by the thermoregulatory effector responses of sweating and alterations in skin blood flow (Sawka and Wenger, 1988).

This chapter reviews human temperature regulation and normal physiological responses to exercise-heat stress. In general, muscular exercise and heat stress interact synergistically and may push physiological systems to their limits in simultaneously supporting the competing metabolic and thermoregulatory demands.

CORE TEMPERATURE RESPONSES TO EXERCISE

During muscular exercise, core temperature initially increases rapidly and subsequently increases at a reduced rate until heat loss equals heat production, and essentially steady-state values are achieved. At the initiation of exercise, the metabolic rate increases immediately; however, the thermoregulatory effector responses for heat dissipation respond more slowly. The thermoregulatory effector responses, which enable sensible (radiative and convective) and insensible (evaporative) heat loss to occur, increase in proportion to the rise in core temperature. Eventually, these heat loss mechanisms increase sufficiently to balance metabolic heat production, allowing achievement of a steady-state core temperature.

During muscular exercise, the magnitude of core temperature elevation is largely independent of the environmental condition and is proportional to the metabolic rate (Gonzalez et al., 1978; Nielsen, 1938, 1970). This concept was first presented by Nielsen (1938) who had three subjects perform exercise at several intensities (up to approximately 3.0 liters oxygen per minute) in a broad temperature range (5° to 36°C with low humidity). Figure 3-1 presents the heat exchange data for one subject during an hour of cycle exercise at a power output of 147 watts and at a metabolic rate of approximately 650 watts. The difference between metabolic rate and total heat loss represents the energy used for mechanical work and heat storage. The total heat loss and, therefore, the heat storage and elevation of core temperature were constant for each environment. The relative contributions of sensible and insensible heat exchange to total heat loss, however, varied with environmental conditions. In the 10°C environment, the large skin-to-ambient temperature gradient facilitated sensible heat exchange, which accounted for about 70 percent of the total heat loss. As ambient temperature increased, this gradient for sensible heat exchange diminished, and there was a greater reliance upon insensible heat exchange. When the ambient temperature was equal to skin temperature, insensible heat exchange accounted for almost all the heat loss. In addition, when the ambient temperature exceeded the skin temperature, there was a sensible heat gain to the body.

Nielsen's finding that the magnitude of core temperature elevation is

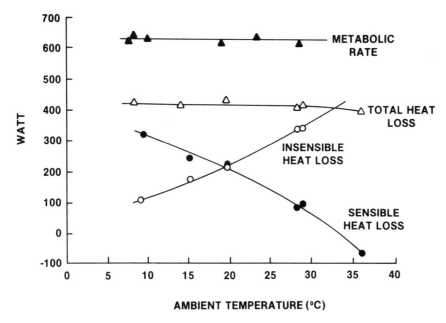

FIGURE 3-1 Heat exchange data averaged over 1 hour for one subject performing constant intensity exercise in a variety of ambient temperatures. The difference between metabolic rate and total heat loss is the sum of mechanical power (147 watts) and mean rate of heat storage. SOURCE: Sawka and Wenger (1988), used with permission. Redrawn from Nielsen (1938).

independent of environmental conditions is inconsistent with the personal experience of most athletes. For example, a runner will experience greater hyperthermia if he or she competes in a 35°C environment (Robinson, 1963). Lind (1963) showed that the magnitude of core temperature elevation during exercise is independent of the environment only within a certain range of conditions or a "prescriptive zone." Figure 3-2 presents a subject's steady-state core temperature responses during exercise performed at three metabolic intensities in a broad range of environmental conditions. The environmental conditions are represented by the "old" effective temperature, which is an index that combines the effects of dry-bulb temperature, humidity, and air motion. Note that during exercise the greater the metabolic rate, the lower the upper limit of the prescriptive zone. In addition, Lind found that even within the prescriptive zone there was a small but significant positive relationship between the steady-state core temperature and the "old" effective temperature. It seems fair to conclude that throughout a wide range of environmental conditions, the magnitude of core temperature elevation during exercise is largely, but not entirely, independent of

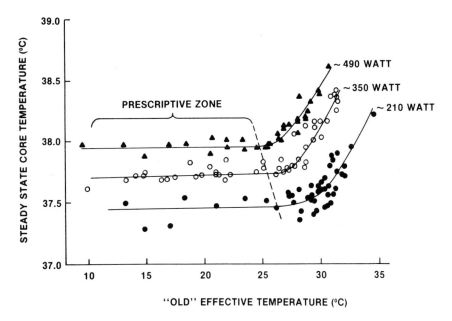

FIGURE 3-2 Relationship of steady-state core temperature responses during exercise at three metabolic rates to the environmental conditions. SOURCE: Sawka and Wenger (1988), used with permission. Redrawn from Lind (1963).

the environment. During exercise with a substantial metabolic requirement, the prescriptive zone might be exceeded, and there is a further elevation of steady-state core temperature.

As stated, within the prescriptive zone, the magnitude of core temperature elevation during exercise is proportional to the metabolic rate (Nielsen, 1938; Saltin and Hermansen, 1966; Stolwijk et al., 1968). Although the relationship between metabolic rate and core temperature is strong for a given individual, it does not always hold well for comparisons between different individuals. Åstrand (1960) first reported that the use of relative intensity (percentage of maximal oxygen uptake), rather than actual metabolic rate (absolute intensity), removes most of the intersubject variability for the core temperature elevation during exercise.

METABOLISM

Metabolic Rate

The effects of acute heat stress on a person's ability to achieve maximal aerobic metabolic rates during exercise have been thoroughly studied. Most investigators find that maximal oxygen uptake is reduced in hot compared to temperate environments (Klausen et al., 1967; Rowell et al., 1969; Saltin et al., 1972; Sen Gupta et al., 1977), but some investigators report no differences (Rowell et al., 1965; Williams et al., 1962). For example, in one study (Sawka et al., 1985) maximal oxygen uptake ($\dot{V}_{O_2 max}$) was 0.25 liter per minute lower in a 49°C, as compared to a 20°C, environment (see Figure 3-3). Clearly, heat stress reduces $\dot{V}_{O_2 max}$ relative to that achieved in a temperate environment. In addition, the state of heat acclimatization did not alter the approximate 0.25 liter per minute decrement in $\dot{V}_{O_2 max}$. The question remains, What physiological mechanism(s) is/are responsible for this reduction in $\dot{V}_{O_2 max}$? It can be theorized that thermal stress might result in a displacement of blood to the cutaneous vasculature, which could (a) reduce the portion of cardiac output perfusing the contracting musculature or (b) result in a decreased effective central blood volume and thus reduce venous return and cardiac output. As skin blood flow can reach 7 liters per minute

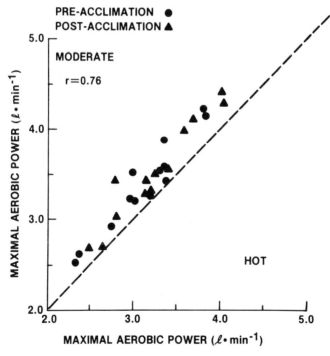

FIGURE 3-3 Maximal aerobic power values (liters per minute) for the pre- and postheat acclimatization tests in a moderate (21°C, 30 percent relative humidity) and a hot (49°C, 20 percent relative humidity) environment. r = Pearson product-moment correlation coefficient. SOURCE: Sawka et al. (1985), used with permission.

TABLE 3-1 Papers Reporting the Effect of Heat on Metabolic Rate During Exercise

Study	Exercise Mode	Metabolic Intensity	Test Environment	Change in Metabolic Rate	Comment
Brouha et al., 1960	Cycle	460 watts	25 vs 32°C 25 vs 37°C	NC* ↓(14%)	—
Consolazio et al., 1961	Treadmill	400 watts	26 vs 40°C 26 vs 41°C 26 vs 40°C 26 vs 41°C	↑(9%) ↑(19%) ↑(8%) ↑(4%)	Acclimated
Consolazio et al., 1963	Cycle	205 watts 545 watts 205 watts 545 watts	21 vs 29°C 21 vs 38°C	NC NC ↑(12%) ↑(11%)	— — — —
Dimri et al., 1980	Cycle	10-90% $\dot{V}_{O_2\,max}$	27 vs 37°C 27 vs 40°C	↑(8%) ↑(18%)	Acclimated ↑LA†
Fink et al., 1975	Cycle	70-85% $\dot{V}_{O_2\,max}$	9 vs 41°C	↑	Unacclimated ↑LA
Peterson and Vejby-Christensen, 1973	Cycle	87-347 watts	24 vs 32°C	↓	Unacclimated ↑LA
Williams et al., 1962	Cycle	—	20 vs 36°C	↓(0.2 liter)	Acclimated ↑LA
Young et al., 1985	Cycle	793 watts	21 vs 49°C	↓(3%)	Unacclimated and Acclimated ↑LA

* NC = No change.
† LA = Plasma lactate.

(Rowell, 1986) during maximal vasodilation, the contracting musculature could receive less perfusion at a given cardiac output level. Rowell et al. (1966) reported that during high-intensity exercise in the heat, cardiac output can be reduced by 1.2 liters per minute below control levels. A reduction in maximal cardiac output by 1.2 liters per minute could account for a 0.25-liter-per-minute decrement in $\dot{V}_{O_2 max}$ with heat exposure, because each liter of blood could deliver about 0.2 liter of oxygen (1.34 ml oxygen per g hemoglobin × 15 g hemoglobin per 100 ml of blood).

Acute heat stress increases resting metabolic rate (Consolazio et al., 1961, 1963; Dimri et al., 1980), but the effect of heat stress on an individual's metabolic rate for performing a given submaximal exercise task is not so clear (see Table 3-1). Such an effect would influence the calculation of the heat balance and might have implications for the nutritional requirements of individuals exposed to hot environments. Many investigators report that to perform a given submaximal exercise task, the metabolic rate is greater in a hot than temperate environment (Consolazio et al., 1961, 1963; Dimri et al., 1980; Fink et al., 1975). Some investigators, however, report lower metabolic rates in the heat (Brouha et al., 1960; Petersen and Vejby-Christensen, 1973; Williams et al., 1962; Young et al., 1985). Heat acclimation state does not account for whether individuals demonstrate an increased or decreased metabolic rate during submaximal exercise in the heat. However, other mechanisms can explain this discrepancy. Most investigators have only calculated the aerobic metabolic rate during submaximal exercise, ignoring the contribution of anaerobic metabolism to total metabolic rate.

Dimri et al. (1980) had six subjects exercise at three intensities in each of three environments. Figure 3-4 presents their subjects' total metabolic rate (bottom) and the percentage of this metabolic rate that was contributed by aerobic and anaerobic metabolic pathways. The anaerobic metabolism was calculated by measuring the postexercise oxygen uptake that was in excess of resting baseline levels. Although there are limitations to this methodology, the study provides useful information. Note that to perform exercise at a given power output, the total metabolic rate increased with the elevated ambient temperature. More importantly, the percentage of the total metabolic rate contributed by anaerobic metabolism also increased with the ambient temperature. The increase in anaerobic metabolic rate exceeded the increase of total metabolic rate during exercise at the elevated ambient temperatures. Therefore, if only the aerobic metabolic rate had been quantified, Dimri et al. (1980) would probably have reported a decreased metabolic rate in the heat for performing exercise at a given power output. Investigations that report a lower metabolic rate during exercise in the heat also report increased plasma or muscle lactate levels (Petersen and Vejby-Christensen, 1973; Williams et al., 1962; Young et al., 1985) or an increased respiratory exchange ratio (Brouha et al., 1960), which also suggests an

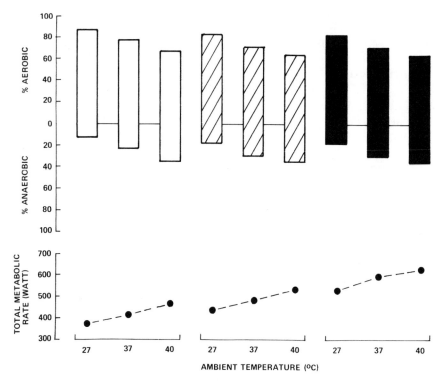

FIGURE 3-4 The total metabolic rate and percentage contribution of aerobic and anaerobic metabolism during exercise at different ambient temperatures. SOURCE: Sawka and Wenger (1988), used with permission. Data from Dimri (1980).

increased anaerobic metabolism. Likewise, other investigators report that plasma lactate levels are greater during submaximal exercise in a hot as compared to a comfortable environment (Dill et al., 1930/1931; Dimri et al., 1980; Fink et al., 1975; Nadel 1983; Robinson et al., 1941).

Interestingly, the oxygen uptake response to submaximal exercise does appear to be affected by heat acclimatization (Sawka et al., 1983). Most reports indicate that oxygen uptake and aerobic metabolic rate during submaximal exercise are reduced by heat acclimatization, although a significant effect is not always observed (see Table 3-2). Large effects (14 to 17 percent reductions) have been reported for stair-stepping (Senay and Kok, 1977; Shvartz et al., 1977; Strydom et al., 1966), but some of the reduction in $\dot{V}_{O_2}$ during stair-stepping can be attributed to increased skill and improved efficiency acquired during the acclimatization program (Sawka et al., 1983). In other studies, although the acclimatization-induced reductions were statistically

TABLE 3-2 Papers Reporting the Effect Heat Acclimatization Has on Metabolic Rate During Exercise

Study	n	Acclimatization (days)	Exercise Mode	Test Environment	Change in Metabolic Rate (ΔM)	%Δ
Cleland et al., 1969	3	7	Treadmill	Hot	NC*	—
Eichna et al., 1950	3	10	Treadmill	Hot	→	4
				Cool		2
Gisolfi, 1973	6	8	Treadmill	Hot	→	12
Jooste and Strydom, 1979	4	7	Treadmill	Hot	→	?
				Cool	→	?
Piwonka and Robinson, 1967	3	4	Treadmill	Hot	NC	—
Robinson et al., 1941	5	10-23	Treadmill	Hot	→	8
Rowell et al., 1967	6	11-12	Treadmill	Hot	NC	—
Sawka et al., 1983	42	6-10	Treadmill	Hot	→	3
				Cool	→	5
Senay and Kok, 1977	5	8	Step	Hot	→	14
				Cool	→	7
Shvartz et al., 1977	7	8	Step	Hot	→	16
				Cool	→	14
	7	8	Step	Hot	→	14
				Cool	→	14
	7	8	Step	Hot	→	10
				Cool	→	9
Strydom et al., 1966	5	12	Step	Hot	→	17
Weinman et al., 1967	5	8	Treadmill	Hot	NC	—
	5	8	Treadmill	Hot	NC	—
Wyndham et al., 1976	4	10	Cycle	Hot	NC	—

*No change.

SOURCE: Modified from Sawka et al. (1983).

significant, the magnitude of the effects was reported to be smaller for treadmill and cycle-ergometer exercise.

Skeletal Muscle Metabolism

Several investigations examined the effects of environmental heat stress on skeletal muscle metabolism during exercise. Fink et al. (1975) had six subjects perform 45 minutes of cycle exercise (70 to 85 percent of $\dot{V}_{O_2 max}$) in a cold (9°C) and a hot (41°C) environment. They found greater plasma lactate levels and increased muscle glycogen utilization during exercise in the heat. Also, muscle triglyceride utilization was reduced during exercise in the heat as compared to the cold. In addition, serum glucose concentration increased, and serum triglyceride concentration decreased during exercise in the heat, compared to the opposite responses during exercise in the cold. During exercise in the heat, the increased muscle glycogen utilization was attributed to an increased anaerobic glycolysis resulting from local muscle hypoxia, caused by a reduced muscle blood flow. Because these investigators (Fink et al., 1975) did not perform control experiments in a temperate environment, it is not known if the differences reported are due partially to the effects of the cold exposure.

Young et al. (1985) had 13 subjects perform 30 minutes of cycle exercise (70 percent of $\dot{V}_{O_2 max}$) in a temperate (20°C) and a hot (49°C) environment. They found skeletal muscle and plasma lactate concentrations were greater during exercise in the heat. There was no difference in muscle glycogen utilization between the two experimental conditions. Young et al. (1985) speculated that during exercise in the heat, an alternative glycolytic substrate might have been utilized, such as blood glucose. Rowell et al. (1968) demonstrated a dramatic increase in hepatic glucose release into the blood during exercise in a hot compared to a temperate environment. Such an increased release of hepatic glucose could account for the elevated serum glucose concentration reported in the hot environment by Fink et al. (1975).

Data from Dimri et al. (1980) and Young et al. (1985) support the concept of increased anaerobic metabolism during submaximal exercise in the heat. Much of the other support for this concept is based on the findings that, during submaximal exercise, the plasma lactate accumulation is greater in a hot than in a comfortable environment. However, any inference about metabolic effects within the skeletal muscle from changes in plasma lactate is open to debate. Plasma lactate concentration reflects the balance between muscular production, efflux into the blood, and removal from the blood. Rowell et al. (1968) have shown that during exercise in the heat the splanchnic vasoconstriction reduced hepatic removal of plasma lactate. Therefore, the greater blood lactate accumulation during submaximal exercise in the heat can be attributed, at least in part, to a redistribution of blood flow away from the splanchnic tissues.

Lactate accumulation in blood and muscle during submaximal exercise is generally found to be reduced following heat acclimatization (Young, 1990). Figure 3-5 shows that heat acclimatization resulted in lower post-exercise muscle lactate concentrations. Muscle lactate concentrations were still higher in the heat than in the cool, and changes in blood lactate concentrations followed exactly the same patterns (Young et al., 1985). King et al. (1985) and Kirwan et al. (1987) observed that heat acclimatization reduced muscle glycogen utilization during exercise in the heat by 40 to 50 percent compared to before acclimatization. Young et al. (1985) also observed a statistically significant glycogen sparing effect due to heat acclimatization, but the reduction in glycogen utilization was small and apparent only during exercise in the cool conditions. Glycogen utilization during exercise in the heat was negligibly affected. The mechanism(s) for the reduction in lactate accumulation during exercise associated with heat acclimatization remains unidentified.

Evaporative Heat Loss

Figure 3-1 illustrates that when ambient temperature increases, there is a greater dependence on insensible (evaporative) heat loss to defend core temperature during exercise. In contrast to most animals, respiratory evaporative cooling is small in humans when compared to total skin evaporative cooling. The use of skin provides the advantage of having a greater surface area available for evaporation. The eccrine glands secrete sweat on the skin surface, which is cooled when the sweat evaporates. The rate of evaporation depends on the wetted area, air movement, and the water vapor pressure gradient between the skin and the surrounding air; the wider the gradient, the greater the rate of evaporation.

For a given person, sweating rate is highly variable and depends on environmental conditions (ambient temperature, dew point temperature, radiant load, and air velocity); clothing (insulation and moisture permeability); and physical activity level (Shapiro et al., 1982). Adolph et al. (1947) reported that for 91 men studied during diverse military activities in the desert, the average sweating rate was 4.1 liters every 24 hours, but values ranged from 1 to 11 liters every 24 hours. The water requirements of soldiers on the modern battlefield may be even greater. The threat of chemical warfare may require military personnel to wear nuclear-biological-chemical (NBC) protective clothing, which prevents noxious agents from reaching the skin. Characterized by low moisture permeability and high insulating properties, NBC clothing prevents the normal dissipation of body heat. As a

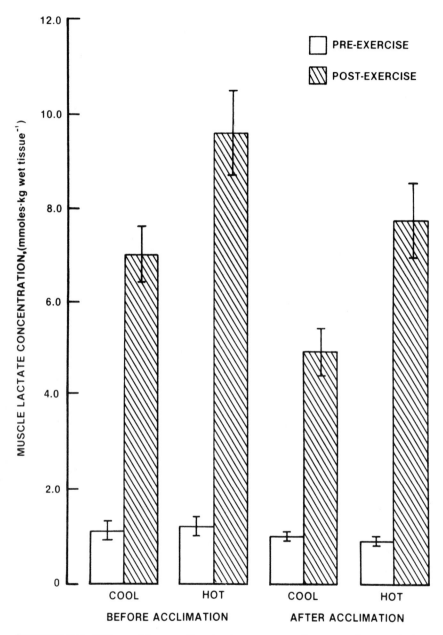

FIGURE 3-5 Effects of heat acclimatization on pre- and postexercise muscle lactate concentration (mean ± standard error) in cool (24°C) and hot (49°C) environments. SOURCE: Young et al. (1985), used with permission.

result, both core and skin temperatures can rise excessively and result in high levels of sweat output, which cannot evaporate within the garments. For example, during light- to moderate-intensity (about 150 to 400 watts) exercise in hot environments, soldiers wearing NBC clothing routinely have sweating rates of 1 to 2 liters per hour (Muza et al., 1988; Pimental et al., 1987).

For athletes, the highest sweating rates occur during prolonged high-intensity exercise in the heat. Figure 3-6 (Sawka and Pandolf, 1990) provides an approximation of hourly sweating rates and, therefore, water requirements for runners based on metabolic rate data from several laboratories. The sweating rates were predicted by the equation developed by Shapiro et al. (1982). The amount of body fluid lost as sweat can vary greatly, and sweating rates of 1 liter per hour are very common. The highest sweating

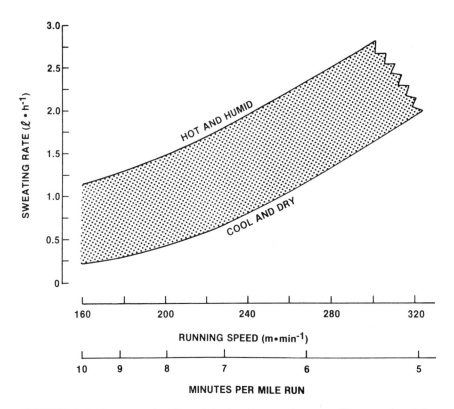

FIGURE 3-6 An approximation of the hourly sweating rates (liters per hour) for runners. Running speed is indicated in meters per minute. SOURCE: Sawka and Pandolf (1990), used with permission.

rate reported in the literature is 3.7 liters per hour, measured for Alberto Salazar during the 1984 Olympic Marathon (Armstrong et al., 1986).

If sweat loss is not fully replaced, the individual's total body water will be decreased (dehydration). Because sweat is more dilute than plasma, dehydration from sweat loss results in an increased plasma tonicity and decreased blood volume, both of which will act to reduce sweat output and skin blood flow (Sawka and Pandolf, 1990). As a result, the body's ability to dissipate heat will be decreased, and dehydration will result in a greater rise in core temperature during exercise-heat stress. In addition, the combination of an elevated core temperature and a reduced blood volume will increase the circulatory strain.

SKIN BLOOD FLOW AND CIRCULATORY RESPONSES

Blood flow from the deep body tissues to the skin transfers heat by convection. When core and skin temperatures are low enough that sweating does not occur, raising skin blood flow brings skin temperature nearer to blood temperature, and lowering skin blood flow brings skin temperature nearer to ambient temperature. This phenomenon allows the body to control sensible (convective and radiative) heat loss by varying skin blood flow and thus skin temperature. In conditions in which sweating occurs, the tendency of skin blood flow to warm the skin is approximately balanced by the tendency of sweating to cool the skin. Therefore, there is usually little change in skin temperature and sensible heat exchange after sweating has begun, and skin blood flow serves primarily to deliver to the skin the heat that is being removed by sweat evaporation. Skin blood flow and sweating thus work in tandem to dissipate heat under such conditions.

During exercise-heat stress, thermoregulatory skin blood flow, although not precisely known, may be as high as 7 liters per minute (Rowell, 1986). The higher skin blood flow will generally, but not always, result in a higher cardiac output, and one might expect the increased work of the heart in pumping this blood to be the major source of cardiovascular strain associated with heat stress. The work of the heart in providing the skin blood flow necessary for thermoregulation in the heat imposes a substantial cardiac strain on patients with severe cardiac disease (Burch and DePasquale, 1962). In healthy subjects, however, the cardiovascular strain associated with stress results mostly from reduced cardiac filling and stroke volume (Figure 3-7), which necessitate a higher heart rate to maintain cardiac output (Nadel et al., 1979; Sawka and Wenger, 1988). This change occurs because the venous bed of the skin is large and compliant and dilates reflexively during heat stress. Therefore, as skin blood flow increases, the blood vessels of the skin become engorged and blood pools in the skin, thus reducing central blood volume and cardiac filling.

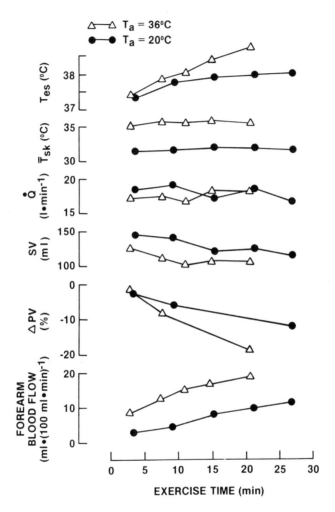

FIGURE 3-7 Thermal and circulatory responses of one subject during cycle exercise at 70 percent $\dot{V}_{O_2 \, max}$ in ambient temperatures (T_a) of 20° and 36°C, showing (from top) esophageal (T_{es}) and mean skin (T_{sk}) temperatures, cardiac output (Q), stroke volume (SV), percentage change in plasma volume (PV), and forearm blood flow. SOURCE: Sawka and Wenger (1988), used with permission. Redrawn from Nadel et al. (1979).

Several reflex adjustments compensate for peripheral pooling of blood and decreases in blood volume to help maintain cardiac filling, cardiac output, and arterial pressure during exercise-heat stress. Splanchnic and renal blood flows are reduced during exercise in proportion to relative exercise intensity (that is, as a percentage of $\dot{V}_{O_2 max}$) (Rowell, 1986). These blood flows also undergo a graded and progressive reduction in subjects who are heated while resting; and in the splanchnic bed, at least, the vasoconstrictor effects of temperature and of exercise appear to be additive, so that at any exercise intensity, the reduction in splanchnic blood flow is greater at a higher skin temperature (Rowell, 1986). Reduction of renal and splanchnic blood flow allows a corresponding diversion of cardiac output to skin and exercising muscle. A substantial volume of blood can thus be mobilized from these beds to help maintain cardiac filling during exercise and heat stress.

During exercise in the heat, the primary cardiovascular challenge is simultaneously to provide sufficient blood flow to exercising skeletal muscle to support metabolism and to provide sufficient blood flow to the skin to dissipate heat. In hot environments, the core-to-skin temperature gradient is less than in cool environments, so that skin blood flow must be relatively high to achieve sufficient heat transfer to maintain thermal balance (Rowell, 1986; Sawka and Wenger, 1988). This high skin blood flow causes pooling of blood in the compliant skin veins, especially below heart level. In addition, as discussed, sweat secretion can result in a net loss of body water, and thereby a reduction in blood volume (Sawka and Pandolf, 1990). Heat stress can reduce cardiac filling through pooling of blood in the skin and through reduced blood volume. Compensatory responses include reductions in splanchnic and renal blood flow; increased cardiac contractility, which helps to defend stroke volume in the face of impaired cardiac filling; and increased heart rate to compensate for decreased stroke volume. If these compensatory responses are insufficient, skin and muscle blood flow will be impaired, possibly leading to dangerous hyperthermia and reduced exercise performance.

SUMMARY

• Acclimatization state, aerobic fitness and hydration level are important factors influencing a person's ability to dissipate body heat to the environment.

• The higher the ambient temperature, the greater the dependence on evaporative heat loss to maintain body heat balance.

• During exercise, the elevation in core temperature is dependent on the metabolic rate, when the environment has sufficient capacity for heat exchange.

• Heat stress reduces a person's ability to achieve maximal metabolic rates during exercise.

• Heat stress increases the total metabolic rate and anaerobic participation during submaximal exercise, and these increases are somewhat abated by heat acclimatization.

• Exercise-heat stress reduces hepatic blood flow and increases hepatic glucose release.

• Individuals routinely have sweating rates of 1 liter per hour when working in hot environments.

• Dehydration from sweat loss increases plasma tonicity and decreases blood volume, both of which reduce heat loss and result in elevated core temperature levels during exercise-heat stress.

• During exercise-heat stress, competing metabolic and thermoregulatory demands for blood flow make it difficult to maintain an adequate cardiac output.

REFERENCES

Adolph, E.F., and associates
1947   Physiology of Man in the Desert. New York: Interscience Publishers.

Armstrong, L.E., and K.B. Pandolf
1988   Physical training, cardiorespiratory physical fitness and exercise-heat tolerance. Pp. 199-226 in Human Performance Physiology and Environmental Medicine at Terrestrial Extremes, K.B. Pandolf, M.N. Sawka, and R.R. Gonzalez, eds. Indianapolis, Ind.: Benchmark Press.

Armstrong, L.E., R.W. Hubbard, B.H. Jones, and J.T. Daniels
1986   Preparing Alberto Salazar for the heat of the 1984 Olympic Marathon. Physician Sportsmed. 14(3):73-81.

Åstrand, I.
1960   Aerobic work capacity in men and women. Acta Physiol. Scand. 49(suppl. 169):64-73.

Brouha, L., P.E. Smith, Jr., R. De Lanne, and M.E. Maxfield
1960   Physiological reactions of men and women during muscular activity and recovery in various environments. J. Appl. Physiol. 16:133-140.

Burch, G.E., and N.P. DePasquale
1962   Hot Climates, Man and His Heart. Springfield, Ill.: Charles C. Thomas.

Cleland, T.S., S.M. Horvath, and M. Phillips
1969   Acclimatization of women to heat after training. Int. Z. Angew. Physiol. 27:15-24.

Consolazio, C.F., R. Shapiro, J.E. Masterson, and P.S.L. McKinzie
1961   Energy requirements of men in extreme heat. J. Nutr. 73:126-134.

Consolazio, C.F., L.O. Matoush, R.A. Nelson, J.A. Torres, and G.J. Isaac
1963   Environmental temperature and energy expenditures. J. Appl. Physiol. 18:65-68.

Dill, D.B., H.T. Edwards, P.S. Bauer, and E.J. Levenson
1930/   Physical performance in relation to external temperature. Arbeitsphysiologie 3:508-
1931   518.

Dimri, G.P., M.S. Malhotra, J. Sen Gupta, T.S. Kumar, and B.S. Aora
1980   Alterations in aerobic-anaerobic proportions of metabolism during work in heat. Eur. J. Appl. Physiol. 45:43-50.

Eichna, L.W., C.R. Park, N. Nelson, S.M. Horvath, and E.D. Palmes
  1950   Thermal regulation during acclimatization in a hot, dry (desert type) environment.
         Am. J. Physiol. 163:585-597.
Fink, W.J., D.L. Costill, and W.J. Van Handel
  1975   Leg muscle metabolism during exercise in the heat and cold. Eur. J. Appl. Physiol.
         34:183-190.
Gisolfi, C.V.
  1973   Work-heat tolerance derived from interval training. J. Appl. Physiol. 35:349-354.
Gonzalez, R.R., L.G. Berglund, and A.P. Gagge
  1978   Indices of thermoregulatory strain for moderate exercise in the heat. J. Appl.
         Physiol. 44:889-899.
Jooste, P.L., and N.B. Strydom
  1979   Improved mechanical efficiency derived from heat acclimation. S. Afr. J. Res.
         Sport Phys. Ed. Rec. 2:45-53.
King, D.S., D.L. Costill, W.J. Fink, M. Hargreaves, and R. A. Fielding
  1985   Muscle metabolism during exercise in the heat in unacclimatized and acclimatized
         humans. J. Appl. Physiol. 59:1350-1354.
Kirwan, J.P., D.L. Costill, H. Kuipers, M.J. Burrell, W.J. Fink, J.E. Kovaleski, and
         R.A. Fielding
  1987   Substrate utilization in leg muscle of men after heat acclimation J. Appl. Physiol.
         63:31-35.
Klausen, K., D.B. Dill, E.E. Phillips, and D. McGregor
  1967   Metabolic reactions to work in the desert. J. Appl. Physiol. 22:292-296.
Lind, A.R.
  1963   A physiological criterion for setting thermal environmental limits for everyday
         work. J. Appl. Physiol. 18:51-56.
Muza, S.R., N.A. Pimental, H.M. Cosimini, and M.N. Sawka
  1988   Portable ambient air microclimate cooling simulated desert and tropic conditions.
         Aviat. Space Environ. Med. 59:553-558.
Nadel, E.R.
  1983   Effects of temperature on muscle metabolism. Pp. 134-143 in Biochemistry of
         Exercise, H.G. Knuttgen, J.A. Vogel, and J. Poortmans, eds. Champaign, Ill.:
         Human Kinetics Publishers.
Nadel, E.R., E. Cafarelli, M.F. Roberts, and C.B. Wenger
  1979   Circulatory regulation during exercise in different ambient temperatures. J. Appl.
         Physiol. 46:430-437.
Nielsen, M.
  1938   Die Regulation der Körpertemperatur bei Muskelarbeit. Skand. Arch. Physiol. 79:193-
         230.
  1970   Heat production and body temperature during rest and work. Pp. 205-214 in Physi-
         ological and Behavioral Temperature Regulation, J.D. Hardy, A.P. Gagge, and
         J.A.J. Stolwijk, eds. Springfield, Ill.: Charles C. Thomas.
Petersen, E.S., and H. Vejby-Christensen
  1973   Effect of body temperature on steady-state ventilation and metabolism in exercise.
         Acta Physiol. Scand. 89:342-351.
Pimental, N.A., H.M. Cosimini, M.N. Sawka, and C.B. Wenger
  1987   Effectiveness of an air-cooled vest using selected air temperature and humidity
         combinations. Aviat. Space Environ. Med. 58:119-124.
Piwonka, R.W., and S. Robinson
  1967   Acclimation of highly trained men to work in severe heat. J. Appl. Physiol. 22:9-12.

Robinson, S.
1963   Temperature regulation in exercise. Pediatrics 32:691-702.
Robinson, S., D.B. Dill, J.W. Wilson, and M. Nielsen
1941   Adaptations of white men and Negroes to prolonged work in humid heat. Am. J. Trop. Med. 21:261-287.
Rowell, L.B.
1986   Human Circulation: Regulation During Physical Strain. New York: Oxford University Press.
Rowell, L.B., J.R. Blackmon, R.H. Martin, J.A. Mazzarella, and R.A. Bruce
1965   Hepatic clearance of indocyanine green in man under thermal and exercise stresses. J. Appl. Physiol. 20:384-394.
Rowell, L.B., H.J. Marx, R.A. Bruce, R.D. Conn, and F. Kusumi
1966   Reductions in cardiac output, central blood volume and stroke volume with thermal stress in normal men during exercise. J. Clin. Invest. 45:1801-1816.
Rowell, L.B., K.K. Kraning II, J.W. Kennedy, and T.O. Evans
1967   Central circulatory responses to work before and after acclimatization. J. Appl. Physiol. 22:509-518.
Rowell, L.B., G.L. Brengelmann, J.B. Blackmon, R.D. Twiss, and F. Kusumi
1968   Splanchnic blood flow and metabolism in heat-stressed man. J. Appl. Physiol. 24:475-484.
Rowell, L.B., G.L. Brengelmann, J.A. Murray, K.K. Kraning, and F. Kusumi
1969   Human metabolic responses to hyperthermia during mild to maximal exercise. J. Appl. Physiol. 26:395-402.
Saltin, B., and L. Hermansen
1966   Esophageal, rectal and muscle temperature during exercise. J. Appl. Physiol. 21:1757-1762.
Saltin, B., A.P. Gagge, U. Bergh, and J.A.J. Stolwijk
1972   Body temperatures and sweating during exhaustive exercise. J. Appl. Physiol. 32:635-643.
Sawka, M.N., and K.B. Pandolf
1990   Effects of body water loss on exercise performance and physiological functions. Pp. 1-38 in Perspectives in Exercise Science and Sports Medicine. Vol. 3, Fluid Homeostasis During Exercise, C.V. Gisolfi and D.R. Lamb, eds. Indianapolis, Ind.: Benchmark Press.
Sawka, M.N., and C.B. Wenger
1988   Physiological responses to acute exercise-heat stress. Pp. 1-38 in Human Performance Physiology and Environmental Medicine at Terrestrial Extremes, K.B. Pandolf, M.N. Sawka, and R.R. Gonzalez, eds. Indianapolis, Ind.: Benchmark Press.
Sawka, M.N., K.B. Pandolf, B.A. Avellini, and Y. Shapiro
1983   Does heat acclimation lower the rate of metabolism elicited by muscular exercise? Aviat. Space Environ. Med. 54:27-31.
Sawka, M.N., A.J. Young, B.S. Cadarette, L. Levine, and K.B. Pandolf
1985   Influence of heat stress and acclimation on maximal aerobic power. Eur. J. Appl. Physiol. 53:294-298.
Sen Gupta, J., P. Midri, and M.S. Malhotra
1977   Metabolic responses of Indians during sub-maximal and maximal work in dry and humid heat. Ergonomics 20:33-40.
Senay, L.C., and R. Kok
1977   Effects of training and heat acclimatization on blood plasma contents of exercising men. J. Appl. Physiol. 43:591-599.

Shapiro, Y., K.B. Pandolf, and R.F. Goldman
    1982   Predicting sweat loss response to exercise, environment and clothing. Eur. J. Appl. Physiol. 48:83-96.
Shvartz, E., Y. Shapiro, A. Magazanik, A. Meroz, H. Birnfeld, A. Mechtinger, and S. Shibolet
    1977   Heat acclimation, physical fitness and responses to exercise in temperate and hot environments. J. Appl. Physiol. 43:678-683.
Stolwijk, J.A.J., B. Saltin, and A.P. Gagge
    1968   Physiological factors associated with sweating during exercise. Aerospace Med. 39:1101-1105.
Strydom, N.B., C.H. Wyndham, C.G. Williams, J.F. Morrison, G.A.G. Bredell, A.J.S. Benade, and M. Von Rahden
    1966   Acclimatization to humid heat and the role of physical conditioning. J. Appl. Physiol. 21:636-642.
Weinman, K.P., Z. Slabochova, E.M. Bernauer, T. Morimoto and F. Sargent II
    1967   Reactions of men and women to repeated exposure to humid heat. J. Appl. Physiol. 22:533-538.
Wenger, C.B.
    1988   Human heat acclimatization. Pp. 153-197 in Human Performance Physiology and Environmental Medicine at Terrestrial Extremes, K. B. Pandolf, M.N. Sawka, and R.R. Gonzalez, eds. Indianapolis, Ind.: Benchmark Press.
Williams, C.G., G.A.G. Bredell, C.H. Wyndham, N.B. Strydom, J.F. Morrison, J. Peter, P.W. Fleming, and J.S. Ward
    1962   Circulatory and metabolic reactions to work in heat. J. Appl. Physiol. 17:625-638.
Wyndham, C.H., G.G. Rogers, L.C. Senay, and D. Mitchell
    1976   Acclimatization in a hot, humid environment: Cardiovascular adjustments. J. Appl. Physiol. 40:779-785.
Young, A.J.
    1990   Energy substrate utilization during exercise in extreme environments. Pp. 65-117 in Exercise and Sport Sciences Reviews, K.B. Pandolf and J.O. Holloszy, eds. Baltimore, Md.: Williams and Wilkins.
Young, A.J., M.N. Sawka, L. Levine, B.S. Cadarette, and K.B. Pandolf
    1985   Skeletal muscle metabolism during exercise is influenced by heat acclimation. J. Appl. Physiol. 59:1929-1935.

4

Effects of Exercise and Heat on Gastrointestinal Function

Carl V. Gisolfi[1]

INTRODUCTION

Compared with cardiorespiratory function, little is known about the effects of exercise-heat stress on gastrointestinal (GI) function. Much of the information is anecdotal, and many of the studies lack adequate controls and quantitation of the exercise response. Most of the information in this area, in recent years, has come from studies on endurance athletes (Brouns et al., 1987; Eichner, 1989; Lorber, 1983; Moses, 1990). This chapter reviews recent prospective studies in this field and the results of a study from this laboratory that evaluated the effects of exercise on intestinal absorption. Because most studies have not isolated the effects of high environmental or internal body temperature per se, the combined effects of exercise and heat stress are discussed. The questions to be addressed include the following:

- What GI symptoms are manifested during exercise-heat stress?
- Are these symptoms intensified with increased exercise intensity, duration, or increased heat stress?
- What are the effects of exercise-heat stress on gastric emptying and intestinal absorption of water?
- What morphological changes occur in the GI system associated with exercise-heat stress?

---

[1] Carl V. Gisolfi, Department of Exercise Science, The University of Iowa, Iowa City, IA 52242

• Do GI symptoms and morphological changes associated with exercise-heat stress persist or do they subside quickly without functional impairment?

GASTROINTESTINAL SYMPTOMS

One of the first and most dramatic accounts of GI distress came from Derek Clayton (Benyo and Clayton, 1979) after he ran the marathon in 2:08:33.6. He commented:

> Two hours later, the elation had worn off. I was urinating quite large clots of blood, and I was vomiting black mucus and had a lot of black diarrhea. I don't think too many people can understand what I went through for the next 48 hours.

Table 4-1 lists the common GI symptoms experienced by runners, although these have also been observed in other athletes (Eichner, 1989).

TABLE 4-1 Gastrointestinal Disturbances Associated with Long-Distance Running

Abdominal cramps
Belching
Gastrointestinal reflux
Flatulence
Bloody stools
Vomiting
Diarrhea
Nausea

They are most often observed with overtraining, dehydration, and the use of aspirin. Another contributing factor may be high ascorbic acid intake (Sharman, 1982). These GI symptoms may be reduced by treatment with cimetidine (Baska et al., 1990) or consumption of an elemental diet (Bounous et al., 1967).

IMPORTANCE OF GI MANIFESTATIONS WITH EXERCISE-HEAT STRESS

Severe heat exposure simulates hemorrhage and intestinal ischemia because blood pools in the cutaneous capacitance vessels, central blood volume and splanchnic blood flow decline, and mean arterial pressure falls because increased heart rate cannot fully compensate for a declining stroke volume that causes cardiac output to fall. Hemorrhage and intestinal ischemia increase capillary permeability (Granger et al., 1981) and have been reported to produce mucosal lesions in the small intestine of humans (Klemperer et al., 1940), dogs (Chiu et al., 1970), rats (Bacalzo et al., 1971), and cats (Haglund and Lundgren, 1973). The pathogenesis of the rise in capillary permeability has been attributed to the production of superoxide radicals (Granger et al., 1981), and the pathogenesis of the mucosal lesions has been attributed to hypoxia (Ahren and Haglund, 1973). Thus, it has been hypothesized that severe hyperthermia (a) produces mucosal lesions in the small intestine from tissue hypoxia, (b) increases capillary permeability, and (c) results in endotoxemia (see Figure 4-1). Systemic endotoxemia has been shown in human heat stroke victims (Coridis et al., 1972; Graber et al., 1971), in ultramarathon runners who collapsed during competition in the heat (Brock-Utne et al., 1988), and following strenuous exercise (Bosenberg et al., 1988).

The diarrhea that occurs in marathon runners, if coincident with bleeding, may be a clinical manifestation of ischemic enteropathy (Bounous and McArdle, 1980). The effects of exercise-heat stress on GI function and performance can range from mild discomfort to serious impairment. For example, GI bleeding, which is often coincident with diarrhea, may be trivial (Eichner, 1989) or lethal (Thompson et al., 1982).

Gaudin et al. (1990) performed a standard endoscopy examination on seven runners 15 minutes before and 12 hours after they performed a maximal distance training run (18 to 50 km). Because the race was not competitive, stress was not considered to be a factor. Mucosal biopsy specimens of the upper digestive track revealed histologically pathological features in all runners (Table 4-2). These features included vascular lesions, ranging from congestion to hemorrhage, and evidence of reduced mucosal secretion (estimated from PAS [para-aminosalicylic acid] staining). The intensity of the lesions was independent of running distance, and a measure of running intensity was not provided. The prevalence of the lesions was independent of clinical symptoms.

Schwartz et al. (1990) studied 41 runners who completed the 1988 Chicago Marathon. Nine of the runners experienced GI bleeding, and three of these consented to esophagogastroduodenoscopy and colonoscopy within 48 hours after the race. Four other runners consented to these procedures 4 to 30 days after the race. Of the three runners examined within 48 hours, two had oozing gastric antral erosions, and the third had patchy areas of hyperemic and eroded mucosa limited to the splenic flexure. The latter portion of the colon is a circulatory watershed area, which suggests that a condition of reduced blood flow may contribute to necrosis of the colonic mucosa. Thus, injury can occur in both upper and lower segments of the GI track. There were no endoscopic findings in the four runners examined three or more days after the race, which suggests that restoration of the

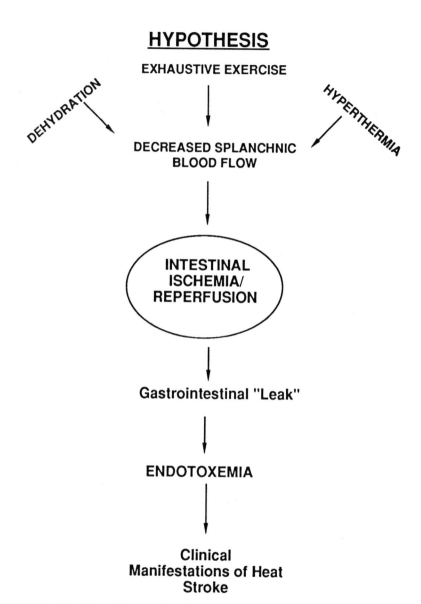

FIGURE 4-1 Flow diagram showing hypothesized mechanisms of endotoxemia and thermal injury associated with exercise-heat stress.

TABLE 4-2 Histological Observations of Runners After a Maximal Distance Training Run (18 to 50 km)

Vascular lesions
   Extravasation
   Petechiae
Reduced mucosal secretion
Reduced mucopolysaccharide epithelial coating
Subepithelial capillary dilation
Edema of lamina propria

SOURCE: Gaudin et al. (1990) and Schwartz et al. (1990).

resting state allows this form of injury to heal quickly. As a cautionary note, the lesions found in this study are similar to those observed with the use of nonsteroidal antiinflammatory drugs (NSAIDs), which are frequently taken by runners with musculoskeletal injuries (Andron, 1991). In the study by Schwartz et al. (1990), 60 percent of the runners in the "bleeding group" used NSAIDs.

The extent of these GI injuries can be more severe. Acute ischemic enteropathy could produce endotoxemia and the cardiovascular manifestations of heat stroke. Of 89 exhausted runners who required admission to the medical tent for treatment in the 1986 Comrades Marathon (89.4 km), 81 percent had endotoxemia that significantly correlated with the occurrence of nausea, vomiting, and diarrhea (Brock-Utne, 1988). It was hypothesized that the intestinal wall was damaged by reduced blood flow, hypoxia, and/or hyperthermia. This damage in turn led to excessive leakage of endotoxin into the portal circulation (Brock-Utne et al., 1988). This hypothesis is supported by the observation that a nonabsorbable antibiotic (kanamycin, 15 mg per kg) administered over a 5-day period to primates before heat exposure prevented the endotoxemia that was observed in control animals heated to a core temperature of 44.5°C (Gathiram et al., 1987).

GASTRIC EMPTYING

Is there any evidence that environmental temperature, or a rise in core body temperature, adversely affects the rate at which the stomach empties? The observation that gastric emptying (GE) is reduced in the heat was first made by Owen et al. (1986). These investigators found that during treadmill exercise (65 percent $V_{O_2 max}$ [maximal oxygen uptake]) in a 25°C environment) subjects emptied 79 percent of the water they ingested (1 liter) com-

TABLE 4-3 Gastric Emptying During Ingestion of Different Beverages

Beverage (environment)	Gastric Residual Volume (ml)	% Drink Emptied
	mean ± SEM	
Glucose polymer (35°C)	487.6 ± 12.3	51.3 ± 1.2
Glucose (35°C)	587.0 ± 98.1*	41.3 ± 9.8*
Water (35°C)	412.1 ± 84.7	58.8 ± 8.5
Water (25°C)	208.8 ± 65.5	79.1 ± 6.5

*Significantly different ($p < 0.05$) from all other runs.

SOURCE: Adapted from Owen et al. (1986).

pared with only 59 percent when they performed the same exercise and ingested the same volume of water in the heat (35°C) (see Table 4-3). Neufer et al. (1989) made a similar observation and found a significant negative correlation between GE and rectal temperature. These investigators also found that hypohydration significantly reduced GE. The mechanism responsible for this reduction is unclear, but it is probably related to the thermal strain associated with hypohydration and exercise-heat stress. Exercise reduces splanchnic blood flow (Rowell et al., 1968) and elevates plasma beta-endorphin levels (Kelso et al., 1984), both of which could reduce GE (Konturek, 1980; Kowalewski et al., 1976). Also, it is known that elevations in core body temperature can reduce stomach and intestinal motility (Tsuchiya and Iriki, 1980; Tsuchiya et al., 1974).

INTESTINAL ABSORPTION

Is there any evidence that intestinal absorption is compromised during exercise-heat stress? Using the plasma accumulation of 3-O-methyl-D-glucose (active) and D-xylose (passive) from a solution ingested orally as measures of intestinal absorption, Williams et al. (1964) found that prolonged (4.5 hour) treadmill exercise (3.0 miles per hour) in the heat (38/27°C dry bulb/wet bulb) reduced active but not passive carbohydrate absorption. Maughan et al. (1990) also found evidence of reduced intestinal absorption during exercise. They measured the rate of plasma D_2O accumulation from a beverage labeled with D_2O and found that exercise at 61 percent $V_{O_2\ max}$ reduced absorption measured at rest, and that absorption at 80 percent $V_{O_2\ max}$ was less than at 42 percent and 61 percent $V_{O_2\ max}$.

Also, Barclay and Tumberg (1988) reported that mild (heart rate = 103 beats per minute) exercise significantly reduced water and electrolyte absorption compared with rest; however, the solution they used contained no carbohydrate, which reduced the rate of intestinal absorption to 2 ml per hour per cm compared with a value of 13 to 15 ml per hour per cm for a carbohydrate-electrolyte solution (Gisolfi et al., 1991).

In contrast to these observations, Fordtran and Saltin (1967) found no effect of exercise (74 percent $V_{O_2 max}$) on either active or passive absorption using the more direct technique of segmental perfusion. Moreover, this author's most recent results (Gisolfi et al., 1991), also using the segmental perfusion technique, show no effect of either exercise intensity (30 to 70 percent $V_{O_2 max}$) or duration (60 to 90 minutes) on fluid absorption (see Figure 4-2 on following page).

PREVENTION AND MANAGEMENT

Although there is much to be learned about GI function during exercise-heat stress, the following suggestions are offered to help prevent or manage GI distress under such conditions:

• GI symptoms, GI bleeding, and endotoxemia seem to be related to exercise intensity, exercise duration, high thermal stress, and sharp increments in training. They also seem to occur among individuals who are poorly trained and who engage in endurance exercise. Thus, it would be prudent to be well conditioned and heat acclimated if thermal stress is anticipated. Also, sharp increments in physical work performed in the heat should be avoided.

• Nonsteroidal antiinflammatory drugs have been known to produce upper GI lesions and should be avoided 12 to 24 hours prior to hard exercise in the heat. Aspirin has a potent and long lasting antiplatelet action and should be avoided for 2 or 3 days prior to severe exercise in the heat. Aspirin is often taken 30 minutes before exercise by individuals with joint pain. If taken immediately before exercise, aspirin can produce marked cramping and related GI discomfort. High doses of ascorbic acid (vitamin C), which are sometimes taken by athletes, can produce diarrhea and should be avoided.

• Prefeeding an elemental semihydrolyzed diet might reduce the incidence and severity of intestinal discomfort in endurance athletes. If gastrids or upper GI ulceration is the source of GI symptoms, therapy with antacids or H_2 blockers may provide relief and allow soldiers to function normally.

• When GI symptoms do occur as a result of exercise per heat stress, they usually abate quickly (within days) with rest.

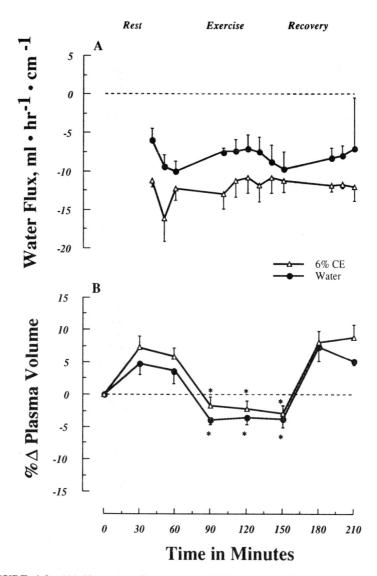

FIGURE 4-2 (A) Net water flux (mean ± SE) across a 40 cm segment of the duodenojejunum during the perfusion (15 ml per min) of water or a 6 percent carbohydrate-electrolyte (CE) solution at rest, during 90 min of exercise at 70 percent $V_{O_2 \, max}$, and during 60 min of recovery. Infusion began at time 0. Negative values indicate absorption. (B) Percent change in plasma volume during rest, exercise, and recovery for perfusion of water and the 6 percent GE solution. Different from rest and recovery values ($p < 0.05$). SOURCE: Gisolfi et al. (1991).

REFERENCES

Ahren, C., and U. Haglund
1973   Mucosal lesions in the small intestine of the cat during low flow. Acta Physiol. Scand. 88:541-550.

Andron, R.I.
1991   Gastrointestinal bleeding in runners. Ann. Intern. Med. 114(5):429.

Bacalzo, L.V., A.L. Cary, L.D. Miller, and W.M. Parkins
1971   Methods and critical uptake volume for hemorrhagic shock in rats. Surgery 70:555-560.

Barclay, G.R., and L.A. Turnberg
1988   Effect of moderate exercise on salt and water transport in the human jejunum. Gut 29:816-820.

Baska, R.S., F.M. Moses, and P.A. Deuste
1990   Cimetidine reduces running-associated gastrointestinal bleeding. Dig. Dis. Sci. 35(8):956-960.

Benyo, R., and D. Clayton
1979   The world's fastest marathoner. Runners World 66-73.

Bosenberg, A.T., J.G. Brock-Utne, S.L. Gaffin, M.T.B. Wells, and G.T W. Blake
1988   Strenuous exercise causes systemic endotoxemia. J. Appl. Physiol. 65(1):106-108.

Bounous, G., and A.H. McArdle
1980   Marathon runners: The intestinal handicap. Med. Hypotheses 33:261-264.

Bounous, G., N.G. Sutherland, A.H. McArdle, and F.N. Gurd
1967   The prophylactic use of an "elemental" diet in experimental hemorrhagic shock and intestinal ischemia. Ann. Surg. 166:312-342.

Brock-Utne, J.G., S.L. Gaffin, M.T. Wells, P. Gathiram, E. Sohar, M.F. James, D.F. Morrell, and R.J. Norman
1988   Endotoxaemia in exhausted runners after a long-distance race. S. Afr. Med. J. 73:533-536.

Brouns, F., W.H.M. Saris, and N.J. Rehrer
1987   Abdominal complaints and gastrointestinal function during long-lasting exercise. Int. J. Sports Med. 8:175-189.

Chiu, C.-J., A.H. McArdle, R. Brown, H.J. Scott, and F.N. Gurd
1970   Intestinal mucosal lesion in low flow states. Arch. Surg. 101:478-483.

Coridis, D.T., R.B. Reinhold, P.W. Woodruff, and J. Fine
1972   Endotoxaemia in man. Lancet 1:1381-1386.

Eichner, E.R.
1989   Gastrointestinal bleeding in athletes. Physician Sportsmed. 17:128-140.

Fordtran, J.S., and B. Saltin
1967   Gastric emptying and intestinal absorption during prolonged severe exercise. J. Appl. Physiol. 23:331-335.

Gathiram, P., M.T. Wells, J.G. Brock-Utne, B.C. Wessels, and S. L. Gaffin
1987   Prevention of endotoxaemia by non-absorbable antibiotics in heat stress. J. Clin. Pathol. 40:1364-1368.

Gaudin, C., E. Zerath, and C.Y. Guezennec
1990   Gastric lesions secondary to long-distance running. Dig. Dis. Sci. 35(10):1239-1243.

Gisolfi, C.V., K.J. Spranger, R.W. Summers, H.P. Schedl, and T. L. Bleiler
1991   Effects of cycle exercise on intestinal absorption in humans. J. Appl. Physiol. 71:2518-2587.

Graber, C.D., R.B. Reinhold, and J.G. Breman
1971   Fatal heatstroke. J. Am. Med.Assoc. 216:1195-1196.

Granger, D.N., G. Rutili, and J.M. McCord
1981   Superoxide radicals in feline intestinal ischemia. Gastroenterology 81:22-29.
Haglund, U., and O. Lundgren
1973   The effects of vasoconstrictor fibre stimulation on consecutive vascular sections of cat small intestine during hemorrhagic hypotension. Acta Physiol. Scand. 88:95-108.
Kelso, T.B., W.G. Herbert, F.C. Gwazdauskas, F.L. Goss and J.L. Hess
1984   Exercise-thermoregulatory stress and increased plasma b-endorphin/b-lipotropin in humans. J. Appl. Physiol. 57:444-449.
Klemperer, P., A. Penner, and A.I. Bernheim
1940   The gastro-intestinal manifestations of shock. Am. J. Dig. Dis. 7:410-413.
Konturek, S.J.
1980   Opiates and the gastrointestinal tract. Am. J. Gastroenterol. 74:285-291.
Kowalewski, K., S. Zajac, and A. Kolodej
1976   Effect of ischemic anoxia on electrical and mechanical activity of the totally isolated porcine stomach. Eur. Surg. Res. 8:12-25.
Lorber, S.H.
1983   Gastrointestinal disorders and exercise. Pp. 279-290 in Exercise Medicine: Physiological Principles and Clinical Applications. New York: Academic Press.
Maughan, R.J., J.B. Leiper, and B.A. McGaw
1990   Effects of exercise intensity on absorption of ingested fluids in man. Exp. Physiol. 75:419-421.
Moses, F.M.
1990   The effect of exercise on the gastrointestinal tract. Sports Med. 9(3):159-172.
Neufer, P.D., A.J. Young, and M.N. Sawka
1989   Gastric emptying during exercise: Effects of heat stress and hypohydration. Eur. J. Appl. Physiol. 58:433-439.
Owen, M.D., K.C. Kregel, P.T. Wall, and C.V. Gisolfi
1986   Effects of ingesting carbohydrate beverages during exercise in the heat. Med. Sci. Sports Exerc. 18(5):568-575.
Rowell, L.B., G.L. Brengelmann, J.R. Blackmon, R.D. Twiss, and F. Kusumi
1968   Splanchnic blood flow and metabolism in heat-stressed man. J. Appl. Physiol. 24:475-484.
Schwartz, A.E., A. Vanagunas, and P.L. Kamel
1990   Endoscopy to evaluate gastrointestinal bleeding in marathon runners. Ann. Intern. Med. 113(8):632-633.
Sharman, I.M.
1982   Gastrointestinal disturbances in runners. Br. J. Sports Med. 16(2):179.
Thompson, P.D., E.J. Funk, and R.A. Carleton
1982   Incidence of death during jogging in Rhode Island from 1975 through 1980. J. Am. Med. Assoc. 247(18):2535-2538.
Tsuchiya, K., and M. Iriki
1980   Effects of spinal cord cooling and heating on gastrointestinal motility in spinal-intact and acutely spinalized dogs. Ital. J. Gastroenterol. 12:255-259.
Tsuchiya, K., E. Kozawa, and M. Iriki
1974   Changes of gastrointestinal motility evoked by spinal cord cooling and heating. Pflugers Arch. 351:275-286.
Williams, J.H., M. Mager, and E.D. Jacobsen
1964   Relationship of mesenteric blood flow to intestinal absorption of carbohydrates. J. Lab. Clin. Med. 63(5):853-863.

DISCUSSION

PARTICIPANT: This damage is associated with running or is it associated with other types of activity as well?

DR. GISOLFI: It is primarily associated with running, but has been observed in triathletes and elite cyclists.

I think it is important that over at least a 90-minute period of intense exercise, we had one subject reach a core temperature of 40°C and observed no reduction in intestinal absorption of either active or passive solutes nor did we observe any change in fluid absorption.

If you exceed 90 minutes of strenuous exercise, especially if it is performed in a warm environment, I don't know the consequences on the GI tract. There is no data.

PARTICIPANT: Would you care to speculate on the differences between indirect and direct evidence on the deuterated water versus the sampling from the intestine?

DR. GISOLFI: This is a good point. Using the direct method of segmental perfusion you are looking at absorption from just a segment of the intestine. Using the indirect method of D_2O accumulation in the blood, you are looking at absorption from the entire intestine.

Some studies have demonstrated that deuterium oxide is taken up by the stomach. How much this contributes to overall absorption is not clear.

When you look at the accumulation of a substance in the blood, you need to know the rate at which the substance is coming into the vascular compartment and the rate at which it is leaving. How is it being distributed to different organs? At what rate is it moving from the vascular compartment into the interstitial fluid compartment and at what rate is it being filtered off by the kidney? Without knowing the dynamics of that situation, it is difficult to say what the accumulation in the vascular compartment really means.

5

Water Requirements During Exercise in the Heat

Carl V. Gisolfi[1]

INTRODUCTION

Water is essential to life. It constitutes the medium in which chemical reactions occur and is crucial to normal function of the cardiovascular system. Water constitutes about 70 percent of body weight in the normal adult. It decreases from 75 percent at birth to 50 percent in old age and is the largest component of the body. Adipose tissue contains less water than lean tissue; thus women have slightly less body water than men. The effects of dehydration occur with as little water loss as 1 percent of body weight and become life threatening at 10 percent (Adolph et al., 1947). Humans cannot adapt to a chronic water deficit, so fluid losses must be replaced if physiological function is to continue unimpaired.

The purpose of this chapter is to review the water requirements of soldiers exercising in the heat. The Desert Shield and Desert Storm operations in 1990 and 1991 made us acutely aware of the importance of military maneuvers in severe heat. Military missions are often 4 to 6 hours in duration and require mild to heavy exercise. This discussion will examine the range of these work loads. Furthermore, chronic water intake is a concern because inadequate water intake over days can lead to water depletion and heat exhaustion.

The requirement for water in the heat is dependent on fluid lost, which

[1] Carl V. Gisolfi, Department of Exercise Science, The University of Iowa, Iowa City, IA 52242

in turn depends on such factors as exercise intensity, exercise duration, environmental conditions, state of training and heat acclimatization, gender, and age. Selected studies are used to illustrate the influence of these different factors rather than to review the literature. Finally, the prediction of sweat losses under a variety of conditions is discussed, as well as the calculation of water requirements under these circumstances.

DISTRIBUTION OF BODY WATER

Total body water constitutes about 70 percent of lean body mass and is most simply divided into two major compartments: (a) intracellular water, which represents 50 percent of body weight or 35 liters in a 70-kg man, and (b) extracellular water, which represents 20 percent of body weight or 14 liters. The latter compartment is subdivided into plasma volume (5 percent body weight) and interstitial fluid volume (15 percent body weight). Intracellular water is not readily measured. It is calculated from measurements of total body water and extracellular fluid volume.

AVENUES OF FLUID LOSS AND GAIN

Table 5-1 gives normal values for daily water intake and output in a healthy adult. However, these values are subject to marked variation. For example, respiratory water loss can range from 200 ml per day when breathing humidified air to 1500 ml per day when exercising at high altitude. Water loss from cutaneous evaporation could range from 500 ml per day at rest in a cool environment to 10 liters per day during exercise in the heat. Fecal losses could range from 100 ml per day when on a mixed diet to 32

TABLE 5-1 Normal Values for Daily Intake and Output of Water in Adults

Intake Source	Amount (ml per day)	Source Output	Amount (ml per day)
Drinking	1200	Urine	1400
Food	900	Lungs and skin	900
Oxidation[*]	300	Feces	100
Total	2400	Total	2400

*Oxidative metabolism produces 0.6 ml water per gram of carbohydrate, 1.09 ml water per gram of fat, and 0.44 ml water per gram of protein.

SOURCE: Gisolfi (1986), used with permission. Data modified from Muntwyler (1968).

liters per day or more in a patient with diarrhea. Obligatory urine volume is limited by the concentrating power of the kidneys, but it can vary from 250 to 1400 ml per day depending on diet. Urine volume is usually 700 ml per day, but a high-protein diet demands more obligatory water to excrete the osmotically active products of protein metabolism.

DETERMINANTS OF SWEAT RATE

Water requirements during exercise in the heat primarily depend on evaporative cooling. Metabolism and environmental heat exchange determine the required evaporative cooling (E_{req}) to achieve thermal balance. Because respiratory water loss contributes little to evaporative cooling in warm or hot environments, cooling must come primarily from cutaneous sweat secretion. The rate of sweating and its regulation are determined by core and skin temperatures, skin wettedness, heat storage, metabolism, and the set point.

WATER REQUIREMENTS

Hot-Wet Versus Hot-Dry Environment

The U.S. military deploys troops to tropical and desert climates, and therefore military men and women are exposed to both wet and dry heat. Figure 5-1 shows the sweat responses as well as the mean changes in rectal temperature, heart rate, and metabolic rate of four distance runners walking 5.6 km per hour in dry heat, in wet heat, and in a cool environment. Experiments were performed 4 to 5 weeks apart and consisted of 4 hours of continuous walking, lunch (30 minutes), followed by another 2 to 3 hours of walking. Water was ingested ad libitum, but the subjects were constantly informed of their weight loss and were successful in maintaining fluid balance. All men walked 6 hours in the neutral and hot-dry environments except one subject who stopped walking after 5.5 hours in dry heat with a rectal temperature of 39°C and a heart rate of 136 beats per minute (bpm). Another subject walked for 7 hours in dry heat and finished with a rectal temperature of 38.3°C and a heart rate of 132 bpm. Sweat rate in the desert environment averaged 1210 ± 56 (x ± SE) ml per hour (Table 5-2).

In the hot-wet environment, sweat rate averaged only 716 ± 56 (x ± SE) ml per hour, which resulted in higher rectal temperatures (39.3°C) and heart rates (132 bpm). The reduced rate of sweating in this environment was associated with sweat gland fatigue (Brown and Sargent, 1965; Hertig et al., 1961; Kerslake, 1972; Nadel and Stolwijk, 1973; Robinson and Gerking, 1947). The mechanism responsible for this phenomenon is not clear, but evidence suggests that it is related to excessive wetting of the skin (Brebner

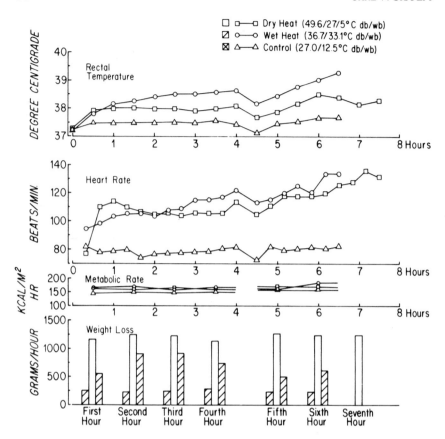

FIGURE 5-1 Rectal temperatures, heart rates, metabolic rates, and weight losses of four highly trained endurance runners during mild treadmill exercise in dry heat, in wet heat, and in a cool ambient temperature. Subjects consumed lunch in the test environment between 4.0 and 4.5 hours. Values are means ± SE. SOURCE: Gisolfi et al. (1977), used with permission.

and Kerslake, 1964; Collins and Weiner, 1962; Nadel and Stolwijk, 1973). These subjects were highly trained and essentially heat acclimatized as a result of their training. Untrained or unacclimatized subjects would have considerably lower sweat rates and would experience much more physiological strain than was shown by these men.

Exercise Intensity and Training

Under constant environmental conditions, skin sweating is a linear function of heat production or exercise intensity (Nielsen, 1969). Training in a neutral environment that results in a significant elevation in maximal oxygen uptake ($V_{O_2 max}$) reduces the core temperature threshold for the onset of sweating (Roberts et al., 1977) but does not necessarily increase total body sweat rate (Taylor, 1986). Sweat rates of male subjects have been found to be positively correlated with aerobic capacity (Greenleaf et al., 1972).

Heat Acclimatization

Maximal sweating capacity can rise from 1.5 liters per hour in a healthy unacclimatized man to as much as 2 to 3 liters per hour in a highly trained acclimatized soldier (Wenger, 1988). One of the highest sweat rates ever observed was recorded on Alberto Salazar during the 1984 Olympic Marathon. Salazar was running at 85 percent of $V_{O_2 max}$ (5.2 meters per second) and had a body weight loss of 5.43 kg (–8.1 percent body weight) despite an estimated fluid ingestion of 1.88 liters. This weight loss was equivalent to a sweat rate of 3.71 liters per hour (Armstrong et al., 1986).

Age and Gender

Military personnel range in age from 18 to 50 years and comprise 14 percent women. The effects of age and gender on thermoregulation, particularly the sweating response to exercise and thermal stress, have been elegantly reviewed by Drinkwater (1986). Contrary to popular opinion, differences in physiological responses to thermal stress cannot be attributed to differences in gender or age. When differences do appear among subjects of

TABLE 5-2 Mean Sweat Rates of Four Highly Trained Endurance Athletes Who Walked (3.5 mph) for 5 to 7 Hours in Hot-Wet, Hot-Dry, and Neutral Climates

Subject	Sweat Rate (liters per hour)		
	Hot-Wet Environment*	Hot-Dry Environment[†]	Neutral Environment[‡]
KM	778	1247	178
JC	659	1198	302
MN	838	1234	272
BC	590	1159	265
Mean ± SE	715 ± 56	1210 ± 20	254 ± 27

*37/33°C dry bulb/wet bulb.
[†]50/28°C dry bulb/wet bulb.
[‡]27/13°C dry bulb/wet bulb.

different age and gender, they are primarily due to differences in aerobic power or heat acclimatization.

In the 1960s, studies of temperature regulation at rest and during exercise in the heat concluded that women were less tolerant of exercise in the heat than were men (Morimoto et al., 1967; Wyndham et al., 1965); however, these investigators did not match their subjects for aerobic power or body weight-to-mass ratio. Weinman et al. (1967) were the first to suggest that gender differences could be explained by differences in physical fitness.

With regard to the effects of age on exercise-heat tolerance, it is well accepted that the aged are more susceptible to thermal injury than their younger counterparts during heat waves. This apparent heat intolerance among the aged has been attributed to a reduction in sweating capacity, a decline in aerobic fitness, or a combination of the two. In a recent review of the effects of exercise and age on thermoregulation, Kenney and Gisolfi (1986) found no evidence that men or women up to 50 to 60 years of age had any impairment in temperature regulation that could be attributed to age per se. This conclusion is also supported by the review of Drinkwater (1986). Robinson et al. (1986) found a decrement in sweating capacity in men 44 to 60 years of age, but this decline in sweating had no adverse effect on the ability of these men to acclimatize to work in a hot-dry (50°C) environment. The decline in heat tolerance associated with men and women 50 to 60 years of age can be readily attributed to reductions in cardiovascular fitness, lack of heat acclimation, or both.

Prediction of Water Requirements

Sweat rate can be predicted from a measure of the overall heat load (E_{req}) and the maximal evaporative cooling capacity of the environment (E_{max}) (Shapiro et al., 1982). The advantage of the latter prediction is that sweat rate (and therefore water required) can be determined from environmental conditions, exercise intensity, and the type of clothing worn without making any physiological measurements (Shapiro et al., 1982). The formula for calculating sweat loss in g per m^2 per hour is

$$\text{sweat loss} = 27.9 \times E_{req}(E_{max})^{-0.455}$$

CONCLUSIONS AND RECOMMENDATIONS

• Water requirements during exercise in the heat depend on fluid loss from sweating. Sweat rate is proportional to metabolic rate and can amount to 3 to 4 liters per hour or as much as 10 liters per day.

• Training and heat acclimatization can increase sweat rate by 10 to 20 percent or 200 to 300 ml per hour.

• Men sweat more than women and require more water, but women show the same physiological responses as men when performing work at the same relative intensity. Well-trained heat-acclimatized women show similar physiological responses to hot-wet and hot-dry heat as men.

• Within the age range of the current U.S. military force (18 to 50 years), there is no decrement in sweating, and therefore the water requirement during exercise in the heat is unchanged.

REFERENCES

Adolph, E.F., and associates
1947   Physiology of Man in the Desert. New York: Interscience Publishers.
Armstrong, L.E., R.W. Hubbard, B.H. Jones, and J.T. Daniels
1986   Preparing Alberto Salazar for the heat of the 1984 Olympic Marathon. Physician Sportsmed. 14(3):73-81.
Brebner, D.F., and D.M. Kerslake
1964   The time course of the decline in sweating produced by wetting the skin. J. Physiol. (Lond.) 175:295-302.
Brown, W.K., and F. Sargent
1965   Hitromeiosis. Arch. Environ. Health 11:442-453.
Collins, K.J., and J.S. Weiner
1962   Observations on arm-bag suppression of sweating and its relationship to thermal sweat-gland fatigue. J. Physiol. (Lond.) 161:538-556.
Drinkwater, B.L., ed.
1986   Female Endurance Athletes. Champaign, Ill.: Human Kinetics Publishers.
Gisolfi, C. V.
1986   Impact of limited fluid intake on performance. Pp. 17-28 in Predicting Decrements in Military Performance Due to Inadequate Nutrition. Washington, D.C.: National Academy Press.
Gisolfi, C.V., N.C. Wilson, and B. Claxton
1977   Work-heat tolerance of distance runners. Ann. N.Y. Acad. Sci. 301:139-150.
Greenleaf, J.E., B.L. Castle, and W.K. Ruff
1972   Maximal oxygen uptake, sweating and tolerance to exercise in the heat. Int. J. Biometeor. 16:375-387.
Hertig, B.A., M.L. Riedesel, and H.S. Belding
1961   Sweating in hot baths. J. Appl. Physiol. 16:647-651.
Kenney, M.J., and C.V. Gisolfi
1986   Thermal regulation: Effects of exercise and old age. Pp. 133-143 in Sports Medicine for the Mature Athlete. Indianapolis, Ind.: Benchmark Press.
Kerslake, D.M., ed.
1972   The Stress of Hot Environments. Cambridge, England: Cambridge University Press.
Morimoto, T., Z. Slabochova, R.K. Naman, and F. Sargent II
1967   Sex differences in physiological reactions to thermal stress. J. Appl. Physiol. 22:526-532.
Muntwyler, E.
1968   Water and electrolyte metabolism and acid-base balance. St. Louis, Mo.: C.V. Mosby.
Nadel, E.R., and J.A.J. Stolwijk
1973   Effects of skin wettedness on sweat gland response. J. Appl. Physiol. 35:689-694.

Nielsen, B.
  1969   Thermoregulation in rest and exercise. Acta Physiol. Scand. Suppl. 323:1-74.
Roberts, M.F., C.B. Wenger, J.A.J. Stolwijk, and E.R. Nadel
  1977   Skin blood flow and sweating changes following exercise and heat acclimation. J.
            Appl. Physiol. 43:133-137.
Robinson, S., and S.D. Gerking
  1947   Thermal balance of men working in severe heat. Am. J. Physiol. 149:476-488.
Robinson, S., H.S. Helding, F.C. Consolazio, S.M. Horvath, and E.S. Turrell
  1986   Acclimatization of older men to work in heat. J. Appl. Physiol. 20:583-586.
Shapiro, Y., K.B. Pandolf, and R.F. Goldman
  1982   Predicting sweat loss response to exercise, environment and clothing. Eur. J. Appl.
            Physiol. 48:83-96.
Taylor, N.A.S.
  1986   Eccrine sweat glands. Adaptations to physical training and heat acclimation. Sports
            Med. 3:387-397.
Weinman, K.P., Z. Slabochova, E.M. Bernauer, T. Morimoto, and F. Sargent II
  1967   Reactions of men and women to repeated exposure to humid heat. J. Appl. Physiol.
            22:533-538.
Wenger, C.B.
  1988   Human heat acclimatization. Pp. 153-197 in Human Performance Physiology and
            Environmental Medicine at Terrestrial Extremes. Indianapolis, Ind.: Benchmark
            Press.
Wyndham, C.H., J.F. Morrison, and C.G. Williams
  1965   Heat reactions of male and female Caucasians. J. Appl. Physiol. 20:357- 364.

DISCUSSION

PARTICIPANT: It is a little unclear. I thought you said that men sweat more but if you expressed it as amount of sweat, provided surface area was the same, but then it looked like in one of the slides it was different.

DR. GISOLFI: No, they are not the same. Even if you express it as percent body surface area, women still sweat less. But the important point is, women are able to maintain the same core body temperature as men when they are at the same relative work load.

PARTICIPANT: And was that formula applicable for both men and women?

DR. GISOLFI: No, the formula was based on men.

PARTICIPANT: Is there any effect from body mass?

DR. GISOLFI: Body fat is going to impede heat loss, certainly, and if you evaluate the impact of body weight to surface area ratio, the heavier person has a greater metabolic heat load and has a smaller surface area to dissipate that heat. These individuals will have more trouble dissipating heat when exposed to a warm environment exercising at the same intensity as an individual who is not carrying that much weight.

PARTICIPANT: Does it affect sweating?

DR. GISOLFI: Not to my knowledge, just having an increased subcutaneous layer of fat does not influence the sweating response.

PARTICIPANT: I have another question about age. Do you have any data on general range?

DR. GISOLFI: There doesn't seem to be a difference in the sweating response up to about 50 or 55. When you get over 60 and it is more clear over 70 years of age, then there is a decrement in the sweating response.

The individuals that Robinson studied (Robinson et al., 1986) were over 60. I think the mean age was something like 61 or 62 years. There was a decrement in the sweating response, but it wasn't reflected in their ability to regulate their body temperature which is, again, the more important point.

PARTICIPANT: Carl, in 1980 Dimri published a review of 55 papers in which he looked at this last point that you mentioned here, the increase in sweating rate during a 7- to 10-day period of heat acclimation (Dimri et al., 1980).

He found in those 55 papers that 15 of them showed no increase in the sweating rate. I know you published a paper at least once that showed no increase in the sweating rate during the deacclimation of 7 to 10 days. Could you comment on that for us?

DR. GISOLFI: I think it depends on the level of fitness of the subject. If you are dealing with a relatively fit individual that you then heat acclimatize, you probably see little change in the sweating response.

If you are dealing with people who are terribly unfit and you heat acclimatize them, you will see a rather substantial elevation in the sweating response.

PARTICIPANT: And also I know you mentioned that in dry environments when you published these studies, for hot, dry and wet, dry environments, there was less of an increase in the sweating range.

PARTICIPANT: At the initiation of exercise, there is an immediate drop or increase in plasma osmolality that doesn't seem to be such in the sweating. That is, there seems to be a movement of fluid from the blood volume to intracellular volume.

I am wondering whether that is due to being acclimatized and unacclimatized and to what extent does that shift in plasma volume affect the sweat rate.

DR. GISOLFI: Initially, I don't think plasma volume and plasma tonicity have a marked influence on sweat rate. The sweating response is being driven primarily by an increase in core body temperature and secondarily by changes in skin temperature.

There are influences from increments in plasma volume and tonicity but compared to an elevation in core body temperature, they are rather small.

DR. GISOLFI: I wanted to make a comment back on sweating, though, on how sweating changes with acclimatization. You must be careful in your interpretation of the literature because if you just look at total body sweating, you get very misleading results.

The magnitude of sweating is related to the rise in body temperature. So if you heat acclimatize a soldier, you will observe increases in sweating early in the process. However, at the end of acclimatization, if you are looking at just total body sweating, you are actually looking at a small rise in body temperature and the same sweating response. The important point is that for a given rise in core temperature, you do have more sweating.

PARTICIPANT: I would like to go back to this prediction equation briefly. That did not take into account obesity or any kind of differences in adiposity amongst individuals; is that right?

DR. GISOLFI: That's correct. The heat required term is based on metabolic rate, which takes body weight into account. Adiposity is not specifically addressed by this equation.

PARTICIPANT: This was done in a military population?

DR. GISOLFI: This was done in the military population, to my knowledge. It is only body weight that is taken into consideration.

PARTICIPANT: So this is a specialized group, then, so it would not necessarily fit across the board; is that what you are saying then?

DR. GISOLFI: Yes. I would also say that I am not familiar with any literature that has indicated that an increase in adiposity reduces the sweating response.

PARTICIPANT: In fact, you showed your men had half the body fat of women and yet their ability to lose heat was equal so adiposity may or may not make any difference, probably not.

6

Energetics and Climate with Emphasis on Heat: A Historical Perspective

Elsworth R. Buskirk[1]

INTRODUCTION

This historical review presents some considerations for supplying military personnel with appropriate nutrition as they operate in different climates. Attention is paid to some of the pertinent investigations undertaken related to energy turnover in the 1930s through the 1960s, with a few comments regarding interpretation of results based on more current knowledge.

EARLY APPRAISALS

Many of the earlier appraisals of the nutritional needs of U.S. Armed Forces personnel were published as reports of the various agencies involved. For the purposes of this presentation, the following agencies are identified:

• Quartermaster Food and Container Institute for the Armed Forces, Chicago, Illinois
• U.S. Army Medical Research and Nutrition Laboratory, Fitzsimmons General Hospital, Denver, Colorado
• Aero Medical Laboratory, Wright Air Development Center, United States Air Force, Wright Patterson Air Force Base, Ohio

---

[1] Elsworth R. Buskirk, Noll Laboratory for Human Performance Research, College of Health and Human Development, The Pennsylvania State University, University Park, PA 16802

TABLE 6-1 Environmental Temperature, Physical Fitness, and Calculated Average Nutrient Intake, U.S. Troops in Pacific Compared with U.S. Troops in North America

Information	Hawaii	Guadal-canal	Guam	Iwo Jima	38th Division, Luzon	Infantry Battalion, Colorado	Training Camps, U.S.*
Mean temperature, °F	+72	+85	+81	+78	+83	+65	Various
Score in fitness test	55	57	70	76	81	71	nd
Nutrient intake, average per man per day							
Kcal per day	3400	3400	3500	3500	3200	3900	3790
Carbohydrate, g	460	450	480	470	430	520	408
Fat, g	124	129	124	129	120	147	178
Protein, g total	110	110	115	115	100	125	125
Protein, g animal	68	65	68	65	58	74	nd

*nd = data not available.

SOURCE: Adapted from Johnson and Kark (1946) based on original data from Howe and Berryman (1945) on 455 messes in U.S. training camps, 1941-1943.

- U.S. Army Medical Research Laboratory, Office of the Surgeon General, Fort Knox, Kentucky
- Quartermaster Climatic Research Laboratory, United States Army, Lawrence, Massachusetts
- U.S. Army Quartermaster Research and Development Center, United States Army, Natick, Massachusetts
- U.S. Army Research Institute of Environmental Medicine, United States Army, Natick, Massachusetts

Those interested in perusing the various investigations conducted by personnel from these agencies should consult their respective report series because not all summaries of the sponsored work have appeared in the open scientific literature. It is hoped that many of the reports remain on file.

Between 1941 and 1946, reliable data were collected of food intakes for physically fit, active ground troops who chose their foodstuffs from the rations provided in temperate, mountain, desert, jungle, arctic, and subarctic areas in North America, Europe, and Asia. Dietary surveys and Army ration trials had been conducted intermittently throughout World War II. Johnson and Kark (1947) summarized these data and presented a brief critical review of the nutrition of U.S. and Canadian soldiers in 1946 based on their more comprehensive report prepared for the U.S. Army's Quartermaster Food and Container Institute for the Armed Forces (Johnson and Kark, 1946). Their summarized nutrient intake data from several studies appear in Table 6-1. A somewhat abbreviated table was subsequently published in 1947 (Johnson and Kark, 1947) (Table 6-2). They clearly demonstrated the inverse relationship of caloric intake with mean local temperature as ascertained from the dietary surveys and ration trials. Groups of from 50 to 200 men were represented in each study. A consistent reduction in voluntary kcal intake per °F over the range −20° to 100°F was found. Their regression equation was: kcal per day = 4660 − 15.9 T (°F) where T is the mean external temperature. The higher the mean environmental temperature the lower the voluntary kcal intake, and the lower the mean environmental temperature the higher the voluntary kcal intake.

Johnson and Kark (1947) concluded that the large difference in caloric intake could not be explained by differences in basal metabolic rate (a difference of 10 to 20 percent at most), body weight, or type of activity because they contended the ground troops carried out similar tasks in each environment. Unfortunately, they had little data to confirm no differences in physical activity by the troops at the several garrisons. Nevertheless, Johnson and Kark stated that the caloric expenditure for a given task was greater in the cold than in warm climates because of the "hobbling effect" of arctic clothing and equipment. They also concluded that more body heat

TABLE 6-2 Body Weight; Kcal Consumption; and Ratio of Protein, Fat, and Carbohydrate Eaten by Representative Groups of Ground Troops in Different Environments

Place and Troops	Environment	Mean Body Weight (kg)	Average Kcal Intake per Man per Day	Percentage of Kcal Provided by:		
				Protein	Fat	Carbohydrate
Canada, mobile force "Musk Ox"	Arctic and subarctic	73.0	4400	11	40	49
U.S.A., ground troops	Temperate	69.0	3800	13	43	44
Colorado Rockies, infantry	Temperate mountain (9000 feet)	69.5	3900	13	34	53
Pacific Islands, ground troops	Tropics	70.0	3400	13	33	54
Luzon, infantry	Tropics	65.5	3200	12	34	54

SOURCE: Adapted from Johnson and Kark (1947).

was required in cold than in warm environments to maintain thermal balance.

A review of Johnson and Kark's additional table clearly shows that the percentage of protein voluntarily chosen was essentially the same in each environment (Table 6-3). Percent fat intake in the warm environments was somewhat less than that in the cold and percent carbohydrate intake somewhat higher. Johnson and Kark's overall conclusion in regard to rations was that essentially the same rations can be supplied regardless of environment, but the colder the environment the more calories are needed. In addition, they emphasized that caloric requirements are in large measure determined by the physical activity in which troops are engaged and that their summary should be regarded as the setting of standards for dietary allowances.

The conclusions of Johnson and Kark, for the most part, appear to be as valid today as when presented in the 1940s. Nutritional knowledge has advanced, food supplies—including military rations—have changed, but many of the tasks required of armed forces personnel still require physical effort, which is the major factor associated with differences in caloric needs. Of consequence, however, is that clothing has been improved, providing better protection in the cold and better potential for allowing heat loss in hot environments. Clothing items are also generally lighter in weight, and various vehicles have somewhat diminished personal load carrying.

As a follow-up to the across-climate comparisons of Johnson and Kark, Quartermaster Research and Development Command and Medical Nutrition Laboratory personnel collaborated on a series of studies in desert, temperate, and arctic environments (Buskirk et al., 1956; Iampietro et al., 1956; Welch et al., 1957a,b, 1958). Caloric intake decreased as ambient temperature decreased, but the regression slope was considerably less than that of Johnson and Kark, when either moderate or relatively heavy work was performed. In fact, the regression slope was also considerably less than that emphasized in 1950 by the Committee of Caloric Requirements of the Food and Agricultural Organization (FAO) of the United Nations (1950):

> The existence of an approximately linear relationship between calorie expenditure and mean annual external temperature was assumed. It is recommended tentatively that for every 10° departure in mean annual temperature from the reference temperature of 10°C, requirements should be adjusted by 5 percent of requirements at the reference level, the 5 percent being subtracted for higher temperatures and added for lower temperatures.

The regressions found in the collaborative study were approximately 4 kcal per °C for both moderate and relatively heavy work. The comparative slopes for FAO were approximately 15 kcal per °C and for Johnson and Kark were 30 kcal per °C. Of interest was that kcal intake was essentially

TABLE 6-3 Voluntary Average Nutrient Intake of North American Ground Troops Who Remained Healthy, Fit, and Efficient in Different Environments

Information	U.S. Training Camps	Camp Carson Trials	Exercise "Musk Ox"	Guam Garrison	Luzon 38th Infantry Division
Type of troops	All	Infantry	Motorized	Garrison	Combat
Type of ration	U.S. garrison	U.S. B supplemented	Canadian arctic	U.S. B supplemented	U.S. New C
Duration of time on ration, weeks	Indefinite	8	12	Indefinite	12
Environment	Temperate	Mountain, summer	Arctic, winter	Moist tropics	Moist tropics
Average intake per man per day					
kcal	3800	3900	4400	3500	3200
protein, g total	125	125	120	115	100
protein, g animal	nd*	75	70	70	60
fat, g	180	145	190	125	120
carbohydrate, g	410	520	520	480	430
percent kcal	43	34	40	32	34
percent kcal, carbohydrate	44	53	49	55	54
percent kcal, protein	13	13	11	13	12

*nd = data not available.

SOURCE: Adapted from Johnson and Kark (1946).

the same in all climates when calculated on the basis of body weight plus clothing and equipment weight manually transported. A kcal intake of 47 to 49 kcal per kg per day was found for moderate work in the three climates. During relatively heavy work, kcal intake increased from 60 to 62 kcal per kg per day (Welch et al., 1958). They concluded that the differences in energy expenditure among environments are largely accounted for by differences in body weight plus weight of clothing and equipment carried during the performance of duties in the respective environments.

A recent field study showed that troops operating in a warm environment and performing moderate work loads consumed an average of between 44.3 and 47.2 kcal per kg per day (Rose and Carlson, 1986), values that agree with those found by Welch et al. (1958).

ENERGY EXPENDITURE: SUBMAXIMAL EXERCISE

An issue that has been investigated over the years with mixed results is the impact of heat on metabolic rate, both during rest and during exercise. A variety of hypothesized causes for different responses of the metabolic rate to exercise in the heat have been proposed and are listed in Table 6-4. The case for a relatively elevated metabolic rate was put forth by Consolazio et al. (1961, 1963, 1970) (Tables 6-5 and 6-6). The primary explanation of the relatively higher energy expenditure in hot compared to cooler environments was the energy expenditure associated with the production and secretion of sweat. Consolazio et al. expanded on the observations of Dill et al. (1931) and Welch et al. (1958). Results from the latter study appear in Table 6-7. Although the differences across climates and locations in the

TABLE 6-4 Differences Among Studies: Hypothesized Causes of Different Responses in Metabolic Rate to Exercise in the Heat

Physical condition of subjects
Extent of heat acclimatization
Skill
Duration of exercise
Exercise intensity
Environmental heat stress
   Type
   Intensity
Hydration state
Febrile state
Clothing worn
Equipment carried

TABLE 6-5 Mean Oxygen Uptake during Rest, Moderate Activity, and Heavy Activity by Young Men ($n = 7$) in a Room Maintained at Different Temperatures

Intensity of Activity	Mean Oxygen Uptake (ml per minute)			
	21.1°C (70°F)	29.4°C (85°F)	37.7°C (100°F)	Percent
Rest	273	282	304*	11.4
Moderate[†]	521	525	590*	13.3
Heavy[‡]	1422	1404	1570*	11.7

*$p \leq 0.05$, i.e., effect of 100°F > 85°F or 70°F.
[†]Fifty minutes on cycle ergometer.
[‡]Fifty minutes on cycle ergometer at 120 watts.

SOURCE: Adapted from Consolazio et al. (1963).

study by Welch et al. were nonsignificant, there appeared to be a trend for a higher energy expenditure during walking in a hot desert environment when expressed either as kcal per hour or kcal per kg per hour, where kg represents total weight transported. However, more recent studies have failed to find significant differences (Klausen et al., 1967; Rowell et al., 1969; Sen Gupta et al., 1977; Shvartz et al., 1977; Young et al., 1985).

Shvartz et al. (1977) clearly indicated little difference in metabolic rate with ergometer exercise prior to heat acclimation (see Table 6-8). Sen Gupta et al. (1977) raised the possibility that although total energy expenditure during submaximal exercise was not different when the exercise was

TABLE 6-6 Oxygen Uptake by Young Men ($n = 7$) Performing Different Types of Exercise* in a Desert Environment, Yuma, Arizona

Exercise Type	Oxygen Uptake (ml per minute)		
	Sun (37.8°C)	Shade (37.8°C)	Indoors (26°C)
Bicycle 1	754[†]	683[†]	641
Bicycle 2	813[†]	751[†]	681
Treadmill	1156	1197[†]	1110
Resting	340[†]	322	314

* Two separate cycle ergometer rides that are indicated here as bicycle 1 and 2.
[†] $p \leq 0.05$.

SOURCE: Adapted from Consolazio et al. (1970).

TABLE 6-7 Partition of Energy Expenditure in Three Climates in 1955

	Climate		
	Cold, Ft. Churchill Canada	Temperate, Natick Massachusetts	Hot, Yuma Arizona
Task	(−22.5°F)	(72°F)	(90.5°)
	8[*]	8[*]	11[*]
Walking (3.41 mph, level terrain)			
kcal per hour	413	318	350
kcal per kg per hour[†]	4.82	5.12	5.26
Resting and sedentary activity,			
kcal × $kg^{0.7}$ per hour[‡]	4.58	4.62	4.40

[*]Number of subjects.
[†]Body weight plus weight of clothing.
[‡]Includes dietary-induced thermogenesis.

SOURCE: Adapted from Welch et al. (1958).

conducted in a hot or comfortable environment, the partitioning of energy expenditure was different, that is, less aerobic expenditure and greater anaerobic expenditure in the hot environment (Table 6-9). The results were subsequently confirmed by Dimri et al. (1980). The hypothesized explanation for this partitioning was the diversion of a significant amount of blood from the muscles to the skin for thermoregulation in hot environments. Although

TABLE 6-8 Mean Oxygen Uptake Responses to Exercise Before (B) and After (A) 8 Days of Heat Acclimation

	Mean Oxygen Uptake (ml per m^2 per minute)					
	41W, 23°C		82W, 23°C		41W, 39.4°C	
Group	B	A	B	A	B	A
Trained ($n = 7$)	623	570*	1075	960*	634	569*
Untrained ($n = 7$)	668	577*	1061	985*	680	586*
Unfit ($n = 7$)	615	531*	1050	932*	618	520*
Control ($n = 5$)	625	578	1068	1030	611	615

NOTE: Heat acclimation regimen = 3 hours of exercise per day at 41 watts, T_{db} = 39.4°C, T_{wb} = 30.3°C, where T_{db} = dry-bulb temperature and T_{wb} = wet-bulb temperature.

*$p \leq 0.05$.

SOURCE: Adapted from Shvartz et al. (1977).

TABLE 6-9   Mean Changes in Aerobic-Anaerobic Fractions of Oxygen
Utilization During Fixed Submaximal Exercise for 5 Minutes in
Comfortable and Hot Conditions

	Mean Change in O_2 Utilization ($\pm$ SD)		
	Comfortable Environment (T_{db} 29.0°C, T_{wb} 21.3°C)	Very Hot Environment (T_{db} 36.5°C, T_{wb} 28.5°C)	Level of Significance
Total $\dot{V}_{O_2}$ (liters)	7.60 ± 1.21	8.06 ± 0.87	n.s.
Aerobic $\dot{V}_{O_2}$ (liters)	5.60 ± 6.50	5.27 ± 0.68	$p < 0.05$
Percentage of total	73.97 ± 6.50	65.40 ± 2.99	$p < 0.02$
Anaerobic $\dot{V}_{O_2}$ (liters)	2.00 ± 0.62	2.78 ± 0.33	$p < 0.01$
Percentage of total	26.03 ± 6.50	34.60 ± 2.99	$p < 0.02$

NOTE: Exercise intensity = 600 kg per min, cycle ergometer; T_{db} = dry-bulb temperature; T_{wb} = wet-bulb temperature.

SOURCE: Adapted from Sen Gupta (1977).

this hypothesis might apply to short periods of exercise such as the 5-minute bouts used by Sen Gupta et al. (1977), it would undoubtedly not apply to longer bouts of exercise, for example, 1 to 8 hours or more when a balance in muscle and skin blood flow would be necessary to sustain the exercise. A relatively elevated anaerobic metabolism and higher blood lactate concentrations would not be present. Thus, the conclusion of Sen Gupta et al. "that during submaximal work in heat, the metabolism becomes more anaerobic and there is reduction in $\dot{V}_{O_2}$ in submaximal and maximal workloads as the heat stress increases" must be qualified at least with respect to duration of submaximal exercise.

Overall, whether energy expenditure is modified during exercise in the heat depends on the circumstances and conditions. Brief intense exercise in a hot environment may elevate energy expenditure by evoking anaerobic processes, but the increment in daily energy expenditure is likely to be negligible. Thus, the earlier investigators posed the problem, but in terms of meeting the daily kcal needs of troops working in a hot environment, the submaximal exercise they perform has no greater impact than if they performed the same tasks in a more comfortable environment.

The possible reasons for either an increase or a decrease in metabolic rate in hot environments are listed in Tables 6-10 and 6-11. A careful appraisal of each military situation would reveal which factors are most important to consider while also bearing in mind the possible causes of different responses previously set forth in Table 6-4.

TABLE 6-10 Possible Reasons for an Increase in Metabolic Rate in Hot Environments

Lack of acclimatization
Inefficient physical activity, psychomotor stress
Q_{10} effect, elevated body temperature
Greater sweat gland activity
Tachycardia
Increased pulmonary ventilation
Increased anaerobic metabolism
    Increased RQ
    Increased O_2 debt
    Increased lactate
    Increased muscle glycogen utilization
    Increased blood glucose utilization
    Lessened skeletal muscle blood flow

NOTE: Q_{10} = adjustment in metabolic rate in relation to temperature change; RQ = respiratory quotient.

TABLE 6-11 Possible Factors That Would Tend to Reduce Metabolic Rate in Hot Environments

Complete acclimatization
Lower basal metabolic rate
Reduced physical activity, particularly intense activity
Lighter-weight clothing
Decreased appetite and associated dietary-induced thermogenesis

ACCLIMATIZATION/ACCLIMATION

A finding that has been repeatedly documented is that unacclimatized personnel suffer the consequences when suddenly exposed to stressful environments, whether the environmental stress is heat, cold, or altitude. The psychological and physical stresses associated with combat only complicate the adverse situation. At issue is inadequate acclimatization, which with sudden exposure to heat, not only perpetrates physiological strain but lessens initiative and appetite, which negatively affects nutritional status including water balance. The acclimatization process with exposure to hot environments proceeds rapidly, being virtually complete in the working soldier within 10 days (Adolph, 1947; Buskirk and Bass, 1957; Dill, 1938). During this time, body weight is invariably lost due to undernutrition, but the weight may be subsequently regained in toto or in part. Johnson (1946), in his review, concluded that following acclimatization, dietary requirements are qualitatively similar in hot and temperate areas but may remain quantitatively lessened in tropical climates by the sustained high loss of sweat and anorexia.

The question of whether heat acclimatization (outdoors or in the field) or acclimation (indoors or in laboratories) has an effect on metabolic rate during rest and exercise has been studied intensively with mixed results. Some pertinent studies are cited from among the many in the literature.

Robinson et al. (1945) and Eichna et al. (1950) found that heat acclimation lowered the metabolic rate associated with exercise in the heat by 4 to 8 percent. Shvartz et al. (1977) studied, using cycle ergometry, several groups of men who varied widely in physical fitness and were exposed to 8 days of heat acclimation. Despite interindividual differences in physical fitness, the postacclimation oxygen uptakes were invariably slightly less in all of the environments studied including a 39.4°C (103°F) environment (see Table 6-8).

Sawka et al. (1983) reevaluated the problem. They concluded that heat acclimation, if it had an effect at all, slightly lowered metabolism associated with performance of exercise in the heat. The conclusion was based not only on their studies of 42 subjects of both genders, but on a review of the literature as well. Young et al. (1985) arrived at essentially the same conclusion (see Table 6-12).

Presumably, the small reduction in metabolism is caused by the lesser respiratory and cardiac work caused by more efficient evaporative cooling, peripheral circulation, regulation, and the lowering of body temperature, although as Sawka et al. (1983) have pointed out, the role of such factors is

TABLE 6-12 Statistical Analysis for Comparison of Main Effects of Heat Acclimation and Environment on Respiratory Measurements of Young Men ($n = 13$)

Variable	Acclimation	Environment
$\dot{V}_{O_2}$, liters per minute	Pre > post*	Cool > hot*
RER[†]	Pre > post*	Cool < hot*
$\dot{V}_E / \dot{V}_{O_2}$	NS	Cool < hot*

NOTE: Environments: Cool—21°C, 30 percent relative humidity; hot—49°C, 20 percent relative humidity. Exercise: 30 minutes of cycle ergometry at 70 percent $\dot{V}_{O_2\,max}$; NS = not significant.

*$p \leq 0.05$

[†]RER = respiratory exchange ratio.

SOURCE: Adapted from Young et al. (1985).

not clear-cut. They suggested further research to investigate the possible role of modification of motor unit recruitment patterns and muscular efficiency—the latter related to phosphorylation efficiency and contractile-coupling efficiency.

Heat acclimatization/acclimation is a valuable physiological adaptation, but the process plays only a minor role in modifying energy turnover and caloric requirements.

APPETITE

Appetite tends to be adversely affected among unacclimatized personnel who are abruptly exposed to a hot environment, a finding that has been recognized for some time. Taylor in 1946, quoted by Mitchell and Edman (1951), suggested the following:

> Hot weather presents no particular problems other than taste, custom and supply. Palatability is essential to combat the prevalent anorexia as assurance of good nutrition.

Kark et al. (1947) recommended maintaining appetite through variety, familiarity, and high quality.

> In providing rations for soldiers at least three considerations are of prime importance. First, a considerable variety of food items should be issued. Second, the food items should be much the same as soldiers are accustomed to in ordinary life, but emphasis should be placed on acceptable foods of high biological value. Third, caloric deficits must be avoided.

Although appetite, hunger, and satiety are complex processes, they must be addressed with regard to hot environments. Hard work in the heat, particularly for the unacclimatized, challenges ration providers and food preparers to offer in sufficient quantity safe, appealing food of good nutritional quality.

RESTING METABOLISM/DIETARY-INDUCED THERMOGENESIS

One of the thoughts perpetuated in the 1930s through the 1950s was that the *specific dynamic action* (SDA) of foods—now commonly identified as the *thermic effect of food* or *dietary-induced thermogenesis*—contributed significantly to daily kcal turnover. Swift and French (1954) reviewed the various studies and concluded that the impact of specific dynamic effect (SDE) was overemphasized, but that it remained a significant minor factor, in the range of 2 to 8 percent of ingested energy. When people consume mixed meals, the relative SDE impact of protein, carbohydrate, or fat becomes indistinguishable.

In an early evaluation of basal metabolism in the tropics, MacGregor and Loh (1941) showed that basil metabolic rate (BMR) declined in certain normal individuals, but not in others. The depression in BMR in those affected appeared to reach a maximum before the end of the first year of residence and was maintained after 2 years in the tropics. Military training for 3 months in the same environment appeared to have no influence on the interindividual patterns of response. Neither alterations in diet nor weight loss accounted for the interindividual differences. The authors concluded that the continued relatively high temperatures and possibly humidities were responsible for the depression of BMR in those susceptible. The environmental conditions in Singapore where the work was done averaged 28.3°C (83°F) during the day and 24.4°C (76°F) at night with frequent high humidity. Others have also reported an impact of environmental temperature on BMR or resting metabolism (for example, Galvao, 1950; Mason, 1934).

To further such observations, an experiment was designed to evaluate the changes in resting metabolism during the day when food and exercise are taken as usual (Buskirk et al., 1957). Comparisons were made across climates varying from a cold (arctic) to a hot (desert) environment. It was concluded that specific dynamic action or dietary-induced thermogenesis assessed by periodic measurements of oxygen consumption was primarily responsible for the upward trend in energy turnover at rest during the day. A small "diurnal" elevation in oxygen consumption occurred during fasting, with or without exercise. Climate per se did not appear to influence the pattern of resting metabolism.

DIETARY DEFICIENCIES

Dietary deficiencies produce various symptoms; however, evidence of gross nutrient deficiency is usually delayed for a considerable period of time unless the deficiency is water, carbohydrate, or total kcal. Johnson summarized the more prominent effects of gross nutrient deficiencies, and his listing was modified by Young (1977) and then adapted here (see Table 6-13). Water deficiency has an almost immediate effect, whereas kcal and carbohydrate deficiency effects are seen in a matter of days. Protein and fat deficiencies produce symptoms within weeks and months, respectively. Based on this early information, attention was paid to water, kcal, and carbohydrate deficiencies in a variety of early studies involving hard work by soldiers in either temperate or warm/hot environments (Grande et al., 1957; Taylor and Keys, 1958). The combination of hypohydration and undernutrition was shown to be particularly compromising with respect to physical performance. Significant nitrogen loss in urine and sweat associated with weight loss and, presumably, skeletal muscle hypotrophy was observed. The nitrogen losses found by Grande et al. (1957) are reported in Table 6-14. Should such nitrogen loss continue, troops would be physically com-

TABLE 6-13 Rate of Onset of Deficiency Syndromes in Working Men Exposed to Complete Deficiency of One or More of the Important Nutrients

Nutrient	Times Before Earliest Effects on Performance Appear in Complete Deficiency	Deficiency Syndrome and End Result
Water	A few hours	Easy fatigue, poor performance, eventual exhaustion of dehydration
Kcal	2 or 3 days	Easy fatigue, poor performance
Carbohydrate	Several days	Easy fatigue; poor performance; eventually, nutritional acidosis
Protein	Probably several weeks	Late result, nutritional edema
Fats	Many months	Earliest effects not known

SOURCES: Adapted from Johnson (1943) and Young (1977).

promised. Unpublished investigations from the University of Minnesota in the 1950s revealed that a loss of 125 g nitrogen was associated with measurable physiological deterioration, including a significant reduction in walking endurance and aerobic power. A review of the effects of prolonged semi-starvation has been set forth in a classic study by Keys et al. (1950). A further discussion of negative nitrogen balance based on the experience of those working at the University of Minnesota was prepared by Taylor and Keys (1958).

Undernutrition is always a problem in military operations for various reasons, among them psychological stress, supply problems, food prepara-

TABLE 6-14 Cumulative Nitrogen Excretion (Urine and Sweat) During 16 Days on a 1000-kcal Carbohydrate Diet

N	Water Allowance	Control Mean Weight (kg)	Nitrogen Excreted, g ($\pm$ SD)		
			Urine	Sweat	Urine + Sweat
6	900 ml per day	75.4	136.72 $\pm$ 10.13	5.02 $\pm$ 0.39	141.74 $\pm$ 20.44
6	1800 ml per day	73.0	109.94 $\pm$ 21.18	5.09 $\pm$ 0.48	115.03 $\pm$ 21.45
13	Ad libitum	69.1	83.79 $\pm$ 14.14	5.41 $\pm$ 1.39	89.20 $\pm$ 14.74

SOURCE: Adapted from Grande et al. (1957).

tion problems, and coping with threats and emergencies. A group led by Sargent and Johnson at the University of Illinois spent considerable time and effort in the 1940s and 1950s working on undernutrition (as well as more normal nutrition). They established fundamental physiological, nutritional bases for an all-environment survival ration (Sargent and Johnson, 1957):

1. Maximal feasible kcal content provided by a balanced mixture of first-class protein, carbohydrate, and fat. The goal should be 2,000 kcal per man per day, of which protein should provide 15 percent of kcal, carbohydrate 52 percent of kcal, and fat 33 percent of kcal.

2. Water allowance as liberal as possible, with a goal of three quarts per man per day for hot weather, and no less than one quart per man per day under any circumstances.

3. An optimal osmotic intake, neither too large nor too small. The goal should be 700 milliosmols per day, provided by the sum of protein and minerals.

4. Within limits set by the recommended proportions of protein, carbohydrate, and fat, minimal ketogenicity, minimal specific dynamic action, and maximal water of oxidation.

Although the focus was on adequate carbohydrate supply during the 1940s and 1950s, largely to avoid the debilitating effects of ketosis, there was also concern about adequate protein and preservation of body tissue including skeletal muscle mass. Mitchell and Edman (1949, 1951) said about protein:

Considering all evidence, it may be concluded that protein requirements may be slightly increased in the tropics by some 5 to 10 grams daily . . . Laboratory experiments show that protein requirements may be increased slightly by (a) a stimulation of tissue catabolism if pyrexia occurs, and (b) by sweat losses of nitrogen uncompensated by diminished losses in the urine.

Consolazio and Shapiro (1964) found in the summary of their studies of men exercising under different climatic conditions that protein intake in the hot climate exceeded the National Research Council's recommended allowance of 100 g per day. In contrast to the conclusion of Mitchell and Edman (1949, 1951), Consolazio and Shapiro felt that increased protein intake in the heat was due not to an innate desire for protein, but to the relatively greater caloric intake. Recently, Paul (1989) suggested that because protein and amino acids contribute from 5 to 15 percent of energy for prolonged exercise—with the higher values perhaps associated with glycogen depletion—adequate protein intake is important when exercising in the heat. He pointed out that urine and sweat urea increase during prolonged, relatively intense exercise. Nevertheless, there appears to be no evidence that protein intakes in excess of from 1 to 1.5 g per kg body weight offer any advantage to the mature military person. One possible disadvantage of high protein intakes is the obligatory urine volume required to excrete protein break-down products, including urea.

A PERSPECTIVE

The comment of D. B. Dill (1985), a former colleague who was well versed in the desert environment, provides a fitting reminder to the readers of this brief historical review.

> In the hot desert even a well trained human can sprint only about half the distance one would guess before collapsing. One should respect the in-credible intensity of the desert, protect oneself with shade, spare water, slow movement, equally-minded partners, then enjoy and relish its beauty.

Unfortunately, military personnel engaged in combat or under the threat of combat may not have the luxury of contemplating beauty, but they never-theless must deal with the "incredible intensity of the desert."

Finally, as the nutritional situation during the recent operations of Desert Shield and Desert Storm is reviewed, a comment by R. M. Kark (1954) comes to mind.

> Field studies have shown that physical deterioration in soldiers may be due to inadequate nutrition, but perhaps what is more important, they have shown that loss of military efficiency through inadequate nutrition is most often due to inadequate planning, catering or supply, and to inadequate training or indoctrination. . . . Maintaining good nutrition is like maintain-ing freedom of speech or democracy. You need eternal vigilance to make it work.

REFERENCES

Adolph, E.F., and associates
    1947   Physiology of Man in the Desert. New York: Interscience Publishers.
Buskirk, E.R., and D.E. Bass
    1957   Climate and Exercise. Technical Report EP-61, U.S. Army Quartermaster Re-search and Development Center, Natick, Mass.
Buskirk, E.R., M. Kreider, R. Brebbia, N. Morana, F. Daniels, B.E. Welch, J.B. Mann, W. Insull, Jr., and T.E. Friedemann
    1956   Caloric Intake and Energy Expenditure in a Sub-Arctic Environment. Report No. EP-33, U.S. Army Quartermaster Research and Development Center, Natick, Mass.
Buskirk, E.R., P.F. Iampietro, and B.E. Welch
    1957   Variations in resting metabolism with changes in food, exercise and climate. Me-tabolism 6:144-153.
Consolazio, C.F., and R. Shapiro
    1964   Energy requirements of men in extreme heat. Pp. 121-124 in Environmental Physi-

ology and Psychology in Arid Conditions: Proceedings of the Lucknow Symposium. Liège, Belgium: United Nations: UNESCO.

Consolazio, C.F., R. Shapiro, J.E. Masterson, and P.S.L. McKinzie
1961   Energy requirements of men in extreme heat. J. Nutr. 73:126-134.

Consolazio, C.F., L.O. Matoush, R.A. Nelson, J.A. Torres, and C.J. Isaac
1963   Environmental temperature and energy expenditures. J. Appl. Physiol. 18:65-68.

Consolazio, C.F., H.L. Johnson, and H.J. Krzywicki
1970   Energy metabolism during exposure to extreme environments. Unnumbered report. U.S. Army Medical Research and Nutrition Laboratory, Fitzsimmons General Hospital. Denver, Colo.

Dill, D.B.
1938   Life, Heat and Altitude. Cambridge, Mass.: Harvard University Press.
1985   The Hot Life of Man and Beast. Springfield, Ill.: Charles C. Thomas.

Dill, D.B., H.T. Edwards, P.S. Bauer, and E.J. Levenson
1931   Physical performance in relation to external temperature. Arbeitsphysiologie 4:508-518.

Dimri, G.P., M.S. Malhotra, J. Sen Gupta, T.S. Kumar, and B.S. Aora
1980   Alterations in aerobic-anaerobic proportions of metabolism during work in the heat. Eur. J. Appl. Physiol. 45:43-50.

Eichna, L.W., C.R. Park, N. Nelson, S.M. Horvath, and E.D. Palms
1950   Thermal regulation during acclimation in a hot dry desert type environment. Am. J. Physiol. 163:585-597.

Food and Agricultural Organization of the United Nations
1950   Caloric Requirements. Report of the Committee on Calorie Requirements. Washington, D.C.: United Nations.

Galvao, E.G.
1950   Human heat production in relation to body weight and body surface. J. Appl. Physiol. 3:21.

Grande, F., J.T. Anderson, and H.L. Taylor
1957   Effect of restricted water intake on urine nitrogen output in man on a low calorie diet devoid of protein. J. Appl. Physiol. 10:430-435.

Howe, P.E., and G.H. Berryman
1945   Average food consumption in the training camps of the United States Army (1941-1943). Am. J. Physiol. 144:558-594.

Iampietro, P.F., J.A. Vaughn, A. MacLead, B.E. Welch, J.G. Marcinek, J.B. Mann, M.P. Grotheer, and T.E. Friedemann
1956   Caloric intake and energy expenditure of eleven men in a desert environment. Report No. EP-40. U.S. Army Quartermaster Research and Development Center, Natick, Mass.

Johnson, R.E.
1943   Nutritional standards for men in tropical climates. Gastroenterology 1:832-840.
1946   Applied physiology. Ann. Rev. Physiol. 8:535-558.

Johnson, R.E., and R.M. Kark
1946   Feeding Problems in Man as Related to Environment. An Analysis of United States and Canadian Army Ration Trials and Surveys. Chicago, Ill.: Quartermaster Food and Container Institute for the Armed Forces.
1947   Environment and food intake in man. Science. 105:378-379.

Kark, R.M.
1954   Studies on troops in the field. Pp. 193-195 in Nutrition Under Climatic Stress, H. Spector and M.S. Peterson, eds. Washington, D.C.: National Academy of Sciences.

Kark, R.M., H.F. Aiton, E.D. Pease, W.B. Bean, C.R. Henderson, R.E. Johnson, and L.M. Richardson
1947   Tropical deterioration and nutrition. Clinical and biochemical observations on troops. Medicine 26:1-40.
Keys, A., J. Brozek, A. Henschel, O. Mickelsen, and H. Taylor
1950   The Biology of Human Starvation, vols. 1-2. Minneapolis, Minn.: University of Minnesota Press.
Klausen, K., D.B. Dill, E.E. Phillips, and D. McGregor
1967   Metabolic reactions to work in the desert. J. Appl. Physiol. 22:292-296.
MacGregor, R.G.S., and G.L. Loh
1941   The influence of a tropical environment upon the basal metabolism, pulse rate and blood pressure in Europeans. J. Physiol. (London) 99:496-509.
Mason, E.D.
1934   The basal metabolism of European women in South India and the effect of change in climate on European and South Indian women. J. Nutr. 8:695.
Mitchell, H.H., and M. Edman
1949   Nutrition and Resistance to Climatic Stress, with Reference to Man. Chicago, Ill: Quartermaster Food and Container Institute for the Armed Forces.
1951   Nutrition and Resistance to Climatic Stress with Particular Reference to Man. Springfield, Ill.: Charles C. Thomas.
Paul, G.L.
1989   Dietary protein requirements of physically active individuals. Sports Med. 8:154-176.
Robinson, S., E.S. Turrell, H.S. Belding, and S.M. Horvath
1945   Rapid acclimatization to work in hot climates. Am. J. Physiol. 140:168-176.
Rose, M.S., and D.E. Carlson
1986   Effects of A-ration meals on body weight during sustained field operations. Report No. T2-87. Natick, Mass.: U.S. Army Research Institute of Environmental Medicine.
Rowell, L.B., G.L. Brengelman, J.A. Murray, K.K. Kraning, and F. Kusumi
1969   Human metabolic responses to hyperthermia during mild to maximal exercise. J. Appl. Physiol. 26:395-402.
Sargent, F., and R.E. Johnson
1957   The Physiological Basis for Various Constituents in Survival Rations. Part 4. An Integrative Study of the All-Purpose Survival Ration for Temperate, Cold and Hot Weather. Wright Air Development Center Technical Report 53-484. Wright-Patterson Air Force Base, Ohio: Wright Air Development Center.
Sawka, M.N., K.B. Pandolf, B.A. Avellini, and Y. Shapiro
1983   Does heat acclimation lower the rate of metabolism elicited by muscular exercise. Aviat. Space Environ. Med. 54:27-31.
Sen Gupta, J., P. Dimri, and M.S. Malhotra
1977   Metabolic responses of Indians during submaximal and maximal work in dry and humid heat. Ergonomics 20:33-40.
Shvartz, E., Y. Shapiro, A. Magazanik, A. Meroz, H. Bernfeld, A. Mechtinger, and S. Shibolet
1977   Heat acclimation, physical fitness, and responses to exercise in temperate and hot environments. J. Appl. Physiol. 43:678-683.
Swift, R.W., and C.E. French
1954   Energy Metabolism and Nutrition. New Brunswick, N.J.: Scarecrow Press.
Taylor, H.L., and A. Keys
1958   Criteria for fitness and comments on negative nitrogen balance. Ann. N.Y. Acad. Sci. 73:465-475.

Welch, B.E., L.M. Levy, C.F. Consolazio, E.R. Buskirk, and T.E. Dee
  1957a   Caloric intake for prolonged hard work in the cold. Report No. 202. U.S. Army
           Medical Nutrition Laboratory, Denver, Colo.
Welch, B.E., J.G. Marcinek, E.R. Buskirk, and P.F. Iampietro
  1957b   Caloric intake and energy expenditure of eight men in a temperate environment.
           Report No.196. U.S. Army Medical Nutrition Laboratory, Denver, Colo.
Welch, B.E., E.R. Buskirk, and P.F. Iampietro
  1958   Relation of climate and temperature to food and water intake in man. Metabolism
           7:141-148.
Young, D.R.
  1977   Physical Performance Fitness and Diet. Springfield, Ill.: Charles C. Thomas.
Young, J.J., M.N. Sawka, L. Levine, B.S. Cadarette, and K.B. Pandolf
  1985   Skeletal muscle metabolism during exercise is influenced by heat acclimation. J.
           Appl. Physiol. 59:1929-1935.

Nutritional Needs in Hot Environments
Pp. 117–135. Washington, D.C.
National Academy Press

7

The Effect of Exercise and Heat on Mineral Metabolism and Requirements

Carl L. Keen[1]

INTRODUCTION

During the last decade there has been increasing interest in the idea that individuals engaged in strenuous exercise may have an increased need for several of the essential minerals. This idea has resulted in the widespread perception that mineral supplements may be advantageous for this subpopulation. The concept is based on two basic perceptions: (a) that individuals engaged in strenuous exercise have a higher requirement for some minerals compared to sedentary individuals due to increased rates of urinary and sweat losses of select minerals and (b) that the perceived inadequate intake of some minerals results in a lowering of endurance capacity and ultimately may lead to the development of some disease states. Although a significant number of athletes, coaches, and professionals in the sports medicine field believe in the salutary effects of mineral supplements, there are remarkably few data supporting a positive effect of dietary mineral supplementation on athletic performance. However, as discussed below, strenuous exercise does influence the metabolism of several minerals, and the amount of minerals lost via sweat (due to either intense heat or exercise) can be significant.

This chapter examines the current understanding of the effects of exercise on mineral metabolism and the potential consequences of these effects. The metabolism of at least eight minerals—copper, chromium, iodine, iron,

[1] Carl L. Keen, Departments of Nutrition and Internal Medicine, University of California, Davis, CA 95616-8669

magnesium, potassium, sodium, and zinc—has been suggested to be influenced by exercise. Due to space constraints, this chapter will focus on four elements—iron, magnesium, zinc, and copper—to exemplify concepts involved in exercise- and heat-induced alterations in mineral metabolism and nutrition. However, prior to this discussion a few comments will be made concerning iodine, selenium, and chromium. The reader is directed to Chapters 12 and 13 for information on exercise- and heat-induced changes in sodium and potassium metabolism.

EFFECTS OF EXERCISE AND HEAT ON IODINE, CHROMIUM, AND SELENIUM METABOLISM

Consolazio (1966) reported that a considerable amount of iodine can be lost via sweat. In that study, 12 adult males were maintained at a temperature of 38.5°C during the day and 33.1°C during the night. During the 24-hour period, the men exercised at a moderate rate on a bicycle ergometer for 1 hour. The average total sweat loss of the men over the 24-hour period was 5576 g, which resulted in an average loss of 146 µg of iodine. Given that the 1989 U.S. recommended dietary allowance (RDA) (NRC, 1989) for iodine for adult men and women is 150 µg per day, and the observation that typical iodine intakes exclusive of iodized salt range from 250 to 170 µg per day for men and women, respectively (Pennington et al., 1989), it is evident that sweat-associated iodine loss can be significant. The above findings suggest that it is critical that iodized salt (which provides ≥70 µg of iodine per g of salt) be consumed when an individual is in an exceptionally hot area and/or engaged in strenuous activity. Studies examining the influence of combined heat exposure and endurance exercise on iodine metabolism are needed.

As with iodine, there is limited literature on the influence of exercise and heat on selenium metabolism, although it has been suggested that athletes may benefit from selenium supplements due to its role in glutathione peroxidase synthesis. Singh et al. (1991) reported that plasma selenium concentrations decreased in men exposed to a 5-day rigorous training program conducted by the U.S. Navy, despite an increase in dietary selenium intake during the program. Singh and colleagues suggested that the decrease in plasma selenium might have reflected a shift in selenium from the plasma pool to tissues requiring increased antioxidant protection. This hypothesis would be consistent with the observation that exercise can result in increased rates of tissue lipid peroxidation (Davies et al., 1982). Although the above observations suggest that selenium metabolism may be influenced by exercise, to date there is no compelling evidence that selenium supplementation is necessary for individuals engaged in endurance activities (Lane, 1989; Lang et al., 1987).

Consolazio et al. (1964) reported an average loss of 340 µg of selenium in sweat over an 8-hour period in men maintained at a temperature of 37.8°C. However, given the observation that typical selenium intakes are only on the order of 100 µg per day (Pennington et al., 1984), the loss reported by Consolazio seems excessive, and may reflect the technical difficulties involved in measuring this element. With the exception of the data by Consolazio, there are no current reports suggesting that selenium requirements are higher in hot environments compared to temperate regions.

Although the metabolic functions of chromium have not been clearly defined, chromium is known to be involved in the regulation of carbohydrate and lipid metabolism, presumably via a role in insulin action. Although not clearly defined in humans, signs associated with marginal chromium status in experimental animals include impaired glucose tolerance, elevated circulating insulin, elevated cholesterol and triglycerides, and increased incidence of aortic plaques (Campbell and Anderson, 1987). The dietary intake of chromium has been reported to be suboptimal for the general population based on dietary survey studies (Anderson and Kozlovsky, 1985). Recent research has indicated that chromium requirements may be influenced by strenuous exercise. Anderson et al. (1984) reported that serum chromium concentrations were increased in adult males immediately after a 6-mile run at near-maximal running capacity. This increase in serum chromium was still evident 2 hours after the completion of the run, and urinary chromium loss was elevated twofold on the run day compared to non-run days. Basal urinary chromium excretions have been shown to be lower in individuals routinely engaged in strenuous activity compared to sedentary controls (Anderson et al., 1988), which suggests either that chronic exercise results in a partial depletion of body chromium stores or that it induces metabolic changes that result in a reduction in urinary chromium excretion. Consistent with the latter idea, Vallerand et al. (1984) reported that, in rats, exercise training is associated with an increase in soft tissue chromium concentrations. In addition to exercise-induced increases in urinary chromium excretion, it would be expected that chromium losses would also be increased with excessive sweating. However, due to analytical difficulties in measuring this element, accurate data on sweat-associated losses of chromium are not currently available. Consolazio et al. (1964) reported that chromium loss in sweat over an 8-hour period averaged 60 µg in men maintained at 37.8°C, a value that would be double that of the typical dietary intake of the element. Studies aimed at better defining the amount of chromium lost in sweat at different amounts of sweat loss are clearly needed.

Chromium deficiency per se has not been accepted as a health problem in endurance athletes. However, it seems prudent, given the above findings, to monitor chromium status of individuals engaged in strenuous activity for prolonged periods of time, particularly if the activity is performed in a hot environment where chromium losses in sweat would be predicted to be high. Studies on the functional consequences of activity-induced changes in chromium metabolism are needed.

EFFECTS OF EXERCISE AND HEAT ON IRON METABOLISM

It is well recognized that iron-deficiency anemia can be associated with a diminished performance in maximal and submaximal physical exercise (Andersen and Barkve, 1970; Edgerton et al., 1981; Gardner et al., 1977; McDonald and Keen, 1988 and references cited therein). However, there is considerable controversy about the extent to which exercise contributes to the development of iron deficiency. Although there is a common perception that athletes as a group tend to have a high incidence of anemia compared to sedentary populations, hematological surveys of elite athletes have typically not supported this idea (Brotherhood et al., 1975; de Wijn et al., 1971; Stewart et al., 1972). Thus, overt iron-deficiency anemia does not appear to be a common complication of chronic intense exercise.

High levels of physical activity have been suggested to cause "sports anemia" (typically defined as a drop in hemoglobin concentration, hematocrit, and red blood cell count; Balaban et al., 1989; Yoshimura, 1970). The phenomenon of sports anemia has been associated with increased erythrocyte destruction, depressed iron absorption, increased sweat loss of iron, and gastrointestinal blood loss (Dressendorfer et al., 1991; Ehn et al., 1980; Frederickson et al., 1983; Paulev et al., 1983; Puhl et al., 1981; Stewart et al., 1984). Although most investigators agree that sports anemia is common in athletes who initiate rigorous training programs, this "anemia" is typically transitory in nature with hematological values often returning to pretraining values within 3 weeks despite continued training (Frederickson et al., 1983). Based on these findings, it has been suggested by some that sports anemia may be in part a consequence of plasma volume expansion and a functional dilution of the red blood cell count because blood volume can increase by as much as 20 percent during training (Brotherhood et al., 1975; Hegenauer et al., 1983).

In recent years there has been interest in the idea that exercise training can result in reduced tissue iron stores. Ehn at al. (1980) reported low bone marrow iron stores and evidence of increased iron absorption in elite distance runners who were characterized by normal hemoglobin and serum iron levels. Low serum ferritin concentrations have been reported by numerous investigators to be a consequence of prolonged, strenuous exercise (primarily when the subject is involved in weight-bearing sports) (Magazanik et al., 1988; Nickerson et al., 1985; Parr et al., 1984; Roberts and Smith, 1990; Snyder et al., 1989). Although there is considerable debate about the extent to which iron supplements may prevent exercise-induced reductions in tissue iron stores, Snyder et al. (1989) and Nickerson et al. (1985) have reported that providing highly bioavailable iron (heme iron in meat) or iron supplements (105 mg per day) can retard the development of low serum ferritin concentrations.

Given the observation that endurance athletes are typically not characterized by a higher than normal frequency of iron-deficiency anemia (see above), many investigators have questioned the significance of the finding of low serum ferritin concentrations in these individuals. However, it is important to note that the occurrence of low tissue iron stores in these individuals could present a problem with regard to recovery from injuries that result in extensive tissue damage or blood loss. It should be noted that marginal iron deficiency resulting in impaired thermoregulation has recently been observed (Beard et al., 1990); thus exercise-induced alterations in iron status may pose particular risks for individuals exposed to extreme temperatures.

As discussed above, an increased rate of sweat loss of iron is thought to contribute to the depletion of iron stores with chronic endurance exercise. Although the loss of iron via sweat is not normally considered to be a major explanation for the iron depletion, sweat iron concentrations can range from 0.1 to 0.3 mg per liter for men and up to 0.4 mg per liter for women (Aruoma et al., 1988; Brune et al., 1986; Lamanca et al., 1988; Paulev et al., 1983). Given these concentrations, sweat can be an appreciable route of iron loss particularly when sweat rates exceed 5 liters per day. The potential interaction between prolonged exposure to high temperatures and vigorous activity with regard to iron status, and an individual's ability to thermoregulate and recover from injury is an area that needs further clarification.

In sum, dietary iron supplementation may in some instances be justified to ensure good health of the individual. However, caution must be used in advocating excessive iron supplementation, given the potential negative side effects that can be associated with its use, including possible gastrointestinal discomfort, and interactions with other metals that have similar physiochemical properties. For example, it has been suggested that high levels of supplemental iron can inhibit the absorption of zinc (Keen and Hackman, 1986; Solomons, 1986). Given that prolonged exposure to a regimen of strenuous exercise and/or exposure to conditions resulting in high rates of sweat loss is associated with marked changes in zinc metabolism (see below), the potential negative effects of excess iron supplementation are clear.

EFFECTS OF EXERCISE AND HEAT ON ZINC METABOLISM

Lichti et al. (1970) first demonstrated that strenuous exercise can result in marked changes in zinc metabolism. They reported a marked increase in plasma zinc concentrations in dogs following short bouts of intense exercise. This observation was extended by Hetland et al. (1975) who found that plasma zinc concentrations in men participating in a 5-hour, 70-km cross-country ski race were 19 percent higher immediately postrace compared to prerace values. However, by day 1 postrace, zinc concentrations were back to control levels. The observation that plasma zinc concentrations can increase significantly during strenuous exercise has since been verified by numerous investigators (Dressendorfer et al., 1982; Lukaski et al., 1984; Ohno et al., 1985; Van Rij et al., 1986). The magnitude of the increase in plasma zinc concentration with exercise is such that it cannot be due to hemoconcentration (Hetland et al., 1975; Lukaski et al., 1984); rather it is thought to reflect the result of muscle leakage of zinc into the extracellular fluid following muscle breakdown (Karlson et al., 1968). Following the cessation of exercise, there is normally a rapid drop in plasma zinc levels back to preexercise concentrations within a short period. It is thought that this rapid postexercise drop in plasma zinc is due to a high urinary excretion of the element coupled with a shift in the distribution of the element from the plasma fraction into the liver (Anderson et al., 1984; Campbell and Anderson, 1987; McDonald and Keen, 1988). The shift of zinc from the plasma into the liver is thought to be in part a consequence of the so-called acute-phase response, which occurs as a consequence of stressors such as infection, inflammation, and trauma. These stressors can result in the elaboration of cytokines, which result in the stimulation of the synthesis of several liver proteins (Cannon and Kluger, 1983; Cousins, 1985; Dinarello, 1989; Keen and Hackman, 1986; Singh et al., 1991). With regard to zinc, one component of the acute-phase response is an increase in liver metallothionein concentration, which can result in a sequestering of zinc in the liver (Cousins, 1985; Whanger and Oh, 1978). (Serum ferritin concentrations can increase as a result of the acute-phase response, a fact that must be considered when collecting samples for assessment of iron status; Singh et al., 1991; Taylor et al., 1987.)

Reductions in plasma zinc concentrations were also observed in men who participated in a 5-day intensive training course conducted by the U.S. Navy (Singh et al., 1991). This reduction in plasma zinc occurred despite an increase in dietary zinc intake during the training period. The authors attributed the reduction in plasma zinc primarily to a redistribution of plasma zinc into liver as a consequence of metallothionein synthesis stimulated by interleukin-6 (IL-6). (The observed increase in plasma IL-6 concentrations was associated with tissue trauma.) Consistent with the above finding, Lichton et al. (1988) observed a reduction in plasma zinc concentrations in male soldiers engaged in a 34-day field exercise at an elevation of 1800 m. The field exercise was simulated combat in which the men performed combat-support activities during both day and night and during which time they lost sleep. Activities included digging foxholes, building lava-stone walls, and walking. During the study, subjects were given a military operational ration, the meal, ready-to-eat (MRE), as their only food. Although the average zinc intake during the field exercise was lower than zinc intakes in a sedentary control group of soldiers who were fed the same food, intakes by both groups were considered adequate. Urinary zinc concentrations in the active soldiers increased from an average basal level of 400 μg per day to about 700 μg per day during the study. Sweat mineral losses were not assessed.

This finding shows that there are short-term effects of exercise on zinc metabolism; however, the immediate physiological consequences of these effects are not known. Dressendorfer and Sockolov (1980) have suggested that a high level of constant exercise can have long-lasting effects on zinc metabolism. This suggestion was based on the observation that a significant number of endurance runners were characterized by low serum zinc concentrations even when tested prior to an exercise bout. This hypozincemia in endurance runners has since been reported by other laboratories (Couzy et al., 1990; Deuster et al., 1986; Dressendorfer et al., 1982; Hackman and Keen, 1986; Haralambie, 1981).

The mechanisms underlying the development of exercise-induced hypozincemia are presumably multifactorial and may include impaired absorption of zinc, excessive sweat and urinary loss of the element, and an altered metabolism of zinc (Anderson et al., 1984; Deuster et al., 1989; Miyamura et al., 1987). Although there is considerable debate about the value of plasma zinc in diagnosing zinc deficiency, most investigators agree that prolonged low plasma zinc concentrations are indicative of suboptimal zinc status. Given that the consequences of a suboptimal zinc status can include behavioral abnormalities, impaired immunocompetence, and reduced rate of recovery from injury (Hambidge, 1989; Keen and Gershwin 1990), it is evident that the functional significance of exercise-induced hypozincemia needs to be defined in future studies. In addition, the interactive effect of prolonged exposure to high temperatures and intense exercise needs to be defined. Exposure to extremes in temperature by itself can result in a stimulation of the acute-phase response with subsequent changes in zinc metabolism (Sugawara et al., 1983; Uhari et al., 1983); sweat losses of zinc can range from 0.5 to 1 mg per liter (Aruoma et al., 1988; Van Rij et al., 1986). Thus a strong synergistic effect of prolonged exposure to exercise and heat would be predicted. To illustrate the above scenario, the following calculations can be made. First, assume a dietary zinc intake of 15 mg, with a typical absorption of 20 percent (King and Turnlund, 1989), resulting in an uptake of 3 mg of zinc. By assuming a sweat zinc concentration of 0.5 mg per liter, it is evident that sweat losses in excess of 8 liters can present a significant problem. In addition, typical urinary zinc losses under conditions of stress will average 0.5 to 0.8 mg per day. Zinc absorption may also be reduced under conditions of stress. Given the above calculations, sustained exercise in a hot environment would be predicted to have a negative impact on an individual's zinc balance. Note that an intermediate value for zinc absorption was used for these calculations. Zinc absorption from typical foods ranges from 10 to 40 percent (King and Turnlund, 1989); thus the type of meal fed will have a significant effect on the zinc balance of individuals exposed to the above conditions.

Given the frequent observation of exercise-induced hypozincemia and the potentially high amounts of the element that can be lost via sweat, there may be a need for zinc supplementation in situations where prolonged exposure to exercise and heat is anticipated. However, as discussed for iron, caution must be used when advocating zinc supplements because this element at high levels can interfere with copper absorption due to the similar physiochemical properties of zinc and copper (Keen and Hackman, 1986). Chronic (more than 6 weeks) consumption of zinc supplements in excess of 50 mg per day has been linked to the induction of copper deficiency in humans (Fischer et al., 1984; Fosmire, 1990; Prasad et al., 1978; Samman and Roberts, 1988). Lower levels of zinc supplementation have not been reported to result in copper deficiency.

INFLUENCE OF EXERCISE AND HEAT
ON MAGNESIUM METABOLISM

There are considerable data demonstrating an effect of exercise on magnesium metabolism. Rose et al. (1970) reported that serum magnesium concentrations in marathon runners immediately following a race were significantly lower than prerace values, a phenomenon that was attributed to sweat losses of the element during the run. The idea that excessive sweating could result in a high loss of magnesium from the body is consistent with the work of Consolazio et al. (1963) who found that, under normal conditions, sweat loss accounted for over 12 percent of the total daily excretion of magnesium in men working in temperatures of 49° to 50°C. (Typical magnesium losses via sweat are on the order of 3 to 4 mg per liter [Beller et al., 1975; Consolazio et al., 1963].) The observed lowering of plasma magnesium with intense exercise has since been verified by numerous investigators (Beller et al., 1975; Deuster et al., 1987; Franz et al., 1985; Haralambie et al., 1981; Laires et al., 1988; Lijnen et al., 1988; Refsum et al., 1973; Stendig-Lindberg et al., 1987, 1989). The typical reduction in plasma magnesium following intense exercise is on the order of 10 percent. Stendig-Lindberg et al. (1989) reported that low plasma magnesium concentrations can be demonstrated in young men for up to 18 days after strenuous exertion (a 70-km march). In addition to an increased loss of magnesium via sweat, urinary magnesium loss can increase by up to 30 percent following a bout of intense exercise (Deuster et al., 1987; Lijnen et al., 1988). Although the reduction in plasma magnesium may be due in part to an increased rate of magnesium loss from the body, redistribution of magnesium from the plasma pool into other sites may also contribute to exercise-induced decreases in plasma magnesium. For example, Costill et al. (1976) reported an increased magnesium content in exercising muscle during prolonged work that paralleled the decline in plasma magnesium. Redistribution of serum magnesium into red blood cells (Abbasciano et al., 1988; Deuster et al., 1987; Lukaski et al., 1983) and into adipocytes (Franz et al., 1985) with exercise has also been reported. Researchers generally agree that prolonged exercise can result in lower than normal plasma magnesium concentrations; however, they have not agreed on the functional consequences of this reduction. Jooste et al. (1979) reported that in some cases the reduction can be severe enough to trigger epileptic-type convulsions in runners. Similarly, Liu et al. (1983) reported a case in which an exercise-induced reduction in plasma magnesium was associated with the induction of carpopedal spasms in a 24-year-old woman. Marginal magnesium deficiency has been associated with the etiology of some cardiac diseases (Rayssiguier, 1984), hypertension (Altura and Altura, 1984), and reduced work capacity (Conn et al., 1986; Keen et al., 1987; Lowney et al., 1990; Lukaski et al., 1983). Marginal magnesium status has also been implicated in a number of human psychiatric disturbances and in chronic fatigue syndrome (Cox et al., 1991).

Given the above reports, it is clear that prolonged strenuous exertion can result in reductions in plasma magnesium concentrations. These reductions can be attributed in part to an increased rate of magnesium loss via sweat, which could be significantly amplified in hot environments. Given the recognition that marginal magnesium deficiency can present a significant health risk to an individual, studies are needed that define the functional consequences of exercise- and heat-induced reductions in plasma magnesium concentrations.

EFFECTS OF EXERCISE AND HEAT ON COPPER METABOLISM

Acute, strenuous exercise has been reported by several investigators to result in a marked increase in plasma copper concentrations, which has been attributed to an increase in plasma ceruloplasmin concentrations (Haralambie, 1975; Ohno et al., 1984; Olha et al., 1982). An increase in ceruloplasmin concentrations is consistent with the induction of an acute-phase response as discussed above. The effects of intense exercise on increasing plasma copper levels can continue for prolonged time periods. Dressendorfer et al. (1982) reported that men engaged in a 20-day, 500-km road race were characterized by plasma copper levels that increased constantly during the first week, after which they remained fairly constant. This increased copper output into the plasma as a result of exercise may have long-lasting effects, as suggested by the observation that plasma copper levels at rest tend to be higher in athletes than in untrained individuals (Haralambie, 1975; Lukaski et al., 1983; Olha et al., 1982).

Given the putative antioxidant properties of ceruloplasmin (Goldstein et al., 1979; Gutteridge, 1986), one explanation for the exercise-induced increase in the concentration of this plasma protein is as a response to tissue injury associated with oxidative damage or to the presence of an increased concentration of free radicals (Alessio et al., 1988; Davies et al., 1982; Jenkins, 1988; Kanter et al., 1986). An additional possibility is that the increased ceruloplasmin output from the liver, and hence increased levels in the plasma, is an adaptive response by the body to an increased requirement for extrahepatic copper. It is known that the higher values of maximal oxygen uptake in trained individuals are correlated to an increase in oxidative enzymes within the cell. One of the enzymes increased is the copper-containing protein, cytochrome oxidase (Terjung et al., 1973). It has been shown that ceruloplasmin copper can be incorporated into cytochrome oxidase, and cell receptor sites for ceruloplasmin have been identified (Stevens et al., 1984). Ceruloplasmin copper has also been demonstrated to be transferred to apo-copper, zinc superoxide dismutase (Percival and Harris, 1991). An increase in cellular copper, zinc superoxide dismutase activity could represent an adaptive response to exercise-induced intracellular oxidative stress (Jenkins, 1988; Lukaski et al., 1990).

In contrast to reports of increased plasma copper concentrations, Anderson et al. (1984) reported that plasma copper concentrations were similar in men prior to and after completing a 6-mile run; Lukaski et al. (1990) reported no influence of training on plasma copper concentrations in elite swimmers, and Singh et al. (1991) observed no change in plasma copper concentrations in men engaged in intense physical activity over a 5-day period. Resina et al. (1990) reported that plasma copper concentrations were lower in long-distance runners than in sedentary controls, and Dowdy and Burt (1980) reported that plasma copper concentrations and ceruloplasmin activity decreased in competitive swimmers over a 6-month period. Uhari et al. (1983) reported that plasma copper concentrations decreased in male and female subjects following exposure to hot temperatures in a sauna bath.

Reasons for the above differences in reported effects of exercise on plasma copper concentrations are various, including differences in copper status of the subjects; type, intensity, and duration of the exercise; physical condition of the individual; and extent of exercise-induced tissue trauma. Presumably, increases in plasma copper occur primarily when there is tissue damage that triggers an acute-phase response. However, note that in the study by Singh et al. (1991), despite evidence of significant tissue damage (see zinc section above), plasma copper concentrations were not elevated.

Additional studies are needed that define the mechanisms underlying exercise-induced increases in plasma copper concentrations.

It is important to point out that the occurrence of high plasma copper concentrations does not necessarily translate into high tissue copper concentrations; indeed, high plasma copper concentrations in some disease states have been correlated to low soft tissue copper concentrations (Clegg et al., 1987; Dubick et al., 1987). Although the interpretation of normal to high plasma copper concentrations with regard to assessing an individual's copper status can be difficult, there is general agreement that low plasma copper concentrations typically reflect a compromised copper status. Thus the report of low plasma copper concentrations in some endurance athletes (see above) is of concern. Although loss of basal copper via sweat is typically considered negligible (Gutteridge et al., 1985; Jacob et al., 1981), Consolazio et al. (1964) reported that the amount of copper lost via sweat can be considerable; men who were maintained at 37.8°C and 50 percent relative humidity lost as much as 1 mg per day in sweat. This value should be contrasted to typical dietary copper intakes, which are on the order of 1 to 2 mg (Pennington et al., 1989). Thus prolonged, excessive loss of copper via sweat during strenuous exercise could result in a marginal copper status. The simultaneous exposure to hot temperatures would be expected to accelerate the development of a marginal copper condition.

CONCLUSIONS

Prolonged strenuous exercise can result in marked changes in chromium, copper, iron, magnesium, and zinc metabolism. Evidence of these changes can persist for several days after the exercise is discontinued. Some of the observed changes in plasma mineral concentrations may be attributed in part to an acute-phase response, which occurs as a result of tissue trauma or stress. Reductions in plasma mineral concentrations may also in part reflect an increased loss of these minerals from the body via urine and sweat. The increased rate of mineral loss that occurs in sweat with exercise is amplified by the simultaneous exposure to hot temperatures.

Given the above observations, the following questions emerge: Do endurance-associated changes in mineral metabolism result in some or all of the following:

- a compromised endurance capacity?
- a compromised immune defense system?
- a compromised antioxidant defense system?
- a slower rate of recovery from injury?

Additional work on the influence of prolonged exposure to strenuous exercise and heat is urgently needed. The influence of diet on the above changes in mineral metabolism, or whether dietary manipulations may attenuate some of the negative consequences of these changes, is an area of research that needs to be expanded.

REFERENCES

Abbasciano, V., F. Levato, M.G. Reali, I. Casoni, M. Patracchini, D. Mazzotta, F. Fagioli, and C. Guglielmini
  1988   Reduction of erythrocyte magnesium concentration in heterozygote β-thalassaemic subjects and in normal subjects submitted to physical stress. Magnesium Res. 1:213-217.
Alessio, H.A., A.H. Goldfarb, and R.G. Cutler
  1988   MDA content increases in fast and slow twitch skeletal muscle with intensity of exercise in a rat. Am. J. Physiol. 255:C874-C877.
Altura, B.M., and B.T. Altura
  1984   Interactions of magnesium and potassium on blood aspects in view of hypertension: Review of present status and new findings. Magnesium 3:175-194.
Andersen, H.T., and H. Barkve
  1970   Iron deficiency and muscular work performance: An evaluation of cardio-respiratory function of iron deficient subjects with and without anemia. Scand. J. Lab. Invest. 25(suppl. 144):1-39.
Anderson, R.A., and A.S. Kozlovsky
  1985   Chromium intake, absorption, and excretion of subjects consuming self-selected diets. Am. J. Clin. Nutr. 41:1177-1183.
Anderson, R.A., M.M. Polansky, and N.A. Bryden
  1984   Strenuous running: Acute effects on chromium, copper, zinc and selected variables in urine and serum of male runners. Biol. Trace Elem. Res. 6:327-336.
Anderson, R.A., N.A. Bryden, M.M. Polansky, and P.A. Deuster
  1988   Exercise effects on chromium excretion of trained and untrained men consuming a constant diet. J. Appl. Physiol. 64:249-252.
Aruoma, O.I., T. Reilly, D. MacLaren, and B. Halliwell
  1988   Iron, copper and zinc concentrations in human sweat and plasma; the effect of exercise. Clin. Chim. Acta 177:81-88.
Balaban, E.P., J.V. Cox, P. Snell, R.H. Vaugh, and E.P. Frenkel
  1989   The frequency of anemia and iron deficiency in the runner. Med. Sci. Sports Exerc. 21:643-648.
Beard, J.L., M.J. Borel, and J. Derr
  1990   Impaired thermoregulation and thyroid function in iron-deficiency anemia. Am. J. Clin. Nutr. 52:813-819.
Beller, G.A., J.T. Maher, L.H. Hartley, D.E. Bass, and W.E.C. Wacker
  1975   Changes in serum and sweat magnesium levels during work in the heat. Aviat. Space Environ. Med. 46:709-712.
Brotherhood, J., B. Brozovic, and L.G.C. Pugh
  1975   Haematological status of middle- and long-distance runners. Clin. Sci. Mol. Med. 48:139-145.
Brune, M., B. Magnusson, H. Persson, and L. Hallberg
  1986   Iron losses in sweat. Am. J. Clin. Nutr. 43:438-443.
Campbell, W.W., and R.A. Anderson
  1987   Effects of aerobic exercise and training on the trace minerals chromium, zinc and copper. Sports Med. 4:9-18.

Cannon, J.G., and M.J. Kluger
1983   Endogenous pyrogen activity in human plasma after exercise. Science 220:617-619.

Clegg, M.S., F. Ferrell, and C.L. Keen
1987   Hypertension-induced alterations in copper and zinc metabolism in Dahl rats. Hypertension 9:624-628.

Conn, C.A., E. Ryder, R.A. Schemmel, P. Ku, V. Seefeldt, and W.W. Heusner
1986   Relationship of maximal oxygen consumption to plasma and erythrocyte magnesium and to plasma copper levels in elite young runners and controls. Fed. Proc. 45:972.

Consolazio, C.F.
1966   Comparisons of nitrogen, calcium and iodine excretion in arm and total body sweat. Am. J. Clin. Nutr. 18:443-448.

Consolazio, C.F., L.O. Matoush, R.A. Nelson, R.S. Harding, and J.E. Canham
1963   Excretion of sodium, potassium, magnesium and iron in human sweat and the relation of each to balance and requirements. J. Nutr. 79:407-415.

Consolazio, C.F., R.A. Nelson, L.O. Matoush, R.C. Hughes, and P. Urone
1964   Trace mineral losses in sweat. Pp. 1-12 in report no. 284 of U.S. Army no. 3A12501A283 (Military Internal Medicine), Subtask no. 03 (Biochemistry), U.S. Army Medical Research and Nutrition Laboratory, Fitzimmons General Hospital, Denver, Colo.

Costill, D.L., R. Cote, and W. Fink
1976   Muscle water and electrolytes following varied levels of dehydration in man. J. Appl. Physiol. 40:6-11.

Cousins, R.J.
1985   Absorption, transport, and hepatic metabolism of copper and zinc: Special reference to metallothionein and ceruloplasmin. Physiol. Rev. 65:238-309.

Couzy, F., P. Lafargue, and C.Y. Guezennec
1990   Zinc metabolism in the athletes: Influence of training, nutrition and other factors. Int. J. Sports Med. 11:263-266.

Cox, I.M., M.J. Campbell, and D. Dowson
1991   Red blood cell magnesium and chronic fatigue syndrome. Lancet 337:757-760.

Davies, K.J.A., A.T. Quintanilha, G.A. Brooks, and L. Packer
1982   Free radicals and tissue damage produced by exercise. Biochem. Biophys. Res. Commun. 107:118-125.

de Wijn, J.F., J.L. de Jongste, W. Mosterd, and D. Willebrand
1971   Haemoglobin, packed cell volume, serum iron and iron binding capacity of selected athletes during training. J. Sports Med. Phys. Fitness 11:42-51.

Deuster, P.A., S.B. Kyle, P.B. Moser, R.A. Vigersky, A. Singh, and E.B. Schoomaker
1986   Nutritional survey of highly trained women runners. Am. J. Clin. Nutr. 45:954-962.

Deuster, P.A., E. Dolev, S.B. Kyle, R.A. Anderson, and E.B. Schoomaker
1987   Magnesium homeostasis during high-intensity anaerobic exercise in men. J. Appl. Physiol. 62(2):545-550.

Deuster, P.A., B.A. Day, A. Singh, L. Douglass, and P.B. Moser-Veillon
1989   Zinc status of highly trained women runners and untrained women. Am. J. Clin. Nutr. 49:1295-1301.

Dinarello, C.A.
1989   The endogenous pyrogens in host-defense interactions. Hosp. Pract. 24:111-128.

Dowdy, R.P., and J. Burt
1980   Effect of intensive, long term training on copper and iron nutriture in man. Fed. Proc. 39:786.

Dressendorfer, R.H., and R. Sockolov
1980   Hypoxincemia in runners. Physician Sports Med. 8:97-100.
Dressendorfer, R.H., C.E. Wade, C.L. Keen, and J.H. Scaff
1982   Plasma mineral levels in marathon runners during a 20-day road race. Physician
         Sports Med. 10:113-118.
Dressendorfer, R.H., C.L. Keen, C.E. Wade, J.R. Claybaugh, and G.C. Timmis
1991   Development of runners' anemia during a 20-day road race: Effect of iron supple-
         ments. Int. J. Sports Med. 12:332-336.
Dubick, M.A., G.C. Hunter, S.M. Casey, and C.L. Keen
1987   Aortic ascorbic acid, trace elements, and superoxide dismutase activity in human
         aneurysmal and occlusive disease. Proc. Soc. Exp. Biol. Med. 184:138-143.
Edgerton, V.R., Y. Ohira, J. Hettiarachchi, B. Senewiratne, G.W. Gardner, and R.J. Barnard
1981   Elevation of hemoglobin and work tolerance in iron-deficient subjects. J. Nutr.
         Sci. Vitaminol. 27:77-86.
Ehn, L., B. Carlmark, and S. Hoglund
1980   Iron status in athletes involved in intense physical activity. Med. Sci. Sports Exerc.
         12:61-64.
Fischer, P.W.F., A. Giroux, and M.R. L'Abbe
1984   Effect of zinc supplementation on copper status in adult man. Am. J. Clin. Nutr.
         40:743-746.
Fosmire, G.J.
1990   Zinc toxicity. Am. J. Clin. Nutr. 51:225-227.
Franz, R.B., H. Ruddel, G.L. Todd, T.A. Dorheim, J.C. Buell, et al.
1985   Physiologic changes during a marathon with special references to magnesium. J.
         Am. Coll. Nutr. 4:187-194.
Frederickson, L.A., J.L. Pulh, and W.S. Runyan
1983   Effects of training on indices of iron status of young female cross-country runners.
         Med. Sci. Sports Exerc. 15:271-276.
Gardner, G.W., V.R. Edgerton, B. Senewiratne, R.J. Barnard, and Y. Ohira
1977   Physical work capacity and metabolic stress in subjects with iron deficiency ane-
         mia. Am. J. Clin. Nutr. 30:910-917.
Goldstein, I.M., H.B. Kaplan, H.S. Edelson, and G. Weissmann
1979   Ceruloplasmin. A scavenger of superoxide anion radicals. J. Biol. Chem. 254:4040-
         4045.
Gutteridge, J.M.C.
1986   Antioxidant properties of the proteins caeruloplasmin, albumin, and transferrin. A
         study of their activity in serum and synovial fluid from patients with rheumatoid
         arthritis. Biochim. Biophys. Acta 869:119-127.
Gutteridge, J.M.C., D.A. Rowley, B. Halliwell, D.F. Cooper, and D.M. Heeley
1985   Copper and iron complexes catalytic for oxygen radical reaction in sweat from
         human athletes. Clin. Chim. Acta 145:267-273.
Hackman, R.M., and C.L. Keen
1986   Changes in serum zinc and copper levels after zinc supplementation in running
         and non-running men. Pp. 89-99 in Sport, Health and Nutrition: 1984 Olympic
         Scientific Congress Proceedings, Vol. 2, F. Katch ed. Champaign, Ill: Human
         Kinetics.
Hambidge, K.M.
1989   Mild zinc deficiency in human subjects. Pp. 281-296 in Zinc in Human Biology,
         C.F. Mills, ed. Great Britain: Springer-Verlag.

Haralambie, G.
1975   Changes in electrolytes and trace elements during long-lasting exercise. Pp. 340-351 in Metabolic Adaptation to Prolonged Physical Exercise, H. Howard and J.R. Poortmans, eds. Basel, Switzerland: Birkhäuser Verlag.
1981   Serum zinc in athletes in training. Int. J. Sports Med. 2:135-138.
Haralambie, G., L. Senser, and R. Sierra-Chavez
1981   Physiological and metabolic effects of a 25 km race in female athletes. Eur. J. Appl. Physiol. 47:123-131.
Hegenauer, J., L. Strause, P. Saltman, D. Dann, J. White, and R. Green
1983   Transitory effects of moderate exercise are not influenced by iron supplementation. Eur. J. Appl. Physiol. 52:57-61.
Hetland, O., E.A. Brubak, H.E. Refsum, and S.B. Stromme
1975   Serum and erythrocyte zinc concentrations after prolonged heavy exercise. Pp. 367-370 in Metabolic Adaptation to Prolonged Physical Exercise, H. Howard and J.R. Poortmans, eds. Basel, Switzerland: Birkhäuser Verlag.
Jacob, P.A., H.H. Sandstead, J.M. Munoz, L.M. Klevay, and D.B. Milne
1981   Whole body surface loss of trace metals in normal males. Am. J. Clin. Nutr. 34:1379-1383.
Jenkins, R.R.
1988   Free radical chemistry. Relationship to exercise. Sports Med. 5:156-170.
Jooste, P.L., J.M. Wolfswinkel, J.J. Schoeman, and N.B. Strydom
1979   Epileptic-type convulsions and magnesium deficiency. Aviat. Space Environ. Med. 50:734-735.
Kanter, M.M., G.R. Lesmes, N.D. Neguin, K.A. Kaminsky, and J.M. Saeger
1986   Serum lipid levels and lipid peroxidation in ultramarathon runners. Ann. Sports Med. 3:39-41.
Karlson, J., R. Diamant, and B. Saltin
1968   Lactic dehydrogenase activity in muscle after prolonged exercise in man. J. Appl. Physiol. 25:88-91.
Keen, C.L., and M.E. Gershwin
1990   Zinc deficiency and immune function. Annu. Rev. Nutr. 10:415-431.
Keen, C.L., and R.M. Hackman
1986   Trace elements in athletic performance. Pp. 51-65 in Sport, Health and Nutrition: 1984 Olympic Scientific Congress Proceedings, vol. 2, F.I. Katch, ed. Champaign, Ill.: Human Kinetics.
Keen, C.L., M.E. Gershwin, P. Lowney, L.S. Hurley, and J.S. Stern
1987   The influence of dietary magnesium intake on exercise capacity and hematological parameters in rats. Metabolism 36:788-793.
King, J.C., and J.R. Turnlund
1989   Human zinc requirements. Pp. 335-350 in Zinc in Human Biology, C.F. Mills, ed. Great Britain: Springer-Verlag.
Laires, M.J., F. Alves, and M.J. Halpern
1988   Changes in serum and erythrocyte magnesium and blood lipids after distance swimming. Magnesium Res. 1:219-222.
Lamanca, J.J., E.M. Haymes, J.A. Daly, R.J. Moffatt, and M.F. Waller
1988   Sweat iron loss of male and female runners during exercise. Int. J. Sports Med. 9:52-55.
Lane, H.W.
1989   Some trace elements related to physical activity: Zinc, copper, selenium, chromium, and iodine. Pp. 301-307 in Nutrition in Exercise and Sports, J.E. Hickson and I. Wolinsky, eds. Boca Raton, Fla.: CRC Press.

Lang, J.K., K. Gohil, L. Packer, and R.F. Burk
1987   Selenium deficiency, endurance exercise capacity, and antioxidant status in rats. J. Appl. Physiol. 63:2532-2535.
Lichti, E.L., M. Turner, M.S. Deweese, and J.H. Henzel
1970   Zinc concentration in venous plasma before and after exercise in dogs. Missouri Med. 67:303-309.
Lichton, I.J., J.B. Miyamura, and S.W. McNutt
1988   Nutritional evaluation of soldiers subsisting on meal, ready-to-eat operational rations for an extended period: Body measurements, hydration, and blood nutrients. Am. J. Clin. Nutr. 48:30-37.
Lijnen, P., P. Hespel, R. Fagard, R. Lysens, E. Vanden Eynde, and A. Amery
1988   Erythrocyte, plasma and urinary magnesium in men before and after a marathon. Eur. J. Appl. Physiol. 58:252-256.
Liu, L., G. Borowski, and L.I. Rose
1983   Hypomagnesemia in a tennis player. Physician Sports Med. 11:79-80.
Lowney, P., J.S. Stern, M.E. Gershwin, and C.L. Keen
1990   Magnesium deficiency and blood 2,3 diphosphoglycerate concentrations in sedentary and exercised male Osborne-Mendel rats. Metabolism 39:837-841.
Lukaski, H.C., W.W. Bolonchuk, L.M. Klevay, D.B. Milne, and H.H. Sandstead
1983   Maximal oxygen consumption as related to magnesium, copper and zinc nutriture. Am. J. Clin. Nutr. 37:407-415.
1984   Changes in plasma zinc content after exercise in men fed a low-zinc diet. Am. J. Physiol. 247:E88-E93.
Lukaski, H.C., B.S. Hoverson, S.K. Gallagher, and W.W. Bolonchuk
1990   Physical training and copper, iron, and zinc status of swimmers. Am. J. Clin. Nutr. 51:1093-1099.
Magazanik, A., Y. Weinstein, R.A. Dlin, M. Derin, S. Schwartzman, and D. Allalouf
1988   Iron deficiency caused by 7 weeks of intensive physical exercise. Eur. J. Appl. Physiol. 57:198-202.
McDonald, R., and C.L. Keen
1988   Iron, zinc and magnesium nutrition and athletic performance. Sports Med. 5:171-184.
Miyamura, J.B., S.W. McNutt, I.J. Lichton, and N.S. Wenkam
1987   Altered zinc status of soldiers under field conditions. J. Am. Diet. Assoc. 87:595-597.
NRC (National Research Council)
1989   Recommended Dietary Allowances, 10th ed. Washington, D.C.: National Academy Press.
Nickerson, H.J., M. Holubets, A.D. Tripp, and W.E. Pierce
1985   Decreased iron stores in high school female runners. Am. J. Dis. Child. 139:1115-1119.
Ohno, H., T. Yahata, F. Hirata, K. Yamamura, R. Doi, M. Harada, and N. Taniguchi
1984   Changes in dopamine-b-hydroxylase, and copper, and catecholamine concentrations in human plasma with physical exercise. J. Sports Med. Phys. Fitness 24:315-320.
Ohno, H., K. Yamashita, R. Doi, K. Yamamura, T. Kondo, and N. Taniguchi
1985   Exercise-induced changes in blood zinc and related proteins in humans. J. Appl. Physiol. 58:1453-1458.
Olha, A.E., V. Klissouras, J.D. Sullivan, and S.C. Skoryna
1982   Effect of exercise on concentration of elements in the serum. J. Sports Med. Phys. Fitness 22:414-425.

Parr, R.B., L.A. Bachman, and R.A. Moss
1984   Iron deficiency in female athletes. Physician Sports Med. 12:81-86.

Paulev, P-E., R. Jordal, and N.S. Pedersen
1983   Dermal excretion of iron in intensely training athletes. Clin. Chim. Acta 127:19-27.

Pennington, J.A.T., D.B. Wilson, R.F. Newell, B.F. Harland, R.D. Johnson, and J.E. Vanderveen
1984   Selected minerals in foods surveys, 1974 to 1981/82. J. Am. Diet. Assoc. 84:771-780.

Pennington, J.A.T., B.E. Young, and D.B. Wilson
1989   Nutritional elements in U.S. diets: Results from the Total Diet Study, 1982 to 1986. J. Am. Diet. Assoc. 89:659-664.

Percival, S.S., and E.D. Harris
1991   Regulation of Cu, Zn superoxide dismutase with copper. Caeruloplasmin maintains levels of functional enzyme activity during differentiation of K562 cells. Biochem. J. 274:153-158.

Prasad, A.S., G.J. Brewer, E.B. Shoomaker, and P. Rabbani
1978   Hypocupremia induced by zinc therapy in adults. J. Am. Med. Assoc. 240:2166-2168.

Puhl, S.H., W.B. Runyan, and S.J. Kruse
1981   Erythrocyte changes during training in high school women cross-country runners. Res. Q. Exerc. Sport 52:484-494.

Rayssiguier, Y.
1984   Role of magnesium and potassium in the pathogenesis of atherosclerosis. Magnesium 3:226-238.

Refsum, H.E., H.D. Meen, and S.B. Stromme
1973   Whole blood, serum and erythrocyte magnesium concentrations after repeated heavy exercise of long duration. Scand. J. Clin. Lab. Invest. 32:123-127.

Resina, A., S. Fedi, L. Gatteschi, M.G. Rubenni, M.A. Giamberardino, E. Trabassi, and F. Imreh
1990   Comparison of some serum copper parameters in trained runners and control subjects. Int. J. Sports Med. 11:58-60.

Roberts, D., and D. Smith
1990   Serum ferritin values in elite speed and synchronized swimmers and speed skaters. J. Lab. Clin. Med. 116:661-665.

Rose, L.I., D.R. Carroll, S.L. Lowe, E.W. Peterson, and K.H. Cooper
1970   Serum electrolyte changes after marathon running. J. Appl. Physiol. 29:449-451.

Samman, S., and D.C.K. Roberts
1988   The effect of zinc supplements on lipoproteins and copper status. Atherosclerosis 70:247-252.

Singh, A., B.L. Smoak, K.Y. Patterson, L.G. LeMay, C. Veillon, and P.A. Deuster
1991   Biochemical indices of selected trace minerals in men: Effect of stress. Am. J. Clin. Nutr. 53:126-131.

Snyder, A.C., L.L. Dvorak, and J.B. Roepke
1989   Influence of dietary iron source on measures of iron status among female runners. Med. Sci. Sports Exerc. 21:7-10.

Solomons, N.
1986   Competitive interaction of iron and zinc in the diet: Consequences for human nutrition. J. Nutr. 116:927-935.

Stendig-Lindberg, G., Y. Shapiro, Y. Epstein, E. Galun, E. Schonberger, E. Graff, and W.E.C. Wacker
1987   Changes in serum magnesium concentration after strenuous exercise. J. Am. Coll. Nutr. 6:35-40.

Stendig-Lindberg, G., Y. Shapira, E. Graff, E. Schonberger, and W.E.C. Wacker
    1989   Delayed metabolic changes after strenuous exertion in trained young men. Magne-
            sium Res. 2:211-218.
Stevens, M.D., R.A. Disilvestro, and E.P. Harris
    1984   Specific receptor for ceruloplasmin in membrane fragments for aortic and heart
            tissue. Biochemistry 23:261-266.
Stewart, G.A., J.E. Steel, A.H. Toyme, and M.J. Stewart
    1972   Observations on the haematology and the iron and protein intake of Australian
            Olympic athletes. Med. J. Austr. 2:1339-1343.
Stewart, J.G., D.A. Ahlquist, D.B. McGill, D.M. Ilstrup, S. Schwartz, and R.A. Owen
    1984   Gastrointestinal blood loss and anemia in runners. Ann. Intern. Med. 100:843-845.
Sugawara, N., C. Sugawara, N. Maehara, T. Sadamato, I. Harabuchi, and K. Yamamura
    1983   Effect of acute stresses on Zn-thionein production in rat liver. Eur. J. Appl. Physiol.
            51:365-370.
Taylor, C., G. Rogers, C. Goodman, R.D. Baynes, T.H. Bothwell, W.R. Bezwoda, F. Kramer,
            and J. Hattingh
    1987   Hematologic, iron-related, and acute-phase protein responses to sustained strenu-
            ous exercise. J. Appl. Physiol 62:464-469.
Terjung, R.L., W.W. Winder, K.M. Baldwin, and J.O. Holloszy
    1973   Effect of exercise on the turnover of cytochrome C in skeletal muscle. J. Biol.
            Chem. 248:7404-7406.
Uhari, M., A. Pakarinen, J. Hietala, T. Nurmi, and K. Kouvalainen
    1983   Serum iron, copper, zinc, ferritin, and ceruloplasmin after intense heat exposure.
            Eur. J. Appl. Physiol. 51:331-335.
Vallerand, A.L., J.-P. Cuerrier, D. Shapcott, R.J. Vallerand, and P.F. Gardiner
    1984   Influence of exercise training on tissue chromium concentrations in the rat. Am. J.
            Clin. Nutr. 39:402-409.
Van Rij, A.M., M.T. Hall, G.L. Dohm, J. Bray, and W.J. Pories
    1986   Changes in zinc metabolism following exercise in human subjects. Biol. Trace
            Element Res. 10:99-106.
Whanger, P.D., and S.H. Oh
    1978   Nutritional and environmental factors affecting metallothionein levels. Experientia
            (Suppl.) 34:281-291.
Yoshimura, H.
    1970   Anemia during physical training (sports anemia). Nutr. Rev. 28:251-253.

DISCUSSION

DR. NESHEIM: Thank you. We will have a few questions before we break for lunch.

PARTICIPANT: Could you elaborate some more on the magnesium uptake by lymphocytes? You mentioned in passing that there could be an increase in uptake by lymphocytes?

DR. KEEN: Yes, this has been suggested by Franz (Franz et al., 1985). And the argument is, although there is no hard data to support it, that for lipolysis, you will have an increase in a lymphocyte magnesium uptake.

While the current data for this idea are not very strong, it is in the literature that it should be considered a possibility.

An exercise-induced erythrocyte uptake of magnesium, has also been argued based on the idea that it is needed for 2,3-diphosphoglycerate synthesis (Lukaski et al., 1983).

However, we have done a study (Lowney et al., 1990) where we looked at the influence of magnesium deficiency on erythrocyte 2,3-diphosphoglycerate production, and it had no influence on 2,3-diphosphoglycerate levels.

PARTICIPANT: How about the endurance study with magnesium deficiency in the animal. Why didn't that continue to go on down as you have a more severe deficiency. Here is a plateau in fact.

DR. KEEN: Yes, it is a plateau. Unfortunately, you can't get animals much more deficient and get meaningful data. We were curious if we could get a dose response using animals fed diets containing less than 50 µg of magnesium per gram, however once pronounced signs of magnesium deficiency occurred, it was difficult to get the males to run.

DR. NESHEIM: Thank you, Carl. That was very interesting and challenging and indeed reports some of the work that needs to be done.

8

The Effect of Exercise and Heat on Vitamin Requirements

Priscilla M. Clarkson[1]

INTRODUCTION

Vitamins are essential nutrients that have a wide variety of functions. The fact that many vitamins play a critical role in energy production has captured the attention of those interested in ways to optimize exercise or work performance. Moreover, increased energy production during exercise could lead to an increased vitamin requirement for those individuals who participate in rigorous physical training.

Because vitamins are essential, generally cannot be manufactured by the body, and must be ingested on a regular basis, it has been tempting to suggest that if a little is good, more is better. This reasoning was perhaps the impetus for many studies that have assessed the effects of vitamin supplementation on physical performance (Robinson and Robinson, 1954). A review of early studies suggested that vitamins were lost to a significant degree in sweat (Robinson and Robinson, 1954). For this reason, exercise—especially in hot environments—was considered to result in vitamin deficiencies. Now it is generally agreed that the vitamin loss in sweat is negligible (Brotherhood, 1984; Mitchell and Edman, 1951; Robinson and Robinson, 1954) (Table 8-1). However, some vitamins have been implicated to have beneficial effects for those individuals living and working in a hot environment.

[1] Priscilla M. Clarkson, Department of Exercise Science, Boyden Building, University of Massachusetts at Amherst, Amherst, MA 01003

TABLE 8-1 Concentration of Vitamins Lost in Sweat

Vitamin	Concentration (µg per 100 ml)
Thiamin	0-15
Riboflavin	0.5-12
Nicotinic acid (total)	8-14
Pantothenic acid	4-30
Ascorbic acid	0-50
Pyridoxine	7
Folic acid (plus metabolites)	0.26

SOURCE: Mitchell and Edman (1951). Data based on ranges reported from several studies completed in the 1940s.

This chapter addresses whether those individuals who expend greater amounts of energy in exercise training or work require greater amounts of vitamins and whether vitamin supplementation will enhance exercise performance. Some of this information has also been covered in a previous paper (Clarkson, 1991). This chapter also examines whether exercise in a hot environment will lead to an increased requirement for certain vitamins and whether vitamin supplements will reduce heat stress.

Vitamins are classified as either water soluble or fat soluble. Water-soluble vitamins are the B complex vitamins and vitamin C. These are stored in relatively small amounts in the body and cannot be retained for long periods. If blood levels of water-soluble vitamins exceed renal threshold, they are excreted into the urine. Most water-soluble vitamins serve major functions of either energy production or hematopoiesis. With the exception of vitamin K, fat-soluble vitamins are stored in greater amounts than the water-soluble vitamins. Fat-soluble vitamins are absorbed and transported in the body in close association with lipids and have roles that are largely independent of energy production.

WATER-SOLUBLE VITAMINS

Vitamin B complex consists of eight vitamins: vitamin B_1 (thiamin), vitamin B_2 (riboflavin), niacin, vitamin B_6 (pyridoxine), vitamin B_{12} (cyanocobalamin), biotin, folic acid, and pantothenic acid. The quantity stored differs among the vitamins. For example, if an individual's diet is deficient in most of the B vitamins, clinical symptoms can sometimes occur in 3 to 7 days (Guyton, 1986). Vitamin B_{12} is an exception because it can be stored in the liver for a year or longer. The B vitamins, except B_{12} and folic acid, primarily serve as coenzymes in the metabolism of glucose and fatty acids. Vitamin C serves many diverse functions in the body. A vitamin C-deficient diet can cause deficiency symptoms after a few weeks and can cause death from scurvy in 5 to 7 months (Guyton, 1986).

In the following discussion, these topics will be addressed for each vitamin: its function, how an individual's status is determined, changes in status by chronic exercise, effects of restriction or supplementation on performance, and relationship to heat stress.

Thiamin

The importance of thiamin ingestion was noted in the late nineteenth century when it was found that adding meat and whole grain to sailors' diets aboard ship prevented the condition known as beriberi (Brown, 1990). Thiamin is absorbed from the small intestine, and some is phosphorylated to form pyrophosphate (the coenzyme form). Pyrophosphate and free thiamin are transported via the blood to tissues, with the highest concentrations occurring in the liver, kidney, and heart. Most thiamin is stored in the pyrophosphate form.

Thiamin plays a role in carbohydrate metabolism. It functions specifically as a coenzyme in the conversion of pyruvate to acetyl coenzyme A (CoA) and alpha-ketoglutarate to succinyl CoA, as well as the transketolase reaction of the pentose phosphate pathway.

A sensitive technique for assessing thiamin status is the use of an erythrocyte enzyme stimulation test performed on blood samples. Erythrocyte transketolase activity is assessed before and after addition of thiamin pyrophosphate (TPP). If a deficiency of TPP exists, then adding TPP to the blood will increase the activity of the enzyme. The level of erythrocyte TPP is also used to determine thiamin status. Sauberlich et al. (1979) reported that urinary excretion of thiamin was a reasonably reliable indicator of thiamin nutritional status, although its use has been questioned (Gubler, 1984).

Whether physical exercise, because of the greater metabolic challenge, will increase the need for thiamin has not been fully established. The few studies that have assessed possible biochemical deficiencies of athletes have reported minimal evidence of thiamin deficiency compared with controls (Cohen et al., 1985; Guilland et al.,1989; Weight et al., 1988). Nijakowski (1966) found that blood levels of thiamin were lower in male athletes compared with a control group, however, it is possible that the lower levels were due to plasma volume expansion in athletes. Athletes were also tested after a 12-km skiing expedition, and thiamin levels showed a further decrease, which Nijakowski (1966) suggested was due to increased bodily requirements.

The National Research Council (1989) recommended that thiamin intake be proportional to caloric intake such that 0.5 mg per 1000 kcal is required. Because of the increased energy demands of exercise, athletes ingest more food. However, many athletes are ingesting a greater proportion of carbohydrates, and it has been shown that some athletes have a high intake of refined carbohydrates with low vitamin content (Brouns and Saris 1989). Furthermore, carbohydrate loading regimens can result in low thiamin intakes. In the 1979 Tour de France, thiamin intakes were found to be too low (0.26 mg per 1000 kcal), which was attributed to the high carbohydrate meals. Van Erp-Baart et al. (1989) also pointed out that when energy intake is high, the amount of refined carbohydrate is high, and the nutrient density of thiamin drops.

Because of the role of thiamin in energy metabolism, it would seem that thiamin deficiency would lead to decrements in exercise performance. However, although thiamin-deficient diets along with deficiencies in other B complex vitamins were shown to adversely affect performance (for review see Van der Beek, 1985), there is some controversy concerning whether thiamin deficiency alone will alter performance (Williams, 1976, 1989). Wood et al. (1980) in a well-controlled study found that performance was not affected by induced thiamin deficiency. They reported no significant difference in time to exhaustion during a cycle ergometry test between subjects who ingested a low-thiamin diet (500 µg thiamin) for 4 to 5 weeks along with a placebo (without thiamin) and subjects who had ingested the same low-thiamin diet along with a thiamin supplement (5 mg thiamin).

Few studies have assessed the effect of thiamin supplementation on exercise performance (see Keith, 1989). In two controlled studies, the effects of thiamin supplements of 5 mg per day for 1 week on an arm endurance task (Karpovich and Millman, 1942) and 0.1 mg daily for 10 to 12 weeks on grip strength and treadmill tests (aerobic and anaerobic work) (Keys et al., 1943) were examined. Both studies found that the supplement had no effect on any measure of work performance.

Mills (1941) studied the effects of heat stress on young rats and found that optimal thiamin intake for growth was increased at high temperature (91°F), although these results were not confirmed by later studies (Edison et al., 1945). Based on his own findings, however, Mills (1941) suggested that thiamin supplements should make workers in boiler or furnace rooms or in other types of heat exposure more resistant to heat effects. Other studies found that an increase in environmental temperature resulted in a decreased thiamin requirement (Edison et al., 1945), and this decrease reflected the decrease in caloric requirements at elevated temperatures. However, the animals in that study were not exercising. It has been shown that exercise in the heat is more metabolically costly perhaps because of the extra energy costs of sweating, circulation, and respiratory mechanisms (Nielsen et al., 1990). If increased caloric intake is needed for those working in a hot environment, then thiamin intake should be increased proportionally.

Thiamin loss in sweat is considered to be around 10 µg per 100 ml (Table 8-1). Working in a hot environment can produce sweat losses of up to 10 liters per day. At this value, the amount of thiamin lost would be about 1.0 mg. Although a well-balanced diet could probably satisfy this need, there should be some concern if the diet is poor or if the thiamin requirement is not increased with an increase in energy intake (to meet the demands of work).

Riboflavin

The coenzyme forms of riboflavin are flavin mononucleotide (FMN) and flavin adenine dinucleotide (FAD). These coenzymes function in cellular oxidation, specifically acting as hydrogen carriers in the mitochondrial electron transport system. Deficiencies in riboflavin are common in many Third World countries and occur invariably with deficiencies in the other water-soluble vitamins (McCormick, 1990).

Riboflavin status can be assessed reliably from blood samples. A sensitive indicator is the measurement of erythrocyte glutathione reductase (EGR) activity (Cooperman and Lopez, 1984). When riboflavin stores are low, EGR loses its saturation with FAD, and its activity drops (Cooperman and Lopez, 1984).

Whether chronic exercise alters riboflavin status is not certain. For the general U.S. population and most athlete groups studied, biochemical deficiencies of riboflavin are rare (Cohen et al., 1985; Guilland et al., 1989; Tremblay et al., 1984). However, one study found inadequate riboflavin status in 8 out of 18 athletes studied (Haralambie, 1976). It has been suggested that exercise training may increase the need for riboflavin. Belko et al. (1983) found that the need for riboflavin in healthy young women (based on an estimation of riboflavin intake required to achieve normal biochemical status) increased when they participated in jogging exercise for 20 to 50 minutes a day. Because biochemical deficiencies in athletes are rare, the increased need for riboflavin probably would be easily met by diet.

Because of the importance of riboflavin to oxidative energy production, performance could be impaired by a riboflavin deficiency. Keys et al. (1944) placed six male students on a riboflavin-restricted diet (99 mg per day or 0.31 mg per 1000 kcal) for 84 days ($n = 3$) and 152 days ($n = 3$). Subjects performed an aerobic walking test (60 minutes) and an anaerobic test (60 seconds) on the treadmill and performed grip strength tests before, every 2 weeks during, and after the restricted-diet period. The low-riboflavin diet did not adversely alter the performance measures. Van der Beek (1985) reviewed other studies on riboflavin restriction and concluded that riboflavin depletion did not alter work performance on submaximal treadmill tests.

Because studies have shown that riboflavin deficiency does not alter exercise performance, it would seem that supplementation should not enhance performance. Belko et al. (1983) studied the effects of riboflavin supplementation in two groups of overweight women who participated in a 12-week exercise program. One group ingested a total of 0.96 mg per 1000 kcal riboflavin per day, and the other group ingested 1.16 mg per 1000 kcal per day. The improvement in aerobic capacity did not differ between groups. Also no difference in exercise performance was found when elite swimmers were supplemented with 60 mg per day of riboflavin for 16 to 20 days (Tremblay et al., 1984).

Tucker et al. (1960) studied the effects of exercise and heat stress on riboflavin excretion into the urine. In one experiment, men walked on a treadmill for 4 to 6 hours per day for six days with the temperature of the heat chamber at 49°C. The men spent a total of 10 hours per day at this temperature. Riboflavin excretion increased gradually over the course of the six days. The authors concluded that there could be a decreased requirement of riboflavin at high temperatures.

The limited data available suggest that the riboflavin requirement may be increased by exercise. However, these needs must be easily met by athletes' diets because athletes have not been shown to have a riboflavin deficiency. The one study concerning exercise and heat stress suggests that there could be a decrease in riboflavin requirement. Further study is needed to confirm this. The amount of riboflavin lost in sweat is small (Table 8-1) and should not be a problem for those working in a hot environment and profusely sweating. The recommended intake of riboflavin is linked to caloric intake (0.6 mg per 1000 kcal), and to be safe, this recommendation should be followed by people living and working in a hot environment.

Niacin

Niacin is the term used to describe nicotinic acid (niacin) and nicotinamide (niacinamide). In the body, niacin is an essential component of two coenzymes: nicotinamide adenine dinucleotide (NAD) and nicotinamide adenine dinucleotide phosphate (NADP). These coenzymes serve as electron carriers or hydrogen donors/acceptors in glycolysis, fatty acid oxidation, and the electron transport system. Severe niacin deficiency results in the condition known as pellagra (raw skin), which was common in the United States in the early 1900s but has virtually disappeared from industrialized countries (Swendseid and Swendseid, 1990).

Two available studies of niacin nutriture of athletes suggest that athletes are not deficient in niacin (Cohen et al., 1985; Weight et al., 1988). These studies used nicotinic acid or niacin levels in the blood to determine status—a questionable assessment technique because niacin and niacin metabolites in the plasma are quite low (Hankes, 1984; Swendseid and Swendseid,

1990). Erythrocyte NAD concentration or levels of 2-pyridone may be more sensitive indicators of niacin depletion (Swendseid and Swendseid, 1990).

Some evidence suggests that exercise may increase the niacin requirement (Keith, 1989). Because most adult athletes have shown no evidence of niacin deficiency, the increased requirement probably is satisfied by the athlete's diet. Chronic ingestion of niacin above the recommended dietary allowance (RDA) (National Research Council, 1989) is not recommended, because large doses are often associated with undesirable side effects, such as flushing, liver damage, increased serum uric acid levels, skin problems, and elevated plasma glucose levels (Hunt and Groff, 1990). Niacinamide in large doses is not harmful. Acute ingestion of nicotinic acid (3 to 9 g per day) has also been shown to prevent the release of fatty acids (Keith, 1989; National Research Council, 1989), which may adversely affect endurance performance.

In a double-blind placebo-controlled experiment, Hilsendager and Karpovich (1964) found that 75 mg of niacin had no effect on arm or leg endurance capacity. Bergstrom et al. (1969) compared the perception of a work load before and after subjects were given niacin, 1 g intravenously and 0.6 g perorally. After the supplementation, the subjects perceived the work load to be heavier. Niacin can decrease free fatty acid mobilization (Carlson and Oro, 1962; Williams, 1989), which may explain the negative effects of the niacin supplement. A decrease in free fatty acid mobilization would force the muscle to rely more on its muscle glycogen stores. In fact, Bergstrom et al. (1969) found that muscle glycogen content was lower in postexercise biopsy samples taken from subjects who had received the niacin supplements than with control subjects.

The only information with regard to niacin requirements in a hot environment comes from an early study that found that nicotinic acid was lost in the sweat in significant amounts (100 µg per 100 ml; Mickelsen and Keys, 1943). However, later studies did not agree with this finding (Mitchell and Edman, 1951; Robinson and Robinson, 1954). Nicotinic acid is considered to be lost in concentrations of 20 µg or less per 100 ml of sweat (Mitchell and Edman, 1951). As with thiamin and riboflavin, niacin intake should be proportional to energy intake (6.6 mg niacin per 1000 kcal). If energy intake is increased to meet the demands of exercise or work in a hot environment, then niacin should be increased as well.

Vitamin B$_6$ (Pyridoxine)

Vitamin B$_6$ is composed of three natural compounds—pyridoxine, pyridoxamine, and pyridoxal (Merrill and Burnham, 1990)—that function in protein and amino acid metabolism; in gluconeogenesis; and in formation of hemoglobin, myoglobin, and cytochromes. The coenzyme form of B$_6$ is pyridoxal 5'-phosphate (PLP) and is used by over 60 enzymes. Glycogen phosphorylase, an enzyme involved in the breakdown of muscle glycogen, requires PLP as a coenzyme. Moreover, glycogen phosphorylase may serve as a reservoir for vitamin B_6 storage (Merrill and Burnham, 1990) and release PLP into the circulation for use by other tissues.

Vitamin B_6 status in blood samples can be assessed in several ways (Driskell, 1984). The method of choice is to assess levels of PLP, the most active form of vitamin B_6 (Driskell, 1984). Chronic exercise does not appear to result in a vitamin B_6 deficiency. Although biochemical deficiencies for vitamin B_6 were found in 17 to 35 percent of male college athletes, similar percentages were found for the control group (Guilland et al., 1989). However, the athletes had a greater intake of vitamin B_6 compared with the control subjects. Adequate vitamin B_6 levels were found from assessments of blood samples of other groups of athletes (Cohen et al., 1985; Weight et al., 1988).

Although it seems that vitamin B_6 status is not altered by chronic exercise, some studies have shown that acute exercise can alter the blood levels. Leklem and Shultz (1983) found that a 4500-m run substantially increased the blood levels of PLP in trained adolescent males. Hatcher et al. (1982) and Manore and Leklem (1988) reported an increase in blood levels of PLP after a 50-minute and after a 20-minute cycling exercise. PLP levels returned to baseline values after only 30 minutes rest (Manore and Leklem, 1988). It was suggested (Leklem and Shultz, 1983; Manore and Leklem, 1988) that PLP may be released from muscle glycogen phosphorylase during exercise so that PLP could be used as a cofactor for gluconeogenesis elsewhere in the body.

Hofmann et al. (1991) also found that prolonged treadmill running (2 hours at 60 to 65 percent of $V_{O_2 \, max}$) resulted in significant increases in blood levels of PLP that were independent of changes in plasma volume, blood glucose, blood free fatty acid levels, and blood enzyme levels. The authors suggested that the increase in plasma PLP could be due to a release of vitamin B_6 from the liver to be used in skeletal muscle to fully saturate glycogen phosphorylase or be used for other critical PLP-dependent reactions (for example, aminotransaminase reactions).

Another study found that 4-pyridoxic acid excretion in urine was significantly lower in trained athletes compared with controls after a vitamin B_6 challenge (Dreon and Butterfield, 1986). The authors suggested that these results reflect a greater storage capacity in athletes so that 4-pyridoxic acid could be available for redistribution with increased need.

Supplementation with vitamin B_6 does not appear to enhance performance. Lawrence et al. (1975a) examined swimming performance of trained swimmers who ingested 51 mg of pyridoxine hydrochloride or a placebo daily for 6 months. No significant difference was found between the groups on 100-yard swimming times.

Because vitamin B_6 is an integral part of the glycogen phosphorylase enzyme, several studies have examined the relationship between carbohydrate intake and vitamin B_6. Hatcher et al. (1982) found that blood levels of PLP and vitamin B_6 after exercise were lower in subjects who had consumed a low-carbohydrate diet compared with a moderate- or high-carbohydrate diet 3 days before the exercise. The authors suggested that on the low-carbohydrate diet gluconeogenesis is accelerated, which increases the need for PLP as a cofactor. In another study from the same laboratory, deVos et al. (1982) reported that vitamin B_6 supplementation may cause a faster depletion of muscle glycogen stores during exercise after ingestion of a low-carbohydrate diet and may accentuate a depletion-loading manipulation used by athletes to increase glycogen stores (glycogen supercompensation). Manore and Leklem (1988) found that vitamin B_6 supplementation, along with increased carbohydrate consumption, resulted in lower free fatty acids during exercise. The authors recommended that athletes who are on a high-carbohydrate diet should not supplement their diets with vitamin B_6 above the RDA level.

Presently there are no data regarding vitamin B_6 requirements in a hot environment. The amount of vitamin B_6 lost in sweat is considered insignificant (Mitchell and Edman, 1951). However, if food intake is increased, then the amount of vitamin B_6 should be increased accordingly. It is recommended that 0.016 mg per g protein of vitamin B_6 be ingested (vitamin B_6 and protein occur together naturally in foods) (National Research Council, 1989).

Pantothenic Acid

Pantothenic acid acts as a structural component of coenzyme A (CoA), an acyl carrier protein. Pantothenic acid is important in transport of acyl groups to the Krebs cycle and in transport of fatty acyl groups across the mitochondrial membrane (Olson, 1990). Pantothenic acid is widely distributed in nature and found in all organisms. Therefore deficiencies are rare. However, during World War II, pantothenic acid deficiency was thought to be responsible for the burning foot syndrome among prisoners in Japan and the Philippines (Fox, 1984).

It is not known whether exercise increases the requirement for pantothenic acid. Nijakowski (1966) found that athletes had higher levels of pantothenic acid in the blood compared to controls. Cycle ergometry exercise of short duration resulted in a decrease in pantothenic acid levels in the blood, but the levels were unchanged after a long-duration exercise of 4 hours. Because plasma volume was not corrected for, it is difficult to interpret these changes.

The effect of pantothenic acid supplementation on exercise performance is equivocal. Compared with the placebo group, highly trained endurance runners who ingested 2-g doses of pantothenic acid per day for 2 weeks showed decreased exercise blood lactate levels and decreased oxygen consumption during prolonged exercise at 75 percent $V_{O_2 max}$ (Litoff et al., 1985). In contrast, Nice et al. (1984), using a controlled double-blind study, examined the effect of pantothenic acid supplementation (1 g per day for 2 weeks) or a placebo on run time to exhaustion in 18 highly trained distance runners. No significant differences were found between groups in run time or any of the standard blood parameters that were assessed (that is, cortisol, glucose, creatine phosphokinase, electrolytes).

There are no data to suggest that the need for pantothenic acid would be increased by living and working in a hot environment. Pantothenic acid is not lost to a significant degree in sweat (Mitchell and Edman, 1951).

Vitamin B_{12} (Cyanocobalamin)

Vitamin B_{12} plays a role in the formation and function of red blood cells (Ellenbogen, 1984) and may also function in protein, fat, and carbohydrate metabolism (Van der Beek, 1985). The condition of pernicious anemia was first described in 1924, and in 1929 a factor in liver was found to act as an antipernicious factor. It was not until 1948 that vitamin B_{12} was isolated and used to treat pernicious anemia (Ellenbogen, 1984).

No information is available on vitamin B_{12} status in athletes. However, it should be noted that athletes who are complete vegetarians may acquire a vitamin B_{12} deficiency because vitamin B_{12} is found mainly in animal products. Red cell vitamin B_{12} levels can indicate vitamin B_{12} status; however, low levels may also indicate a folate deficiency (Herbert, 1990). Several other tests are available to discern the two deficiencies; these are detailed elsewhere (Herbert, 1990).

Existing evidence suggests that vitamin B_{12} supplementation has no effect on performance (Williams, 1976). Montoye et al. (1955), in a double-blind study, placed 51 adolescent boys (ages 12 to 17) into either an experimental group that consumed 50 μg of vitamin B_{12} daily, a placebo group, or a control group. No significant difference was found after 7 weeks between the supplemented group or the placebo group in the time to run 0.5 mile or in the Harvard step-test score (Montoye et al., 1955). Tin-May-Than et al. (1978) studied performance capacity in 36 healthy male subjects before and after injection of 1 mg cyanocobalamin given 3 times a week for 6 weeks. They found no significant improvement in $V_{O_2 max}$, grip strength, pull-ups, leg lifts, or standing broad jump performance.

There is no information concerning the effects of heat stress on vitamin B_{12} status. Recent studies have shown that megadoses of vitamin C (500 mg) may detrimentally affect the availability of vitamin B_{12} from food (Herbert, 1990). Doses of vitamin C of 3 g per day may even result in vitamin B_{12} deficiency disease. How this occurs is still unclear, but Herbert (1990) states that nutritionists should advise persons taking megadoses of vitamin C to have their blood checked regularly for vitamin B_{12} status. These findings should be taken into account with regard to the use of vitamin C to reduce heat stress (see section on vitamin C).

Folic Acid (Folate) and Biotin

Folic acid (pteroylglutamic acid) and folate (pteroylglutamate) are involved with DNA synthesis and nucleotide and amino acid metabolism, and they are especially important in tissues undergoing rapid turnover, such as red blood cells. Folic acid deficiency has been suggested to be the most common vitamin deficiency in humans and can result in anemia (Keith, 1989). No studies have assessed the relationship of folic acid status and exercise performance or the effect of folic acid supplementation on performance.

Biotin acts as a coenzyme for several carboxylase enzymes that are important in supplying intermediates for the Krebs cycle and for amino acid metabolism. It is also important in fatty acid and glycogen synthesis. Biotin deficiencies are rare in individuals consuming a nutritionally sound diet. One study found no difference in blood biotin levels in athletes compared with controls (Nijakowski, 1966). No studies have examined the effect of biotin supplementation on performance.

B Complex Vitamins

Many studies have shown that a deficiency of more than one of the B complex vitamins could lead to a decrease in physical performance capacity (for detailed reviews, see Van der Beek, 1985; Williams, 1989). Deficiency of a combination of several B vitamins produced subjective symptoms of fatigue, loss of ambition, irritability, and pain and loss of efficiency during normal work (see Van der Beek, 1985). Most of the studies that evaluated the effects of depletion of several B vitamins were done in the 1940s. More recently, Van der Beek et al. (1988) placed 12 men on a thiamin-, riboflavin-, vitamin C-, and vitamin B_6-poor diet for 8 weeks. After 8 weeks, this diet caused borderline or moderately deficient blood levels of the four vitamins. These deficiencies were associated with a 9.8 percent decrease in $V_{O_2 \, max}$ and a 19.6 percent decrease in anaerobic threshold. Thus, a restricted diet of 21.3 to 32.5 percent of the Dutch RDA of these B vitamins and vitamin C led to decreased endurance capacity within a few weeks. This decrease was most probably due to the deficiency in the B vitamins rather than vitamin C (see section on vitamin C).

Because deficiencies of several B vitamins will lead to performance decrements, it is reasonable to assume that supplementation with a combination of B vitamins would enhance performance. Several studies have evaluated the effects of vitamin B complex supplementation (an excellent and detailed review can be found in Williams, 1989). Using a controlled, crossover design, Keys and Henschel (1941) examined the effect of supplementation with 100 mg nicotinic acid amide, 5 mg thiamin chloride, and 100 mg ascorbic acid daily for 4 weeks. Subjects were eight infantry men, and the exercise test was a 15-minute submaximal treadmill test (marching) where the subjects carried a pack and rifle. Compared with the placebo, the supplementation did not result in improved physiological parameters during exercise. In a follow-up study, Keys and Henschel (1942) examined the effects of a supplement containing 5 to 17 mg thiamin, 10 mg riboflavin, 100 mg nicotinic acid, 10 to 100 mg vitamin B_6, 20 mg calcium pantothenate, and 100 to 200 mg ascorbic acid for 4 to 6 weeks. Subjects were 26 soldiers, and the exercise test was a strenuous treadmill run. Like their first study, Keys and Henschel found no beneficial effects on performance, so that endurance and resistance to fatigue were unaltered.

The effect of B complex supplementation on endurance capacity during a treadmill test was examined in physically active male college students (Read and McGuffin, 1983). The supplement contained 5 mg thiamin, 5 mg riboflavin, 25 mg niacin, 2 mg pyridoxine, 0.5 μg vitamin B_{12}, and 12.5 mg pantothenic acid. After 6 weeks of supplementation, there was no significant improvement in endurance capacity.

Early and Carlson (1969) suggested that vitamin B complex supplementation could enhance exercise in the heat because these water-soluble vitamins may be lost via sweating. They studied the effect of one dose of a vitamin B supplement, which contained 100 mg thiamin, 8 mg riboflavin, 100 mg niacinamide, 5 mg pyridoxine, 25 mg cobalamin, and 30 mg pantothenic acid. High school males were given either the supplement or a placebo 30 minutes before running 10 50-yard dashes during hot weather. The running times were recorded for each trial. The group that received the supplement showed less fatigue (drop-off in running time) over the trials. These authors suggested that the amount of supplement and the combination of ingredients may be important for a supplement to be effective. They stated that the lower dosages of vitamins used in previous studies may not have been adequate to fulfill the additional vitamin requirement because of sweat loss and heightened metabolic activity with exercise in the heat.

Henschel et al. (1944a) examined the effects of a supplement containing 200 mg ascorbic acid or 0.5 mg thiamin, 10 mg riboflavin, and 100 mg nicotinamide ingested for 3 days prior to exposure to heat for 2 to 4 days. During the heat exposure, the temperature was 110° to 120°F in the day and 85° to 90°F at night. The vitamin supplementation had no effect on sweat composition, water balance, strength tests, or exercise performance and recovery. Thus, the vitamin supplementation did not affect the rate and degree of acclimatization, the incidence of heat exhaustion, and the ability to perform work in the hot environment (Mayer and Bullen, 1960).

Although studies are equivocal with regard to whether supplementation of several of the B complex vitamins will enhance performance in a hot environment, these studies mainly assessed the effects of a short period of supplementation and a short exposure to exercise in the heat. Because exercise in the heat may increase energy expenditure (Consolazio, 1963), it is possible that a deficiency in B complex vitamins could occur if the dietary intake is not increased accordingly. This is especially true because of the loss of several of the B complex vitamins in sweat. Although the loss is small, if the intake of these vitamins is also compromised, a deficiency could occur. If caloric intake should be increased by work in a hot environment, then the intake of these vitamins would increase accordingly. Thus, for adults, 0.5 mg thiamin per 1000-kcal diet, 0.6 mg riboflavin per 1000-kcal diet, 0.016 mg vitamin B_6 per g protein, and 6.6 mg niacin per 1000-kcal diet are recommended (National Research Council, 1989).

Vitamin C (Ascorbic Acid)

Scurvy was identified as far back as the ancient Greeks and Romans. This condition proved to be a scourge to armies, navies, and explorers until the early 1900s when Albert Szent-Gyorgyi first identified a substance that was later named vitamin C and used to prevent scurvy (Sauberlich, 1990). Vitamin C has numerous functions, including the biosynthesis of collagen, catecholamines, serotonin, and carnitine. It also plays a role as an antioxidant and is needed for nonheme iron absorption, transport, and storage (Keith, 1989).

Vitamin C is probably one of the most studied vitamins and one of the most controversial. The popularly believed benefits of vitamin C supplementation range from curing or preventing the common cold to reducing fatigue, wound healing, preventing injury, and enhancing performance capacity (Jaffe, 1984; Keith, 1989; National Research Council, 1989; Pike and Brown, 1984). Vitamin C is widely distributed throughout the body with highest concentrations in the pituitary, adrenals, and leukocytes. Major concentrations also are found in skeletal muscle, brain, and liver.

Ascorbic acid can be measured in the serum or plasma, leukocytes, and urine; however, levels in the plasma or serum are most commonly used (Sauberlich, 1990). Of several groups of athletes studied, most had adequate or above adequate blood levels of vitamin C (for review see Clarkson, 1991). These data provide no evidence to suggest that chronic exercise creates a vitamin C deficiency.

Acute exercise appears to increase blood levels of ascorbic acid. Plasma and lymphocyte ascorbic acid levels increased in nine men who completed a 21-km race (Gleeson et al., 1987). This study also found that the increase in plasma ascorbic acid levels correlated significantly with an increase in plasma cortisol. The authors suggested that exercise may cause ascorbic acid to be released from the adrenal glands into the circulation along with the release of cortisol. Normally, vitamin C inhibits adrenocorticotropic hormone synthesis (Strydom et al., 1976). If chronic stress increases the release of vitamin C from the adrenals, an abnormal release of adrenocorticotropic hormones could occur followed by a "fatigue" of the adrenal glands. At this point the adrenals could not function adequately in another stress situation (Strydom et al., 1976).

Van der Beek et al. (1990) assessed the effect of vitamin C restriction on physical performance in 12 healthy men. The subjects ingested a diet providing only 10 mg per day of vitamin C for 3 weeks and 25 mg per day for 4 weeks. During this time, vitamin C levels in the blood decreased significantly. However, no effect of the vitamin C restriction was found on $\dot{V}_{O_2 \text{ max}}$ or the onset of blood lactate accumulation. The marginal vitamin C deficiency did not alter exercise performance.

Excellent and comprehensive reviews of studies concerning the effects of ascorbic acid supplementation on performance can be found elsewhere (Keith, 1989; Williams, 1989). Keith (1989) cited 19 studies, many from outside the United States, that have shown a positive effect, and 18 that have shown no effect, of vitamin C supplementation on performance. Although several studies have shown that vitamin C supplementation will enhance performance (for example, Howald et al., 1975), these studies are flawed by poor designs, or the subjects may have been deficient in vitamin C. There are equally as many studies, and often better controlled ones, to demonstrate that vitamin C supplementation has no effect (for example, Keith and Merrill, 1983; Keren and Epstein, 1980).

Smokers have been shown to have a greater requirement for vitamin C, and the RDA for smokers is set at a minimum of 100 mg of vitamin C per day (compared with 60 mg per day for nonsmokers) (National Research Council, 1989). Keith and Driskell (1982) examined whether vitamin C supplementation of 300 mg per day for 3 weeks improved measures of lung function, resting and exercise heart rate, resting and exercise blood pressure, and the amount of work performed during a treadmill test in chronic smokers and nonsmokers. They concluded that vitamin C supplementation had little effect on lung function and exercise performance in either smokers or nonsmokers.

One study examined the effect of vitamin C supplementation on injury rate as well as on performance. Gey et al. (1970) placed 286 U.S. Air Force officers into two groups: officers in one group received 1000 mg vitamin C and officers in the other received a placebo daily for 12 weeks during moderate training. After 12 weeks, the groups showed no differences in improvement of performance on the Cooper 12-minute walk-run test (Gey et al., 1970). Also, the group taking vitamin C supplements had no reduction in injury rate compared with the group without supplementation.

Vitamin C also acts as an antioxidant to protect cells from free radical damage (see vitamin E section) (Machlin and Bendich, 1987). Because muscle soreness after exercise may result from muscle tissue damage (Ebbeling and Clarkson, 1989), it could be hypothesized that vitamin C supplementation may affect the development of soreness. Staton (1952) examined whether vitamin supplementation of 100 mg per day for 30 days would affect the performance of sit-ups on the second day of performance of the sit-ups (assuming that subjects were sore from the first day of sit-ups). The number of fewer repetitions the subjects were able to perform on the second day was taken to indicate the amount of soreness experienced. Vitamin C did not affect the number of sit-ups that could be performed, and Staton (1952) concluded that vitamin C had no effect on soreness. Whether the criterion score reflected an individual's soreness is uncertain. Also, because the exercise used in this study may not have produced significant muscle damage, especially with regard to the generation of free radicals, further study of the relationship of vitamin C and exercise-induced muscle damage is warranted.

In 1942, Holmes reviewed the use of vitamin C during World War II. He stated that "under certain severe conditions soldiers may need dietary supplements of certain vitamins. This is especially true of vitamin C, ascorbic acid, of which the United States used 17 tons in 1940 and may soon reach an annual output (synthetic) of 100 tons." Although Holmes provides citations to support the loss of vitamin C in appreciable quantities in sweat, this claim has not been substantiated by other studies. For example, one study found that at a sweat secretion of 700 ml per hour or more, the loss in vitamin C would not exceed 3 mg per day (Mitchell and Edman, 1951). However, Holmes stated that "the function of the vitamin C may go beyond mere replacement of the amount lost. It may combat heat shock." He also suggested that vitamin C may play a role in the healing of fractures and other wounds.

An interesting letter (Poda, 1979) regarding vitamin C intake and heat stroke appeared in a medical journal in 1979 and is excerpted below:

> In 1951, a salesman with an Indiana-Illinois district sustained "heat stroke." Thereafter, if the temperature rose to more that 29.5°C he got "sick," very weak, and shocklike. He thus missed most of his summer saleswork, since air conditioned cars were not common then. On a hunch, from an old army

tale from World War II, I had him take 100 mg of vitamin C (ascorbic acid) three times daily during the summer months. Even though temperatures stayed at 32°C and higher (up to 40.6°C), he was able to drive his non-air-conditioned car and function. If he forgot to take his vitamin C, he got "sick."

In an early study, Henschel et al. (1944b) studied men who (a) were on a rigidly controlled vitamin C-restricted diet or on a vitamin C-supplemented (500 mg per day) diet for 4 to 7 days and who (b) were exercising in the heat for 2 hours per day for 4 days. The criterion measures were pulse rate at rest, pulse rate during exercise, and rectal temperature. No differences were found between the restricted and the supplemented conditions. Heat exhaustion occurred with equal frequency in each condition.

Strydom et al. (1976) reevaluated the Henschel et al. (1944b) study and noted that the authors had acknowledged that the vitamin C-supplemented condition showed a slight advantage with regard to rectal temperature. Furthermore, Henschel et al. (1944b) had studied only 4 days of heat stress, which may not have been sufficient to determine the effects of vitamin C supplementation. Therefore, Strydom et al. (1976) decided to further investigate whether vitamin C ingestion would affect the rate and degree of acclimatization to heat stress. In a study done in South Africa, they placed 60 mining recruits into three groups and administered a placebo, vitamin C (250 mg per day), or vitamin C (500 mg per day) for 10 days. During the supplementation period, the subjects were exposed to temperatures of 33.9°C for 4 hours per day while working at an intensity of 35 watts. Measurement of rectal temperature showed that vitamin C supplementation enhanced the rate and degree of acclimatization, with no difference between the two levels of supplementation. No effect of the supplement was found on sweat rates or heart rate response to the work. The initial blood levels of vitamin C for the three groups were 0.48 mg per 100 ml (placebo group), 0.60 mg per 100 ml (250-mg ascorbic acid group), and 0.43 mg per 100 ml (500-mg ascorbic acid group). These levels are considered adequate (Hunt and Groff, 1990), but at the low end of normal (Strydom et al., 1976).

In a subsequent study from the same laboratory (Kotze et al., 1977), a similar experiment was performed, but blood ascorbic acid levels were also assessed daily during the 10 days of heat stress. Resting blood ascorbic acid levels increased by the same amount in subjects receiving either the 250-mg or the 500-mg vitamin C supplement, and blood levels reached the saturation point between the third and the fifth day. The increase in blood ascorbic acid levels was associated with a reduction in rectal temperature and a reduction in total sweat output (which was independent of the reduction in rectal temperature). The maximum beneficial effect of the supplements in reducing rectal temperature occurred over the first 3 days of heat stress.

Thus, the supplements were more effective when heat stress was relatively high and blood levels of vitamin C had not reached the saturation point.

Although vitamin C status was adequate for the subjects in both of the studies cited above, the status was probably lower than in the normal healthy population, and the vitamin C supplementation raised blood levels of vitamin C to that found in healthy, well-fed individuals. However, blood levels of 0.43 to 0.60 mg per 100 ml may not be uncharacteristic of many lower socioeconomic groups, especially those who have poor diets, do not take supplements, and are smokers. In fact, Woteki et al. (1986) reported that in a 1976-1980 survey, about 5 percent of young adult American males were found to have blood vitamin C levels below 0.25 mg per 100 ml. Thus it could be expected that a sizable proportion of those individuals rapidly mobilized into military service may have suboptimal vitamin C status (between 0.43 and 0.60 mg per 100 ml).

Some data show that vitamin C status may be compromised by living and working in a hot environment for an extended period of time (see Scott, 1975). Visagie et al. (1974) found among mine workers in South Africa a high incidence of vitamin C deficiency during the first 3 months of employment. This deficiency occurred despite diets adequate in vitamin C.

Hindson (1970) examined vitamin C levels in the white blood cells of apparently healthy Europeans living in the tropics, a subject population consisting of British forces and their families living in Singapore. Anyone taking vitamin C supplements was excluded. Results showed a significant drop in vitamin C levels for the men but only a modest fall for the women. Although vitamin C is not lost in sweat to a significant degree in acclimatized individuals, vitamin C is needed in increased quantities for the process of sweating. Hindson (1970) concluded that vitamin C supplements should be taken by men who are working in the tropics. Also, vitamin C has been shown to be beneficial in treating prickly heat, a common disease of sweat glands for those living in the tropics (Hindson, 1970).

Recently, Chen et al. (1990) developed a sports drink especially for athletes training in hot environments. Made from *Actinidia sinensis* Planch (ASP; also known as kiwifruit), the drink contained several minerals and 48 mg per 100 ml vitamin C (Chen et al., 1990). During the summer of 1982, elite Chinese soccer and track athletes were tested at their training site. Environmental temperatures were 26.6° to 31.5°C. Athletes drank 500 to 1200 ml of ASP 10 minutes prior to a 1.5- to 2.7-hour normal training session and again halfway through the training session. On a separate occasion (training session), subjects drank an equivalent volume of a placebo drink. Vitamin C content in the athletes' urine averaged 132 mg per day when ingesting the ASP drink and 44 mg per day when ingesting the placebo. The authors concluded that vitamin C status of athletes ingesting the

ASP drink was improved. However, when the body's pool of vitamin C is greater than 1500 mg, the efficacy of kidney reabsorption decreases, and vitamin C is excreted into the urine (Hunt and Groff, 1990). Thus, increased vitamin C in the urine may simply indicate that the athletes had high levels of vitamin C already, and the excess "spilled over" into the urine.

FAT-SOLUBLE VITAMINS

Vitamins A, D, E, and K are fat-soluble vitamins, and these can be stored in appreciable amounts in the fat stores of the body. Because vitamin D is involved in calcium metabolism and vitamins A and E can function as antioxidants, these supplements may be important to exercise or work performance. Because no studies have been uncovered that examined the relationship of vitamin K (a vitamin necessary for blood clotting) with exercise performance or heat stress, this vitamin will not be discussed in the following sections.

Vitamin A

Night blindness was recognized by the ancient Egyptians and was treated by adding liver to the diet or by topically applying liver extract to the eyes (J. A. Olson, 1990). In 1914 the compound now known as vitamin A was found to prevent night blindness. Interestingly, the early Egyptian remedies had been lost over the years so that in the nineteenth century, night blindness plagued armies throughout the world (J. A. Olson, 1990).

Vitamin A designates a group of compounds including retinol, retinaldehyde, and retinoic acid. The body's need for vitamin A can be met by intake of preformed retinoids with vitamin A activity, which are generally found in animal products (National Research Council, 1989). Also, the need can be met by ingesting carotenoid precursors of vitamin A (beta-carotene, alpha-carotene, and cryptoxanthin) commonly found in plants (National Research Council, 1989). The primary function of vitamin A is for maintenance of vision. Vitamin A is also involved in the growth process and the body's immune response. Beta-carotene, the major carotenoid precursor of vitamin A, plays a role as an antioxidant.

Blood levels of vitamin A (retinol) provide a relatively good index of total body stores. When the liver stores of vitamin A are low, the plasma levels fall (Olson, 1984). The few studies that have examined vitamin A status of athletes found no deficiencies (Guilland et al., 1989; Weight et al., 1988). The absence of deficiencies is most probably due to the body's relatively large storage capacity for vitamin A.

Only one study has examined the effect of vitamin A supplementation on exercise performance. Five men were placed on a vitamin A-deficient diet (100 IU per day) for about 6 months followed by vitamin A supplementation (25,000 to 75,000 IU per day) for 6 weeks (Wald et al., 1942). No significant difference in run to exhaustion on a treadmill was found between the deficient and supplemented condition. Because the subjects had supplemented their diets with 75,000 IU for 30 days prior to the depletion phase of the experiment, the 6-month period of vitamin deficiency may not have been long enough to deplete the body's stores of vitamin A. However, it seems that vitamin A stores are generally adequate to meet the demands of exercise.

An antioxidant supplement containing 10 mg beta-carotene, 1000 mg vitamin C, and 800 IU of vitamin E was given to subjects before a downhill running exercise on a treadmill (Viguie et al., 1989). Although the details of the study are not available because this was a published abstract, it seems that the subjects performed the same exercise twice, the first time without the supplement and the second time with the supplement. Results showed that the supplement enhanced glutathione status (antioxidant status) and reduced indicators of exercise-induced muscle damage. However, other studies have shown that when the same damage-inducing exercise was repeated, the indices of damage were always reduced on the second bout regardless of any treatment (Clarkson and Tremblay, 1988). Further studies of the effects of beta-carotene as an antioxidant to reduce muscle damage from strenuous exercise are warranted. Presently there is no information on the effects of heat stress on vitamin A requirements.

Vitamin D

In the seventeenth century, rickets was scientifically described as resulting from a dietary deficiency (Norman, 1990). Later vitamin D was found to be synthesized by the body when skin was exposed to sunlight. The major function of vitamin D is its action as a hormone in the mineralization of bones and teeth (Keith, 1989). When the skin is exposed to ultraviolet radiation of the sun, a sterol (7-dehydrocholesterol) is converted into vitamin D (cholecalciferol). Eventually vitamin D is converted to its hormone forms, 25-hydroxycholecalciferol ($25(OH)D_3$) and 1,25-dihydroxycholecalciferol ($1,25(OH)_2D_3$), by the liver and kidney, respectively. Also, vitamin D is obtainable from a few food sources including fortified milk and milk products.

Biochemical status of vitamin D is generally assessed from measurement of $25(OH)D_3$ in the blood; however, blood levels do not fully reflect the extent of storage. Although few studies have examined biochemical status of vitamin D in athletes (Adams et al., 1982; Cohen et al., 1985), vitamin D deficiencies generally are believed to be rare for those individuals with adequate milk consumption and exposure to sunlight.

Because vitamin D is involved with calcium metabolism, it could be thought to be related to exercise performance. However, existing evidence suggests that vitamin D supplementation does not affect work performance (Keith, 1989). Unique findings have been reported by Bell et al. (1988) who showed that blood levels of Gla-protein, an indicator of bone formation, and vitamin D were higher in subjects involved in muscle building training compared to controls. The authors suggested that the muscle building exercises stimulated (a) osteoblastic bone formation and (b) the production of vitamin D, possibly to provide calcium for newly forming muscle tissue. Whether these data indicate a greater vitamin D requirement for strenuous work where large loads are carried or moved is not known, and the question warrants further investigation.

Exposure to sunlight in a hot environment should be sufficient to prevent a vitamin D deficiency. In fact one study found no cases of vitamin D deficiency rickets in a survey of 224 African infants (Kendall, 1972). Because the mothers spent time in sunlight, and breast feeding is universal in the African population studied, babies get sufficient vitamin D. Also, it has been suggested that tropical vegetable foods contain appreciable amounts of vitamin D (Kendall, 1972).

Vitamin E

The major symptom of vitamin E deficiency in animals, which was identified in 1922, is a damping of the reproductive ability. However, muscle wasting or dystrophic muscles have also been noted in vitamin E-deficient animals (Bieri, 1990). It was not until the 1950s that vitamin E was shown to be important for humans as well as other animals.

Vitamin E comprises at least four compounds known as tocopherols. The most active and well known of these is alpha-tocopherol. Vitamin E has been shown to function as an antioxidant of polyunsaturated fatty acids in cellular membranes (Machlin and Bendich, 1987). In this role, vitamin E serves as a free radical scavenger to protect cell membranes from lipid peroxidation. Free radicals are chemical species with one or more unpaired electrons in their outer orbit, which makes them highly reactive. Because strenuous exercise can increase lipid peroxidation (Kanter et al., 1988; Maughan et al., 1989), vitamin E may have important implications for exercise or work capacity.

Plasma or serum tocopherol levels can provide a relatively good index of vitamin E status (Machlin, 1984). Although few studies have assessed vitamin E status of athletes (Cohen et al., 1985; Guilland et al., 1989; Weight et al., 1988), vitamin E deficiencies are considered rare (Kagen et al., 1989). Vitamin E intake among athletes is considered to be more than sufficient (Buskirk, 1981; Clarkson, 1991). High vitamin E intakes were routinely used by athletes in the Mexico City and Munich Olympic Games (Buskirk, 1981).

Acute exercise has been shown to affect blood levels of tocopherol. Pincemail et al. (1988) found that plasma tocopherol levels were significantly increased in nine men during intense cycle ergometer exercise. The authors suggested that tocopherol was mobilized from adipose tissue into the blood and distributed to exercising muscles. At the muscle level, tocopherol could act to prevent lipid peroxidation induced by the exercise. However, because this study did not correct for hemoconcentration, and the small increase in plasma tocopherol was back to baseline after 10 minutes of rest, the results may simply be due to plasma volume changes induced by exercise.

To study the effects of vitamin E deficiency, Bunnell et al. (1975) fed subjects who were employed in jobs of hard physical labor a low vitamin E diet for 13 months. Although vitamin E levels dropped significantly during the study, subjects did not perceive any muscle weakness, pain, or cramps. Work capacity was not assessed.

Results from several well-controlled experiments have shown that vitamin E supplementation had no effect on the following:

• The performance of standard exercise tests, including bench step tests, 1-mile run, 400-m swim, and motor fitness tests in adolescent male swimmers given 400 mg of alpha-tocopherol daily for 6 weeks (Sharman et al., 1971).

• $\dot{V}_{O_2 \, max}$ or muscle strength in college swimmers given 1200 IU daily for 85 days (Shephard et al., 1974).

• $\dot{V}_{O_2 \, max}$ in ice hockey players given 1200 IU daily for 50 days (Watt et al., 1974).

• A swimming endurance test and blood lactate in competitive swimmers given 900 IU daily for 6 months (Lawrence et al., 1975a,b).

• Motor fitness tests, cardiorespiratory efficiency during cycle ergometry exercise and bench stepping, and 400-m swim times in male and female trained swimmers given 400 mg daily for 6 weeks (Sharman et al., 1976).

• 100- or 400-m swim performance in swimmers given 1600 IU daily for 5 weeks (Talbot and Jamieson, 1977).

Because of the role of vitamin E as an antioxidant, two studies examined the effect of vitamin E supplementation on performance at high altitudes, where oxygen availability may be compromised. Nagawa et al. (1968) reported that supplementation of 300 mg per day for at least 4 to 5 weeks had a moderate effect on several exercise tests, including cycle ergometry exercise and running sprints, performed at altitudes of 2700 and 2900 m. Using a better controlled design, Kobayashi (1974) examined the effect of vitamin E supplementation of 1200 IU daily for 6 weeks on submaximal cycle ergometry exercise. Testing was done at altitudes of 1525 m (5000 feet) and 4570 m (15,000 feet). Submaximal oxygen intake, oxygen debt, and blood lactate levels were significantly lower in the vitamin E-supplemented group compared with the placebo group. At the higher altitudes, the decreased availability of oxygen may increase lipid peroxidation of the red blood cell and muscle cell membranes and thereby enhance their destruction. Williams (1989) suggested that increased levels of vitamin E could counteract this effect. A recent study by Simon-Schnass and Pabst (1988) showed that lipid peroxidation was lower in a group of mountain climbers supplemented with vitamin E.

Vitamin E may play an antioxidant role in reducing muscle damage from strenuous exercise (Ebbeling and Clarkson, 1989). Exhaustive exercise that produces muscle damage also results in an increase in free radical activity (Kanter et al., 1988; Maughan et al., 1989). However, results are equivocal on whether muscle damage is reduced by vitamin E supplementation. Helgheim et al. (1979) found that vitamin E (447 IU per day) supplementation for 6 weeks did not reduce the leakage of muscle enzymes into the blood following strenuous exercise. Also, muscle soreness, a general indicator of muscle damage, was not reduced in subjects taking vitamin E supplements (600 IU per day) for 2 days before performing a strenuous exercise (Francis and Hoobler, 1986). Although Sumida et al. (1989) found that 4 weeks of vitamin E supplementation (447 IU per day) resulted in a reduced serum enzyme response to exercise, a balanced design was not used. Rather, subjects performed the same exercise before supplementation and then again after supplementation. It has been well documented that serum enzyme response is substantially reduced the second time an exercise regimen is performed (Clarkson and Tremblay, 1988; Ebbeling and Clarkson, 1989). However, Goldfarb et al. (1989) examined the effect of 800 IU of vitamin E per day for 4 weeks on lipid peroxidation in blood samples taken after a run at 80 percent $\dot{V}_{O_2 \, max}$. Compared to the placebo group, the vitamin E-supplemented group showed reduced levels of lipid peroxidation at rest and after running.

There is currently no information concerning vitamin E supplementation for exercise in the heat. Vitamins A, C, and E are all antioxidants and may have significant roles in reducing muscle damage (via lipid peroxidation) induced by strenuous exercise. It has been suggested that work in the heat could create a hypoxic condition in the muscle due to the redistribution of blood from the muscle to the skin, although there is some question whether this occurs (Young, 1990). While no studies have examined lipid peroxidation during exercise in the heat, it is possible that hypoxia, dehydration, or other changes induced by heat stress could exacerbate lipid peroxidation in exercising muscle. If so, the antioxidant vitamins may be useful in the reduction of heat stress. Further research in this area seems warranted.

CONCLUSIONS AND RECOMMENDATIONS

The requirement for B vitamins does not seem to be increased by living and working in a hot environment. Although loss of these vitamins in sweat is minimal, a deficiency could occur over time from profuse sweating coupled with an insufficient dietary intake. Because thiamin, riboflavin, niacin, and vitamin B_6 are important to energy metabolism, the level of vitamin intake should be related to the amount of food consumed. Thus, for adults, 0.5 mg of thiamin per 1000-kcal diet, 0.6 mg of riboflavin per 1000-kcal diet, 0.016 mg of vitamin B_6 per g protein, and 6.6 mg of niacin per 1000-kcal diet are recommended (National Research Council, 1989). If calorie intake is not sufficient to meet the demands of exercise in the heat, then the vitamin intake will be compromised as well.

Folic acid and vitamin B_{12} are not linked to energy production, and their intake should be that of the 1989 RDA. There is no information to suggest that exposure to a hot environment would increase their need above levels recommended by the National Research Council.

Since World War I, vitamin C has received popular attention as a nutrient that can reduce heat stress. More recent studies have generally confirmed the anecdotal studies. Increased vitamin intake of 250 mg seems to have a positive effect on reducing heat stress during acclimatization in those individuals with adequate but low vitamin C levels. Some data have shown that vitamin C status may be compromised by long-term exposure to a hot environment. Thus, vitamin C supplements may be useful for those individuals who live and work in a hot environment. However, intakes of greater than 250 mg per day are not recommended because high doses of vitamin C can adversely affect the absorption of vitamin B_{12}.

The one study (Bell et al., 1988) suggesting that vitamin D may be related to muscle building induced by strenuous resistance exercise is interesting and warrants further attention. However, at this time, there is no reason to recommend vitamin D supplements for people who work in the heat. Exposure to sunlight probably is sufficient for adequate vitamin D status.

Vitamins A, C, and E are antioxidants and may be useful in the reduction of lipid peroxidation induced by exercise stress. However, there have been no studies to examine whether lipid peroxidation is exacerbated by exercise in a hot environment. Further studies on whether these vitamins will be important as antioxidants for people living and working in a hot environment are warranted.

The following recommendations are made:

• Thiamin, riboflavin, vitamin B_6, and niacin should be linked to changes in food consumption as recommended by the RDAs (National Research Council, 1989). Insufficient data exist to recommend otherwise.

• The RDA of folic acid and vitamin B_{12} should be sufficient to meet the body's requirement. Insufficient data exist to recommend otherwise.

• Further studies should be done to determine the effects on vitamin status of long-term exposure to living and working in the heat.

• During acclimatization, vitamin C intake should be about 250 mg per day to reduce heat stress and enhance acclimatization in those people who have adequate but low vitamin C status. Further study is warranted to confirm this recommendation and to determine whether supplementation may be effective in reducing heat stress in people with optimal vitamin C status.

• Existing data show that vitamin C supplements may be needed for extended periods of living and working in hot environments. Further studies are needed to confirm this finding and to determine the amount of vitamin C needed to prevent a decrease in status.

• There is no need to supplement vitamin D in hot environments.

• Vitamin A (beta-carotene), vitamin C, and vitamin E function as antioxidants and may be useful as supplements in a hot environment. Further research is needed for confirmation.

REFERENCES

Adams, M.M., L.P. Porcello, and V.M. Vivian
  1982   Effect of a supplement on dietary intakes of female collegiate swimmers. Physician Sportsmed. 10:122-134.
Belko, A.Z., E. Obarzanek, H.J. Kalwarf, M.A. Rotter, S. Bogusz, D. Miller, J.D. Haas, and D.A. Roe
  1983   Effects of exercise on riboflavin requirements of young women. Am. J. Clin. Nutr. 37:509-517.
Bell, N.H., R.N. Godsen, D.P. Henry, J. Shary, and S. Epstein
  1988   The effects of muscle-building exercise on vitamin D and mineral metabolism. J. Bone Miner. Res. 3:369-373.
Bergstrom, J., E. Hultman, L. Jorfeldt, B. Pernow, and J. Wahren
  1969   Effect of nicotinic acid on physical working capacity and on metabolism of muscle glycogen in man. J. Appl. Physiol. 26:170-176.
Bieri, J.G.
  1990   Vitamin E. Pp. 117-121 in Present Knowledge in Nutrition, M.L. Brown, ed. Washington, D.C.: International Life Sciences Institute.
Brotherhood, J.R.
  1984   Nutrition and sports performance. Sports Med. 1:350-389.
Brouns, F., and W. Saris
  1989   How vitamins affect performance. J. Sports Med. Phys. Fitness 29:400-404.
Brown, M.L.
  1990   Thiamin. Pp. 142-144 in Present Knowledge in Nutrition, M.L. Brown, ed. Washington, D.C.: International Life Sciences Institute.
Bunnell, R.H., E. DeRitter, and S.H. Rubin
  1975   Effect of feeding polyunsaturated fatty acids with a low vitamin E diet on blood levels of tocopherol in men performing hard physical labor. Am. J. Clin. Nutr. 28:706-711.

Buskirk, E.R.
1981   Some nutritional considerations in the conditioning of athletes. Ann. Rev. Nutr. 1:319-350.
Carlson, L.A., and L. Oro
1962   The effect of nicotinic acid on the plasma free fatty acids. Acta Med. Scand. 172:641-645.
Chen, J.D., Z.Y. Yang, S.H. Ma, and Y.C. Zhen
1990   The effects of *Actinidia sinensis* Planch (kiwi) drink supplementation on athletes training in hot environments. J. Sports Med. Phys. Fitness 30:181-184.
Clarkson, P.M.
1991   Vitamins and trace minerals. Pp. 21-42 in Perspectives in Exercise Science and Sports Medicine, vol. 4: Ergogenics: Enhancement of Performance in Exercise and Sport, D.R. Lamb and M.H. Williams, eds. Dubuque, Iowa: W. C.B. Brown and Benchmark.
Clarkson, P.M., and I. Tremblay
1988   Rapid adaptation to exercise induced muscle damage. J. Appl. Physiol. 65:1-6.
Cohen, J.L., L. Potosnak, O. Frank, and H. Baker
1985   A nutritional and hematological assessment of elite ballet dancers. Physician Sportsmed. 13:43-54.
Consolazio, C.F.
1963   The energy requirements of men living under extreme environmental conditions. 3. Extremely hot environments. Pp. 65-77 in World Review of Nutrition and Dietetics, vol. 27, G.H. Bourne, ed. New York: Hafner Publishing.
Cooperman, J.M., and R. Lopez
1984   Riboflavin. Pp. 299-327 in Handbook of Vitamins. Nutritional, Biochemical and Clinical Aspects, L.J. Machlin, ed. New York: Marcel Dekker.
deVos, A.M., J.E. Leklem, and D.E. Campbell
1982   Carbohydrate loading, vitamin B_6 supplementation, and fuel metabolism during exercise in man. Med. Sci. Sports Exerc. 14:137 (abstract).
Dreon, D.M., and G.E. Butterfield
1986   Vitamin B_6 utilization in active and inactive young men. Am. J. Clin. Nutr. 43:816-824.
Driskell, J.A.
1984   Vitamin B_6. Pp. 379-401 in Handbook of Vitamins. Nutritional, Biochemical and Clinical Aspects, L. J. Machlin, ed. New York: Marcel Dekker.
Early, R.G., and B.R. Carlson
1969   Water-soluble vitamin therapy in the delay of fatigue from physical activity in hot climatic conditions. Int. Z. angew. Physiol. 27:43-50.
Ebbeling, C.B., and P.M. Clarkson
1989   Exercise-induced muscle damage and adaptation. Sports Med. 7:207-234.
Edison, A.O., R.H. Silber, and D.M. Tennent
1945   The effect of varied thiamine intake on the growth of rats in tropical environment. Am. J. Physiol. 144:643-651.
Ellenbogen, L.
1984   Vitamin B_{12}. Pp. 497-547 in Handbook of Vitamins. Nutritional, Biochemical and Clinical Aspects, L.J. Machlin, ed. New York: Marcel Dekker.
Fox, H.M.
1984   Pantothenic acid. Pp. 437-457 in Handbook of Vitamins. Nutritional, Biochemical and Clinical Aspects, L.J. Machlin, ed. New York: Marcel Dekker.
Francis, K.T., and T. Hoobler
1986   Failure of vitamin E and delayed muscle soreness. J. Med. Assoc. Alabama 55:15-18.

Gey, G.O., K.H. Cooper, and R.A. Bottenberg
1970   Effect of ascorbic acid on endurance performance and athletic injury. J. Am. Med. Assoc. 211:105.

Gleeson, M., J.D. Robertson, and R.J. Maughan
1987   Influence of exercise on ascorbic acid status in man. Clin. Sci. 73:501-505.

Goldfarb, A.H., M.K. Todd, B.T. Boyer, H.M. Alessio, and R.G. Cutler
1989   Effect of vitamin E on lipid peroxidation at 80 percent $V_{O_2 max}$. Med. Sci. Sports Exerc. 21:S16 (abstract).

Gubler, C.J.
1984   Thiamin. Pp. 245-297 in Handbook of Vitamins. Nutritional, Biochemical and Clinical Aspects, L.J. Machlin, ed. New York: Marcel Dekker.

Guilland, J., T. Penaranda, C. Gallet, V. Boggio, F. Fuchs, and J. Klepping
1989   Vitamin status of young athletes including the effects of supplementation. Med. Sci. Sports Exerc. 21:441-449.

Guyton, A.C.
1986   Textbook of Medical Physiology, 7th ed. Philadelphia: W.B. Saunders.

Hankes, L.V.
1984   Nicotinic acid and Nicotinamide. Pp. 329-377 in Handbook of Vitamins. Nutritional, Biochemical and Clinical Aspects, L.J. Machlin, ed. New York: Marcel Dekker.

Haralambie, G.
1976   Vitamin B_2 status in athletes and the influence of riboflavin administration on neuromuscular irritability. Nutr. Metab. 20:1-8.

Hatcher, L.F., J.E. Leklem, and D.E. Campbell
1982   Altered vitamin B_6 metabolism during exercise in man: Effect of carbohydrate modified diets and vitamin B_6 supplements. Med. Sci. Sports Exerc. 14:112 (abstract).

Helgheim, I., O. Hetland, S. Nilsson, F. Ingjer, and S.B. Stromme
1979   The effects of vitamin E on serum enzyme levels following heavy exercise. Eur. J. Appl. Physiol. 40:283-289.

Henschel, A., H.L. Taylor, O. Mickelsen, J.M. Brozek, and A. Keys
1944a   The effect of high vitamin C and B intake on the ability of man to work in hot environments. Fed. Proc. 3:18.

Henschel, A., H.L. Taylor, J. Brozek, O. Mickelsen, and A. Keys
1944b   Vitamin C and ability to work in hot environments. Am. J. Trop. Med. Hyg. 24:259-264.

Herbert, V.
1990   Vitamin B-12. Pp. 170-178 in Present Knowledge in Nutrition, M. L. Brown, ed. Washington, D.C.: International Life Sciences Institute.

Hilsendager, D., and P. Karpovich
1964   Ergogenic effect of glycine and niacin separately and in combination. Res. Q. 35:389-392.

Hindson, T.C.
1970   Ascorbic acid status of Europeans resident in the tropics. Br. J. Nutr. 24:801-802.

Hofmann, A., R.D. Reynolds, B.L. Smoak, V.G. Villanueva, and P.A. Duester
1991   Plasma pyridoxal and pyridoxal 5'-phosphate concentrations in response to ingestion of water or glucose polymer during a 2-h run. Am. J. Clin. Nutr. 53:84-89.

Holmes, H.N.
1942   Vitamin C in the war. Science 96:384-386.

Howald, H., B. Segesser, and W.F. Korner
1975   Ascorbic acid and athletic performance. Ann. N.Y. Acad. Sci. 258:458-463.

Hunt, S.M., and J.L. Groff
1990   Advanced Nutrition and Human Metabolism. St. Paul, Minn.: West Publishing.
Jaffe, G.M.
1984   Vitamin C. Pp. 199-244 in Handbook of Vitamins. Nutritional, Biochemical and Clinical Aspects, L. J. Machlin, ed. New York: Marcel Dekker.
Kagen, V.E., V.B. Spirichev, and A.N. Erin
1989   Vitamin E, physical exercise, and sport. Pp. 255-278 in Nutrition in Exercise and Sport, J.E. Hickson and I. Wolinsky, eds. Boca Raton, Florida: CRC Press.
Kanter, M.M., G.R. Lesmes, L.A. Kaminsky, J. La Ham-Saeger, and N.D. Nequin
1988   Serum creatine kinase and lactate dehydrogenase changes following an eighty kilometer race. Eur. J. Appl. Physiol. 57:60-63.
Karpovich, P.V., and N. Millman
1942   Vitamin B_1 and endurance. N. Engl. J. Med. 226:881-882.
Keith, R.E.
1989   Vitamins in sport and exercise. Pp. 233-253 in Nutrition in Exercise and Sport, J.E. Hickson and I. Wolinsky, eds. Boca Raton, Florida: CRC Press.
Keith, R.E., and J.A. Driskell
1982   Lung function and treadmill performance of smoking and nonsmoking males receiving ascorbic acid supplements. Am. J. Clin. Nutr. 36:840-845.
Keith, R.E., and E. Merrill
1983   The effects of vitamin C on maximal grip strength and muscular endurance. J. Sports Med. 23:253-256.
Kendall, A.C.
1972   Rickets in the tropics and sub-tropics. Cent. Afr. J. Med. 18:47-49.
Keren, G., and Y. Epstein
1980   The effect of high dosage vitamin C intake on aerobic and anaerobic capacity. J. Sports Med. 20:145-148.
Keys, A., and A.F. Henschel
1941   High vitamin supplementation (B_1, nicotinic acid and C) and the response to intensive exercise in U.S. Army infantrymen. Am. J. Physiol. 133:350-351.
1942   Vitamin supplementation of U.S. Army rations in relation to fatigue and the ability to do muscular work. J. Nutr. 23:259-269.
Keys, A., A.F. Henschel, O. Mickelsen, and J. M. Brozek
1943   The performance of normal young men on controlled thiamine intakes. J. Nutr. 26:399-415.
Keys, A., A.F. Henschel, O. Mickelsen, J.M. Brozek, and J.H. Crawford
1944   Physiological and biochemical functions in normal young men on a diet restricted in riboflavin. J. Nutr. 27:165-178.
Kobayashi, Y.
1974   Effect of vitamin E on aerobic work performance in man during acute exposure to hypoxic hypoxia. Ph.D. dissertation. University of New Mexico, Albuquerque.
Kotze, H.F., W.H. van der Walt, G.G. Rogers, and N.B. Strydom
1977   Effects of plasma ascorbic acid levels on heat acclimatization in man. J. Appl. Physiol. 42:711-716.
Lawrence, J.D., J.L. Smith, R.C. Bower, and W.P. Riehl
1975a   The effect of alpha-tocopherol (vitamin E) and pyridoxine HCl (vitamin B_6) on the swimming endurance of trained swimmers. J. Am. Coll. Health Assoc. 23:219-222.
Lawrence, J.D., R.C. Bower, W.P. Riehl, and J.L. Smith
1975b   Effects of alpha-tocopherol acetate on the swimming endurance of trained swimmers. Am. J. Clin. Nutr. 28: 205-208.

Leklem, J.E., and T.D. Shultz
  1983   Increased plasma pyridoxal 5'-phosphate and vitamin B_6 in male adolescents after a 4500-meter run. Am. J. Clin. Nutr. 38:541-548.
Litoff, D., H. Scherzer, and J. Harrison
  1985   Effects of pantothenic acid supplementation on human exercise. Med. Sci. Sports Exerc. 17:287 (abstract).
Machlin, L.J.
  1984   Vitamin E. Pp. 99-145 in Handbook of Vitamins. Nutritional, Biochemical and Clinical Aspects, L.J. Machlin, ed. New York: Marcel Dekker.
Machlin, L.J., and A. Bendich
  1987   Free radical tissue damage: Protective role of antioxidant nutrients. Fed. Am. Soc. Exp. Biol. J. 1:441-445.
Manore, M.M., and J.E. Leklem
  1988   Effect of carbohydrate and vitamin B_6 on fuel substrates during exercise in women. Med. Sci. Sports Exerc. 20: 233-241.
Maughan, R.J., A.E. Donnelly, M. Gleeson, P.H. Whiting, and K.A. Walker
  1989   Delayed-onset muscle damage and lipid peroxidation in man after a downhill run. Muscle Nerve 12:332-336.
Mayer, J., and B. Bullen
  1960   Nutrition and athletic performance. Physiol. Rev. 40:369-397.
McCormick, D.B.
  1990   Riboflavin. Pp. 146-154 in Present Knowledge in Nutrition, M.L. Brown, ed. Washington, D.C.: International Life Sciences Institute.
Merrill, Jr., A.H., and F.S. Burnham
  1990   Vitamin B-6. Pp. 155-162 in Present Knowledge in Nutrition, M. L. Brown, ed. Washington, D.C.: International Life Sciences Institute.
Mickelsen, O., and A. Keys
  1943   The composition of sweat with special reference to the vitamins. J. Biol. Chem. 149: 479-490.
Mills, C.A.
  1941   Environmental temperatures and thiamine requirements. Am. J. Physiol. 133:525-532.
Mitchell, H.H., and M. Edman
  1951   Nutrition and Climatic Stress. Springfield, Ill.: Charles C. Thomas.
Montoye, H.J., P.J. Spata, V. Pinckney, and L. Barron
  1955   Effects of vitamin B_{12} supplementation on physical fitness and growth of young boys. J. Appl. Physiol. 7:589-592.
Nagawa, T., H. Kita, J. Aoki, T. Maeshima, and K. Shiozawa
  1968   The effect of vitamin E on endurance. Asian Med. J. 11:619-633.
National Research Council
  1989   Recommended Dietary Allowances, 10th ed. Washington, D.C.: National Academy Press.
Nice, C., A.G. Reeves, T. Brinck-Johnsen, and W. Noll
  1984   The effects of pantothenic acid on human exercise capacity. J. Sports Med. 24:26-29.
Nielsen, B., G. Savard, E.A. Richter, M. Hargreaves, and B. Saltin
  1990   Muscle blood flow and muscle metabolism during exercise and heat stress. J. Appl. Physiol. 69:1040-1046.
Nijakowski, F.
  1966   Assays of some vitamins of the B complex group in human blood in relation to muscular effort. Acta Physiol. Pol. 17:397-404.

Norman, A.W.
  1990   Vitamin D. Pp. 108-116 in Present Knowledge in Nutrition, M. L. Brown, ed.
          Washington, D.C.: International Life Sciences Institute.
Olson, J.A.
  1984   Vitamin A. Pp. 1-43 in Handbook of Vitamins. Nutritional, Biochemical and Clinical
          Aspects, L. J. Machlin, ed. New York: Marcel Dekker.
  1990   Vitamin A. Pp. 96-107 in Present Knowledge in Nutrition, M. L. Brown, ed.
          Washington, D.C.: International Life Sciences Institute.
Olson, R.E.
  1990   Pantothenic acid. Pp. 208-211 in Present Knowledge in Nutrition, M. L. Brown,
          ed. Washington, D.C.: International Life Sciences Institute.
Pike, R.L., and M.L. Brown
  1984   Nutrition, An Integrated Approach, 3rd ed. New York: Macmillan.
Pincemail, J., C. Deby, G. Camus, F. Pirnay, R. Bouchez, L. Massaux, and R. Goutier
  1988   Tocopherol mobilization during intensive exercise. Eur. J. Appl. Physiol. 57:189-
          191.
Poda, G.A.
  1979   Vitamin C for heat symptoms? Ann. Intern. Med. 91(4):657.
Read, M.H., and S.L. McGuffin
  1983   The effect of B-complex supplementation on endurance performance. J. Sports
          Med. 23:178-184.
Robinson, S., and A.H. Robinson
  1954   Chemical composition of sweat. Physiol. Rev. 34:202-220.
Sauberlich, H.E.
  1990   Ascorbic acid. Pp. 132-141 in Present Knowledge in Nutrition, M.L. Brown, ed.
          Washington, D.C.: International Life Sciences Institute.
Sauberlich, H.E., Y.F. Herman, C.O. Stevens, and R.H. Herman
  1979   Thiamin requirement of the adult human. Am. J. Clin. Nutr. 32:2237-2248.
Scott, M.L.
  1975   Environmental influences on ascorbic acid requirements in animals. Ann. N.Y.
          Acad. Sci. 258:151-155.
Sharman, I.M., M.G. Down, and R.N. Sen
  1971   The effects of vitamin E and training on physiological function and athletic perfor-
          mance in adolescent swimmers. Br. J. Nutr. 26:265-276.
Sharman, I.M., M.G. Down, and N.G. Norgan
  1976   The effects of vitamin E on physiological function and athletic performance of
          trained swimmers. J. Sports Med. 16:215-225.
Shephard, R.J., R. Campbell, P. Pimm, D. Stuart, and G.R. Wright
  1974   Vitamin E, exercise, and the recovery from physical activity. Eur. J. Appl. Physiol.
          33:119-126.
Simon-Schnass, I., and H. Pabst
  1988   Influence of vitamin E on physical performance. Internat. J. Vit. Nutr. Res. 58:49-
          54.
Staton, W.M.
  1952   The influence of ascorbic acid in minimizing post-exercise muscle soreness in
          young men. Res. Q. 23:356-360.
Strydom, N.B., H.F. Kotze, W.H. Van der Walt, and G.G. Rogers
  1976   Effect of ascorbic acid on rate of heat acclimatization. J. Appl. Physiol. 41:202-
          205.
Sumida, S., K. Tanaka, H. Kitao, and F. Nakadomo
  1989   Exercise-induced lipid peroxidation and leakage of enzymes before and after vita-
          min E supplementation. Int. J. Biochem. 21:835-838.

Swendseid, J., and M.E. Swendseid
 1990   Niacin. Pp. 163-169 in Present Knowledge in Nutrition, M. L. Brown, ed. Washington, D.C.: International Life Sciences Institute.
Talbot, D., and J. Jamieson
 1977   An examination of the effect of vitamin E on the performance of highly trained swimmers. Can. J. Appl. Sport Sci. 2:67-69.
Tin-May-Than, Ma-Win-May, Khin-Sann-Aung, and M. Mya-Tu
 1978   The effect of vitamin B_{12} on physical performance capacity. Br. J. Nutr. 40:269-273.
Tremblay, A., B. Boilard, M.F. Breton, H. Bessette, and A.G. Roberge
 1984   The effects of riboflavin supplementation on the nutritional status and performance of elite swimmers. Nutr. Res. 4:201-208.
Tucker, R.G., O. Mickelsen, and A. Keys
 1960   The influence of sleep, work, diuresis, heat, acute starvation, thiamine intake and bed rest on human riboflavin excretion. J. Nutr. 72:251-261.
Van der Beek, E.J.
 1985   Vitamins and endurance training: Food for running or faddish claims? Sports Med. 2:175-197.
Van der Beek, E.J., W. van Dokkum, J. Schrijver, M. Wedel, A.W.K. Gaillard, A. Wesstra, H. van de Weerd, and R.J.J. Hermus
 1988   Thiamin, riboflavin, and vitamins B-6 and C: Impact of combined restricted intake on functional performance in man. Am. J. Clin. Nutr. 48:1451-1462.
Van der Beek, E.J., W. van Dokkum, J. Schrijver, A. Wesstra, C. Kistemaker and R.J.J. Hermus
 1990   Controlled vitamin C restriction and physical performance in volunteers. J. Am. Coll. Nutr. 9:332-339.
Van Erp-Baart, A.M.J., W.M.H. Saris, R.A. Binkhorst, J.A. Vos, and J.W.H. Elvers
 1989   Nationwide survey on nutritional habits in elite athletes. Part 2. Mineral and vitamin intake. Int. J. Sports Med. 10:S11-16.
Viguie, C.A., L. Packer, and G.A. Brooks
 1989   Antioxidant supplementation affects indices of muscle trauma and oxidant stress in human blood during exercise. Med. Sci. Sports Exerc. 21:S16 (abstract).
Visagie, M.E., J.P. Du Plessis, G. Groothof, A. Alberts, and N.F. Laubscher
 1974   Changes in vitamin A and C levels in Black mine workers. S. African Med. J. 48:2502-2506.
Wald, G., L. Brouha, and R.E. Johnson
 1942   Experimental human vitamin A deficiency and the ability to perform muscular exercise. Am. J. Physiol. 137:551-556.
Watt, T., T. T. Romet, I. McFarlane, D. McGuey, C. Allen, and R.C. Goode
 1974   Vitamin E and oxygen consumption. Lancet 2:354-355 (abstract).
Weight, L.M., T.D. Noakes, D.Labadarios, J. Graves, P. Jacobs, and P.A. Berman
 1988   Vitamin and mineral status of trained athletes including the effects of supplementation. Am. J. Clin. Nutr. 47:186-191.
Williams, M. H.
 1976   Nutritional Aspects of Human Physical and Athletic Performance. Springfield, Ill.: Charles C. Thomas.
 1989   Vitamin supplementation and athletic performance, an overview. Int. J. Vitam. Nutr. Res. 30:161-191.
Wood, B., A. Gijsbers, A. Goode, S. Davis, J. Mulholland, and K. Breen
 1980   A study of partial thiamin restriction in human volunteers. Am. J. Clin. Nutr. 33:848-861.

Woteki, C., C. Johnson, and R. Murphy
  1986   Nutritional status of the U.S. population: Iron, vitamin C, and zinc. Pp. 21-39 in
          What is America Eating? Proceedings of a Symposium, Food and Nutrition Board,
          National Research Council. Washington, D.C.: National Academy Press.
Young, A.J.
  1990   Energy substrate utilization during exercise in extreme environments. Pp. 65-117
          in Exercise and Sport Sciences Reviews, vol. 18, K. E. Pandolf, ed. Baltimore,
          Md.: Williams & Wilkins.

DISCUSSION

DR. NESHEIM: Thank you, Dr. Clarkson. We have a few minutes for questions or comments.

DR. EVANS: Well, we have one paper that we published in January and two more that are about to be published in which we have looked at the effects of vitamin E supplementations on skeletal muscle damage, circulating and skeletal muscle cytokine (CK) levels, and neutrophil generation.

And it appears that vitamin E has a profound effect in subjects that are over 60 in terms of altering all of their responses so that they look like young people in terms of CK release and neutrophil generation and monocyte function.

But it has very little effect in young people in all of those things and it may well be that membrane function is very different in old people as compared to young people.

But the other thing that vitamin E does is that it causes almost a total suppression of interleukin-1 (IL-1) production which may also have some very interesting effects. If IL-1 is necessary for adaptation to increased use, vitamin E may have some not such great effects.

PARTICIPANT: Dr. Clarkson, I was particularly interested in how you arrived at the quantitative figure of 250 milligrams (mg) for vitamin C.

DR. CLARKSON: That is what Strydom (Strydom et al., 1976) actually used in his paper. He used 250 milligrams as a supplement as well as 500 mg.

PARTICIPANT: Did he titrate the dose or was that just something that he chose?

DR. CLARKSON: I believe he based it on the Henshel et al. earlier study, (Henschel et al., 1944b) and it was no different. That graph depicting the 250 mg and the 500 mg dose showed no difference between the two doses. So 250 mg seems to be sufficient.

PARTICIPANT: You know it seems to be striking that all of the potential effects on vitamin supplementation have been measured just using a gross measure in a $V_{O_2 max}$. Maybe you can comment on that.

It seems to me that there are so many other potentially more sensitive measurements that we can make of metabolic responses to exercise that have been ignored for the most part because $V_{O_2 max}$ is easy to measure.

DR. CLARKSON: I agree. Many studies that we find have used $V_{O_2 max}$, but there are also several studies that used submaximal exercise and studies that used strength.

These are easy to measure. I think that is why they are used. Also, except for vitamin C where I only showed you three representative studies, mostly all the studies that are available were presented here. So it is not that there are a hundred other studies out there.

I think that more people should be involved in looking at the effects of vitamins on performance. I think one of the problems why people aren't involved in looking at vitamins is that it is hard to measure in the blood and therefore difficult to determine initial status.

PARTICIPANT: My question is specifically in terms of looking at measurements as opposed to plasma or sweat loss. What about some other measure—urine or something else.

DR. CLARKSON: Well, urine levels are hard to interpret because what happens is, as soon as you reach a threshold level the nutrient spills over, so you are not quite sure what urinary secretion means.

Does increased excretion mean you need less? Perhaps for a non-exercising person this is true. I am not ready to really believe that for an exercising person. In this case when you get an increased excretion it is not clear what this really means.

If I gave a sedentary individual large doses of a particular vitamin and it increases in the urine, then we would say, yes, the status is adequate and the person does not need a supplement.

However, when you add stressors like heat and exercise, I am not really sure what an increase in urinary levels of vitamins means.

PARTICIPANT: I just wanted to follow up one comment you had made on niacin. There are two papers—certainly submitted—in those studies Evelyn Stephasson(?) had administered niacin supplementation to individuals and had them exposed to heat and attempted exercise.

She found a very profound dilation and increased incidence of syncopy. So niacin supplementation in heat could actually reduce performance.

DR. CLARKSON: Yes, I mentioned the flushing.

PARTICIPANT: In the Strydom (Strydom et al., 1976) paper, do you happen to recall whether he assessed what the vitamin C status was before he did the supplementation?

DR. CLARKSON: No, on the second paper they did check vitamin C levels.

PARTICIPANT: And they were adequate before this?

DR. CLARKSON: Yes, but low.

PARTICIPANT: Based on plasma concentrations?

DR. CLARKSON: Yes.

PARTICIPANT: I just want to make a comment. I don't know if anyone noticed, about a week or two ago in *Science* magazine, there was just a short note on Dr. Linus Pauling who is still at age 90 consuming 18 grams per day of vitamin C. I don't know what type of effects that would have on absorption and interference that you talk about.

And the other thing, I was also interested in the work in the South Africans on vitamin C apparently accelerating the acquisition of acclimation. Do you know of any other papers that have followed that up? That was mid-1970s; correct?

DR. CLARKSON: Yes, and that is it. I found that one.

PARTICIPANT: I could offer a technical comment. My thesis was on vitamin B_{12} chemistry and I did study some of the interactions of vitamin C and B_{12} and so has Victor Herbert (RDA, ninth edition). And a lot of these effects are an artifact of the analytical techniques. I don't take that too seriously.

It turns out that vitamin C plus certain forms of B_{12} will be generating singlet oxygen and will destroy the chromophore in the test tube. So if you don't prevent this artifact—it is a pro-oxidant when you add it to iron usually.

So a lot of the studies are flawed because they didn't prevent this. You have high C levels carried over in your serum when you are doing analysis in B_{12}.

DR. CLARKSON: In his (Herbert, 1990) recent review of literature on vitamin B_{12}, Herbert suggests that vitamin C does have an effect on absorption of vitamin B_{12}.

PARTICIPANT: Just a comment on vitamin B_{12}. I would think it would be rather unlikely that you would see a B_{12} deficiency if you were to put adults on a low intake for a period of time. It is going to take a long long time to get a deficiency.

Actually, I did my thesis work on B_{12} requirements in baby pigs and the only way we could ever produce a B_{12} requirement in those pigs was to put the dams on a low or almost no B_{12} intake and then take the pigs away from the dam almost immediately after birth and put them on a vitamin B_{12}-free diet and then we could produce a deficiency and, as a matter of fact, we produced it very quickly.

But if we let them have the colostrum milk for even four or five days, it just went a long time to ever produce a B_{12} deficiency.

PARTICIPANT: I would like to comment that there is some data that I think has appeared in the literature now by Doris Calloway and colleagues who were involved in a three-country study—Mexico, Kenya, and Egypt—and were looking at growth and other performance parameters in children.

They appeared to be finding an impact of animal protein intake per day in terms of the growth and development of these young children and they are looking very hard at trying to get data on the actual B_{12} content of these diets.

It is a possibility, since these populations tend to be very much on a vegetarian type of program—very little meat in these poorer populations—that you are seeing some of it (vitamin B_{12} deficiency) in the military.

But then again, I think it is highly unlikely that we would see a B_{12} deficiency as it relates to that.

PARTICIPANT: Just maybe one other comment. Haven't there been some reported vitamin D deficiencies in Middle Eastern countries in which women, in fact, have very little skin exposure to the sun?

I mean, it is a complicating factor. In a desert environment, many people have kind of an ironic effect of D deficiency because their skin doesn't see the sun.

PARTICIPANT: I seem to recall reading some comments to that but I don't know of any specific literature.

DR. EVANS: We are in the process of conducting some studies in vitamin D deficiencies in older people but vitamin D deficiency is very present. They don't drink milk and they don't see the sun very much and it may be associated with a profound muscle weakness due to a calcium metabolism problem.

DR. CLARKSON: There might also be vitamin D deficiencies in some athlete groups like dancers who don't drink milk, because quite a few of them do have a low consumption of milk and they do not spend much time in the sunlight.

PARTICIPANT: I was going to ask a question, and this relates to the microorganisms in the GI tract and the vitamin C. I wonder, has anyone done any studies and looked at the types of microbes that are in the GI tract, the possibility of infection (subclinical infections) that occur in long-distance runners? Has anyone ever done that type of work?

PARTICIPANT: If anything, there was one paper that suggested that too much vitamin C might contribute to some of the lesions that have been observed in the GI tract in athletes.

PARTICIPANT: You would have to take in a large amount, wouldn't you?

DR. EVANS: With some athletes, apparently they do take in quite a bit.

DR. NESHEIM: Thank you very much for your interesting comments.

Nutritional Needs in Hot Environments
Pp. 173–185. Washington, D.C.
National Academy Press

9

Heat as a Factor in the Perception of Taste, Smell, and Oral Sensation

Barry G. Green[1]

INTRODUCTION

Because all biological systems are to some extent sensitive to temperature, heat can be expected to affect the perception of taste. Although thermal influences on taste perception have been confirmed in numerous studies, much remains to be learned about the range of temperature-taste interactions that occur, their relevance to food preferences and nutrition, and the mechanisms that underlie them. As this review of the available data will illustrate, most of what has been learned pertains to simple chemosensory "model" stimuli, rather than to foods, and to the effects of stimulus temperature alone rather than to the effects of both environmental and stimulus temperature. The extent to which existing data are relevant to real-world perceptions of food in a hot environment is therefore difficult to assess.

To place what is known about temperature-taste effects in the correct context, it is helpful to review the sensory innervation of the oronasal region and the terminology used to describe the perception of foods and beverages. In common usage, the term *taste* refers to the oral experience produced during the ingestion of a food or beverage. In fact, this experience derives from several different sensory systems, only one of which actually conveys information about taste (gustation) per se. As currently defined, taste sensations fall into four, or possibly five, categories: sweet, sour, salty,

---

[1] Barry G. Green, Monell Chemical Senses Center, 3500 Market Street, Philadelphia, PA 19104-3308

and bitter; many Japanese researchers also argue that the taste of monosodium glutamate (MSG), which they refer to as *umami*, is unique and "basic" (for example, Nakamura and Kurihara, 1991; Rogers and Blundell, 1990). All other sensations associated with the ingestion of foods derive from other sensory systems that innervate the oral and nasal cavities. In particular, the qualities that we frequently use to describe how something tastes— such as chocolate, vanilla, strawberry, and orange—are actually odors detected retronasally via the opening between the oropharynx and the nasal cavity. Qualities such as creaminess and crunchiness derive from mechanical stimulation and thus are mediated by the sense of touch. The "burn" or "heat" of chili pepper, mustard, alcohol, and other irritants is mediated at least in part by the pain and thermal senses (Green, 1991; Green and Lawless, 1991). Thus, the term *taste* should be reserved for the limited range of gustatory sensations, and the term *flavor* should be used to describe the totality of oral sensations—taste, smell, touch, temperature, and chemical irritation (pain)—that accompany eating.

To evaluate thermal effects on flavor therefore requires more than merely measuring the modulation of sweet, sour, salty, and bitter tastes under conditions of changing stimulus temperature. The present chapter reviews the current literature on thermal effects in all four of the above-mentioned modalities and suggests future research.

SENSORY EFFECTS OF TEMPERATURE

Taste

The effect of temperature on the perception of taste has been studied scientifically for over a century (for review see Green and Frankmann, 1987; Pangborn et al., 1970). However, because temperature-taste effects were usually measured in piecemeal fashion (that is, testing only one or two taste stimuli at a time) in different laboratories using different experimental methods, few generalizations could be gleaned from the early experiments. The only reliable finding seemed to be that the threshold for detecting the four basic tastes tended to vary in a U-shaped manner as a function of temperature, having a minimum somewhere in the range between 20° and 30°C. The temperature at which the minimum occurred varied across taste stimuli (see McBurney et al., 1973 for example), which means that, in general, when foods or beverages are heated to temperatures above 30°C (about 86°F), detecting weak tastes becomes more difficult.

Interestingly, the pattern of thermal effects at threshold does not extend to suprathreshold concentrations, when tastes are unambiguously present. At these higher concentrations, the perception of some taste stimuli continues to be affected by temperature while the perception of others is relatively unaffected. In particular, Green and Frankmann (1987, 1988) showed that the perceived sweetness of sucrose (Figure 9-1), fructose, and glucose increased in intensity when the temperature of the solution was increased between 20° and 36°C, but to a degree that was inversely related to the concentration of the taste stimulus; the stronger the taste stimulus, the smaller was the effect of temperature. The same result had been observed earlier for sucrose alone (Bartoshuk et al., 1982; Calvino, 1986). Green and Frankmann (1987) also reported that the bitterness of caffeine grew stronger at warmer temperatures, whereas the sourness of citric acid and the saltiness of NaCl were not significantly altered (Figure 9-2). Overall, therefore, as temperature rises, perceptions of sweetness and bitterness tend to intensify, and perceptions of sourness and saltiness tend to remain the same. Because the effect of temperature is not uniform across compounds, it can be expected that the taste "profile" of a food will change as its temperature changes. If all else is equal, at hot temperatures bitter and sweet tastes should dominate salty and sour ones.

From a practical standpoint, these thermal effects are not particularly large. Although Green and Frankmann (1987) noted changes in the perceived intensity of sweetness as great as 100 percent, these perceptions only occurred when the temperature of the tongue—not just the temperature of the solution—had been changed by 16°C (from 36° to 20°C). Large changes in tongue temperature are difficult to produce under normal circumstances because of the tongue's abundant vascularization. Furthermore, these effects were obtained by cooling the tongue. Although other studies have shown that the trends observed for sweetness and bitterness between 20° and 36°C persist at solution temperatures above normal oral temperature (for example, Bartoshuk et al., 1982; Paulus and Reisch, 1980), the relationship between temperature and perceived intensity at very hot temperatures (for example, greater than 45°C or 113°F) has not been clearly worked out.

Touch

The "feel" of a food or beverage, produced by mechanical stimulation and mediated by the tactile sense, is an important but often overlooked aspect of flavor. The perception of food devoid of its tactile properties is difficult to imagine; foods would literally be intangible substances, and flavor would be rendered a disembodied sensory quality. It is consequently of interest to know if the temperature of a food affects its perceived tactile characteristics. Although no data exist that address this issue directly, it has been established that, in a manner similar to taste, the tactile sensitivity of the tongue changes as its temperature changes. In general, the sensitivity to so-called high-frequency vibration (greater than 100 Hz) varies directly with temperature between 20° and 36°C (Green, 1987). In contrast, the sensitiv-

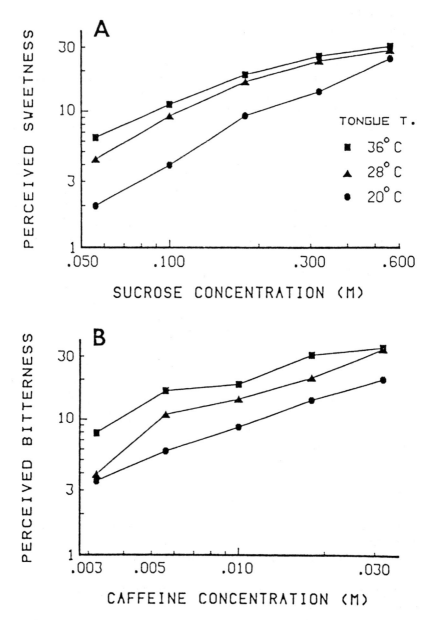

FIGURE 9-1 The effect of tongue temperature on perceptions of (A) the sweetness of sucrose and (B) the bitterness of caffeine. The parameter is the temperature of the tongue and the taste solutions. SOURCE: Green and Frankmann (1987), used with permission.

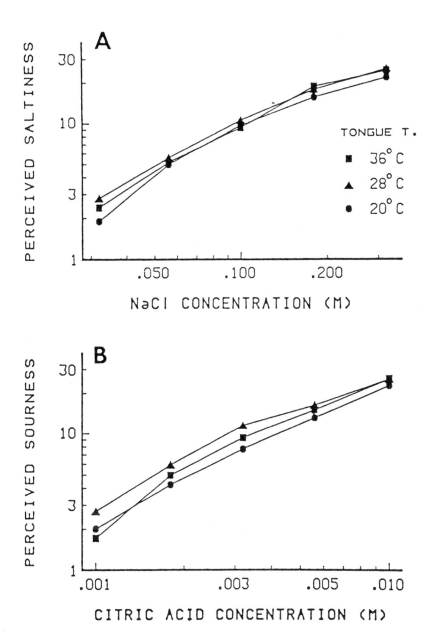

FIGURE 9-2 The effect of tongue temperature on perceptions of (A) the saltiness of NaCl and (B) the sourness of citric acid. Note that neither taste stimulus yielded a significant effect of temperature on perceived intensity. SOURCE: Green and Frankmann (1987), used with permission.

ity to low-frequency vibration remains independent of temperature. The sensitivity to vibration is important because virtually every mechanical stimulus—particularly those produced by complex forces like those associated with chewing—sets up vibrations in the skin. The differential effect of temperature across frequencies means that changing temperature does not simply blunt tactile sensitivity; rather, the quality as well as the quantity of the tactile sensation is likely to change. We can therefore expect that the texture of foods changes as their temperature does. A study of the effect of temperature on the perception of surface roughness perceived by the fingertip supports this hypothesis (Green et al., 1979).

In addition to its effects on the high-frequency components of mechanical stimulation, temperature probably also modulates the sensitivity of the mouth to simple pressure. Studies of the tactile sensitivity of the hand have shown that cooling blunts pressure sensitivity, and warming enhances it (Stevens et al., 1977). There is no reason to believe that the same trend does not occur in the oral mucosa.

Another, opposite, temperature-touch interaction also needs to be considered. It has long been known that when rested on the skin, cool objects are perceived as heavier than warm objects (Stevens and Green, 1978). This phenomenon, known as the Weber illusion, could well play a role in the perception of the mechanical characteristics of foods and beverages. Unlike the numbing effect of cooling the skin itself, cooling the stimulus tends to heighten (at least briefly) the mechanical component of sensation. Perhaps the initial pressure components of warm or hot oral stimuli are reduced relative to cool or cold stimuli.

How these various changes in tactile sensitivity affect the perception of foods and beverages has never been studied directly. What is required are experiments designed specifically to measure the effect of object and oral temperature on the perception of such dimensions as smoothness, creaminess, thickness, and roughness.

Chemical Irritation

Of the three forms of oral stimulation subject to thermal modulation, chemical irritation, or "chemesthesis" (Green, 1991; Green and Lawless, 1991), is the most vulnerable. By their nature, the sensory endings that mediate chemical irritation (nociceptors) are temperature sensitive. As a consequence, changing the temperature of the stimulus and tongue can drastically affect the sensitivity to an irritant. This effect has been most clearly demonstrated for capsaicin, the pungent compound in chili pepper (Green, 1986; Szolcsanyi, 1977). As shown in Figure 9-3, the burning sensation produced by capsaicin varies directly with the temperature of the solution

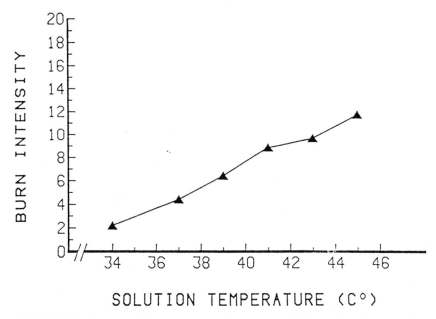

FIGURE 9-3 Perceived intensity of the burning sensation produced by capsaicin as a function of the temperature of the test solution. SOURCE: Green (1986), used with permission.

that contains it. In fact, by cooling the tongue to only about 25°C, the burning sensation induced by a moderate concentration of capsaicin can be completely eliminated (Green, 1986). This effect is readily apparent whenever one sips a cool beverage to quell the burning sensation produced by an overly "hot" spicy food; the burn is reduced almost instantly but rebounds after the beverage is swallowed and the mouth warms to its normal temperature.

Thermal effects are not limited to capsaicin. Although the effect may vary in magnitude across compounds, they have also been observed with piperine (black pepper), ethanol, and even the irritation produced by high concentrations of salt (Green, 1990). There is no doubt, therefore, that consuming foods that contain "hot" spices in a hot environment will increase the sensory impact of those foods. What effect this may have on consumption will likely vary markedly across individuals because of the wide range of individual differences in liking for "chemical heat" (Rozin and Schiller, 1980; Rozin et al., 1982). Hot spices do, however, trigger additional salivary flow (Lawless, 1984), which might prove to be a positive factor in a hot, dry environment.

Smell (Olfaction)

Despite the significant role odor plays in the formation of flavor, the effect of temperature on the perception of retronasal odors has not been studied. Based strictly on thermodynamics, one would expect that heating a food would increase the olfactory component of flavor by increasing the release of volatile compounds. Indeed, it is apparent in everyday experience that heating heightens the appreciation of odors sensed orthonasally; it would be very surprising if the same were not true of odors that originate in the mouth.

The effect on hedonics of thermal modulation of odors is more difficult to predict and would almost certainly depend on both the food being consumed and the preferences of the consumer. Too much of any odor can in theory become undesirable, and as appears to be the case with taste, touch, and probably chemesthesis, differential effects of temperature on the components of a complex odor would likely change the quality as well as the quantity of the olfactory experience.

PHYSIOLOGICAL AND PSYCHOLOGICAL EFFECTS OF TEMPERATURE

In addition to affecting the transduction and conduction of sensory information about foods, the thermal environment can also influence the flavor of foods indirectly via physiological and psychological factors. Given the paucity of information about direct thermal effects on flavor and flavor preference, it is not surprising that even less is known about possible indirect effects on these variables. What little is known suggests that physiological and psychological responses to extreme temperatures (in both the environment and the food) could, under some circumstances, be more important than sensory factors in determining flavor, hedonic tone, and eating behavior.

Serious consideration should be given, for example, to possible effects of heat-induced electrolyte imbalances on the perception of taste. Extreme sodium depletion has been shown to affect sensitivity to and preference for NaCl and salty foods (Beauchamp et al., 1990); however, such depletions are likely to occur only under the most dire circumstances, when survival itself is at stake. In general, studies that have investigated nutritional and metabolic effects on taste perception have usually found significant effects only when deficiencies of vitamins (for example, vitamin A or vitamin B) or minerals (for example, zinc) have been extreme (as in disease states) and associated with some form of lesion or tissue atrophy (Mattes and Kare, in press). But the occurrence of depletion effects under extreme, acute conditions at least raises the possibility that less severe depletions suffered over longer intervals might cause changes in the preference for and/or sensitivity to tastes or flavors.

Psychological factors can also play an important role in changes in taste preferences associated with changes in the temperature of foods. It is common experience that the temperature at which a food is consumed affects it liking (Brown et al., 1985; Zellner et al., 1988), and it has been shown that the temperature preferences that underlie these effects are largely a product of experience (Zellner et al., 1988). Thus, warm beer is less liked by consumers who normally drink chilled beer, whereas those who have always drunk it warm prefer it that way. However, the same study that demonstrated the importance of experience and expectation on the liking of foods and beverages (Zellner et al., 1988) also showed that the effect of temperature can be partially offset merely by changing consumers' expectations about the temperature of the comestible. The latter fact suggests that, given sufficient time and exposure, it should be possible to change temperature preferences to suit changing environmental needs. This is an important hypothesis; the extent to which it is true will determine how severe and long lasting the effects of a very hot (or very cold) environment may be on the perception and liking of foods.

SUMMARY AND SUGGESTIONS FOR FUTURE RESEARCH

The available data clearly show that temperature can be an important variable in flavor perception. However, its importance in real-world situations undoubtedly depends on numerous factors, including how extreme the thermal stimulus is, what kind of food is being consumed, the physiological condition of the individual, and the psychological "mind-set" he or she brings to the situation. Furthermore, the likelihood that complex interactions take place among these variables makes it very difficult to evaluate the importance of each. Future research should therefore seek to evaluate the effect of combining these variables in different ways and in different degrees.

Listed below are some of the issues relevant to the possible effects of extreme environmental temperatures on flavor perception that have not been addressed experimentally:

• What are the purely psychological effects of eating foods in unusually warm (or cold) environments (for example, does preferred serving temperature vary inversely with environmental temperature)?

• How, if at all, does environmental temperature (independent of serving temperature) affect the perception of the temperature of foods (for example, are there contrast or assimilation effects)?

• Does acclimatization to a harsh thermal environment produce changes in flavor preferences (that is, should different foods and beverages be made available before versus after acclimatization)?

• What might the combined effects on flavor perception be of reduced salivary flow (due to dehydration) and unusually high serving and environmental temperatures? Can salivary stimulants offset these effects?

• Should spicy, "hot" foods be avoided in very hot environments because of the heightened perception of oral heat they invoke?

• Could peppers be used to create the illusion of thermal heat when meals cannot be heated in the field? Conversely, might foods that contain artificial cooling agents, such as menthol, improve the experience of eating in hot environments by creating the illusion of coolness?

• Do foods that have strong flavors (that is, intense olfactory components) at cool ambient temperatures become less preferred in hot environments and at high serving temperatures?

A notable feature of most of these questions is that they can only be addressed in experiments conducted under conditions in which environmental temperature is controlled (for example, in an environmental chamber). Although the requirement of conducting experiments under controlled climatic conditions—or even on site in extreme environments—limits the number of investigators who would be able to undertake them, the hypotheses that have been generated in simple psychophysical studies must eventually be tested under realistic circumstances. This is particularly true given that the measurements of interest may well be influenced by psychological and physiological factors that are unique to thermally stressful environments.

ACKNOWLEDGMENT

Preparation of this paper, and some of the research reported in it, was supported by a research grant from the National Institutes of Health (DC00249).

REFERENCES

Bartoshuk, L.M., K. Rennert, H. Rodin, and J.C. Stevens
   1982   Effects of temperature on the perceived sweetness of sucrose. Physiol. Behav.
           28:905-910.
Beauchamp, G.K., M. Bertino, D. Burke, and K. Engelman
   1990   Experimental sodium depletion and salt taste in normal human volunteers. Am. J.
           Clin. Nutr. 51:881-889.
Brown, N.E., M.M. McKinley, L.E. Baltzer, and C.F. Opurum
   1985   Temperature preferences for a single entree. J. Am. Diet. Assoc. 85:1339-1341.
Calvino, A.M.
   1986   Perception of sweetness: The effects of concentration and temperature. Physiol.
           Behav. 36:1021-1028.

Green, B.G.
1986   Sensory interactions between capsaicin and temperature in the oral cavity. Chem. Sens. 11:371-382.
1987   The effect of cooling on the vibrotactile sensitivity of the tongue. Percept. Psychophys. 42:423-430.
1990   Effects of thermal, mechanical, and chemical stimulation on the perception of oral irritation. Pp. 171-192 in Chemical Senses. Vol. 2, Irritation, B.G. Green, J. R. Mason, and M.R. Kare, eds. New York: Marcel Dekker.
1991   Oral chemesthesis: The importance of time and temperature for the perception of chemical irritants. Pp. 107-123 in Sensory Science Theory and Applications in Foods, H.T. Lawless, and B.P. Klein, eds. New York: Marcel Dekker.
Green, B.G., and S.P. Frankmann
1987   The effect of cooling the tongue on the perceived intensity of taste. Chem. Sens. 12:609-619.
1988   The effect of cooling on the perception of carbohydrate and intensive sweeteners. Physiol. Behav. 43:515-519.
Green, B.G., and H.T. Lawless
1991   The psychophysics of somatosensory chemoreception in the nose and mouth. Pp. 235-253 in Smell and Taste in Health and Disease, T.V. Getchell, R.L. Doty, L.M. Bartoshuk, and J.B. Snow, eds. New York: Raven Press.
Green, B.G., S.J. Lederman, and J.C. Stevens
1979   The effect of skin temperature on the perception of roughness. Sens. Proc. 3:327-333.
Lawless, H.T.
1984   Oral chemical irritation: Psychophysical properties. Chem. Sens. 9:143-157.
Mattes, R.D., and M.R. Kare
In   Nutrition and the chemical senses. In Modern Nutrition in Health and Disease,
press   M.E. Shils, J.A. Olson, and M. Shike, eds. Philadelphia: Lea & Febiger.
McBurney, D.H., V.B. Collings, and L.M. Glanz
1973   Temperature dependence of human taste response. Physiol. Behav. 11:89-94.
Nakamura, M., and K. Kurihara
1991   Canine taste nerve responses to monosodium glutamate and disodium guanylate: Differentiation between umami and salt components with amiloride. Brain Res. 541:21-28.
Pangborn, R.M., R.B. Chrisp, and L.L. Bertolero
1970   Gustatory, salivary, and oral-thermal responses to solutions of sodium chloride at four temperatures. Percept. Psychophys. 8:69-75.
Paulus, K., and A.M. Reisch
1980   The influence of temperature on the threshold values of primary tastes. Chem. Sens. 5:11-21.
Rogers, P.J., and J.E. Blundell
1990   Umami and appetite: Effects of monosodium glutamate on hunger and food intake in human subjects. Physiol. Behav. 48:801-804.
Rozin, P., and D. Schiller
1980   The nature and acquisition of a preference for chili pepper by humans. Motiv. Emot. 4:77-101.
Rozin, P., L. Ebert, and J. Schull
1982   Some like it hot: A temporal analysis of hedonic responses to chili pepper. Appetite 3:13-22.
Stevens, J.C., and B.G. Green
1978   Temperature-touch interaction: Weber's phenomenon revisited. Sens. Proc. 2:206-219.

Stevens, J.C., B.G. Green, and A.S. Krimsley
  1977   Punctate pressure sensitivity: Effects of skin temperature. Sens. Proc. 1:238-243.
Szolcsanyi, J.
  1977   A pharmacological approach to elucidation of the role of different nerve fibres and
         receptor endings in mediation of pain. J. Physiol. (Paris) 73:251-259.
Zellner, D.A., W.F. Stewart, P. Rozin, and J.M. Brown
  1988   Effect of temperature and expectations on liking for beverages. Physiol. Behav.
         44:61-68.

DISCUSSION

DR. NESHEIM: Questions for Dr. Green?

PARTICIPANT: The point of the distinction of sour and sweet from pain was illustrated by comments from a number of soldiers about the hot sauce they were provided. They liked the hot sauce very much but many of them thought it was too sour. They didn't like the vinegar in it and they asked for just dry red pepper, as an alternative to the hot sauce.

DR. GREEN: Cayenne is basically capsaicin, and although it does have flavor components, one of the interesting things about capsaicin is that it has virtually no taste. It is therefore an ideal food additive, in that sense, because you can add a sensory dimension without also adding possibly negative flavors—like sourness.

PARTICIPANT: Are there individuals who are particularly sensitive to some of these food additives? Some people tell me that they are sensitive to pepper, for example. Is there a danger if we cook these items in the food rather than let the individual add it to the food that people many not like the food?

DR. GREEN: Absolutely. We see it in the laboratory. That is one of the difficulties in studying capsaicin. There are large individual differences in the tolerance and their liking capsaicin.

Some people come into the lab eager to be tested; others won't agree to do the study even for pay because they simply don't eat hot and spicy foods.

So yes, I think including capsaicin or cayenne as something that could be added to the food rather than already in the food is critical.

I also think the ability to have control over a flavor component may also be very important in fighting the monotony issue.

PARTICIPANT: Are you saying, then, with menthol you would have a similar figure that indicated people perceived greater coolness as temperature decreased?

DR. GREEN: Yes, we have done those studies. The difference in the cooling effect doesn't vary much with temperature, which means that menthol has a reasonably strong impact even at room temperature.

And of course, even if you eat a relatively hot food that has menthol in it, once it coats your oral cavity, just breathing through your mouth produces evaporative cooling. Menthol enhances the effect of evaporative cooling; it is as though you are breathing cooler air.

PARTICIPANT: Is that what menthol does in cigarettes?

DR. GREEN: Yes. However, I am told by experts at the tobacco companies that people don't like menthol in cigarettes to counteract the heat as much as they merely enjoy it as another sensory dimension.

PARTICIPANT: It has been published that when people have to drink volumes of water for sweat fluid replacement—that is to say, between 12 and 18 quarts a day—that the preferred temperature is somewhere between 14° and 17°C (55° to 60 °F).

My own experience from the southwestern deserts of the United States, is that this temperature estimate is a bit high. Do you have any feeling or could you make any comments?

DR. GREEN: The only feeling I have about it is that you are speaking about field tests in an extreme climate. One of the things that needs to be done—perhaps it has been done for thirst—is to look at possible effects of acclimatization on preferred temperatures. Perhaps once you become acclimatized to a hot environment, you prefer to avoid a sharp, cold contrast in favor of a more mild coolness.

PARTICIPANT: Are there any systematic racial or gender differences?

DR. GREEN: With regard to the basic tastes, I know of no significant racial or gender differences.

There is a gender effect with irritants in the nose but not in the mouth; females tend to be more sensitive than males. There are also some data which suggest that odor sensitivity varies across the menstrual cycle.

A bigger factor in each of these modalities, though, is individual differences. There are large individual differences in the chemical senses.

PARTICIPANT: Do sour stimuli give any sensations of coolness?

DR. GREEN: Not that I am aware of.

People have, in the past, tried to associate tastes with temperatures the same way that colors have been associated with temperature. For example, sweetness is thought of as being warm, salt as being less warm. I don't know where sourness might fit in.

DR. NESHEIM: Thank you, Barry.

10

Effects of Heat on Appetite

C. Peter Herman[1]

INTRODUCTION

Hot environments induce efforts to stay cool. This chapter addresses the issue of how one's food intake is adjusted to compensate for environmental heat. Common knowledge suggests that people eat less when it is hot, and that they eat "lighter" and "cooler" foods. (This impression is reinforced by a casual survey of newspaper and magazine suggestions for summer meal planning.) As with most impressions derived from common knowledge, systematic evidence is needed to support these assertions. What does the scientific literature have to say about the effects of heat on food intake and food selection? What follows is a review of the available scientific literature on the effects of heat on appetite. This literature has been supplemented by a survey designed specifically for this chapter (consumer survey, University of Toronto, unpublished data, 1991). Because of the anticipation that the scientific literature, especially on humans, might be skimpy, a questionnaire was sent to a number of restaurant and grocery chains in the metropolitan Toronto area asking about shifts in customer purchasing behavior as a function of environmental heat. This survey is by no means scientific, but it reflects the accumulated experience of merchants whose livelihood depends to some extent on accurately assessing how people's food purchases vary with the heat.

---

[1] C. Peter Herman, The Department of Psychology, University of Toronto, 100 St. George Street, Toronto, Ontario, CANADA M5S 1A5

Before examining the available data on the effects of heat on appetite, some preliminary considerations require attention, including a definition of terms. *Heat* can be defined in number of ways. Environmental temperature varies seasonally in the moderate climates in which most of the research is done, so one may ask whether appetite differs in summer and winter. Even within the seasons, of course, there may be considerable variability in temperature; does appetite suffer during a summer heat wave as compared to normal summer weather? Even more acute variations in temperature are available for examination, owing to the prevalence of air-conditioning. If, during a summer heat wave, one eats in an air-conditioned dining room, is appetite controlled by the outdoor or indoor temperature? Aside from temperature changes in the normal environment, one might also want to look at changes of environment. A winter trip to the tropics probably represents a greater short-term shift in temperature than might be encountered if one stayed put; how does it affect appetite?

To further complicate matters, how hot one feels is not simply a matter of the environment; one's own activity may generate heat, so that being active may be functionally equivalent to raising the environmental temperature. Indeed, eating itself has thermogenic effects, so that not only does heat affect appetite, but appetite may affect heat.

The meaning of *appetite* should also be clarified. There is tremendous variability in what scientists mean when they use the term (Herman and Vaccarino, 1992). Ordinarily, to achieve some clarity, one must distinguish among three terms that are often used interchangeably and confusingly. Appetite refers to the subjective desire to eat, whereas *hunger* usually refers to a more objective deprivation state. These terms are not unrelated, but it is preferable to think of hunger as a true need that often produces a felt desire (appetite). Distinguishing between hunger and appetite becomes useful when considering the possibility that one may desire to eat something even in the absence of a need for it. Conceivably, one might also be hungry without recognizing it or feeling a desire to eat, as is allegedly the case with some anorexia nervosa patients.

The third appetite-related term requiring attention is *intake*. In the scientific literature, food intake is often taken to be an operationalization of appetite, especially in nonhuman species where the animal's desires must be inferred from its behavior. In humans, it is quite possible to distinguish between what the person wants (appetite) or needs (hunger), on the one hand, and what the person eats (intake), on the other. People sometimes eat when they experience neither hunger nor appetite. Conversely, people sometimes refrain from eating despite experiencing hunger or appetite or both. For instance, Rolls et al. (1990) found, in a study related to temperature that is reviewed below, almost no relationship between how hungry or sated people claimed to be, on the one hand, and how much they subsequently ate, on the other. In this chapter, owing to the fact that the literature largely ignores the distinctions just suggested, the effect of heat on appetite, hunger, and intake is considered collectively, with the awareness that heat may affect one of these without affecting the others. Use of the term *appetite* in a general or unqualified sense should be understood to refer to all three constructs.

One final preliminary caution. The mandate here was to examine the effect of heat on appetite in humans. For perhaps understandable reasons, a high proportion of the scientific research on appetite and on heat effects has been conducted on nonhumans. In what follows, preference will be given to human studies. Caution is urged in extrapolating from rats and other species to humans, but the paucity of human data requires reference to animal studies for clues as to how human appetite is affected by heat.

ENVIRONMENTAL TEMPERATURE, EATING, AND THERMOREGULATION

Any discussion of the effects of heat on eating must begin with a recognition that eating represents the basic means of securing energy for humans. Most analyses of heat and eating go one step further and point out that a major physiological concern of humans is thermoregulation—the maintenance of an appropriate body temperature—and that eating provides a major contribution to maintaining body heat (Brobeck, 1948). Indeed, it may be that "the important factor in regulation of food intake is not its energy value, but rather the amount of extra heat released in its assimilation" (Strominger and Brobeck, 1953). Thus, this "thermostatic hypothesis" of feeding argues that the total energy content of the food is not the determining factor in regulation. Energy that becomes stored as fat does not control feeding; rather, it is the direct heating effect of food intake that is monitored and that provides a regulatory mechanism.

According to this view, if the environment is cold, the resultant heat loss demands compensatory strategies, including notably increased food intake for its thermic effect. By extension, if the ambient temperature is warm, and heat loss is not an issue, there ought to be a reduced caloric demand. And should the environment become significantly hot—which changes the concern from how to obtain energy to how to dissipate it—a suppression of caloric intake should be expected. "At a high temperature where loss of heat is difficult, food intake should be low, lest by eating and assimilating food the body acquire more heat than it can dispose of" (Brobeck, 1948). This temperature-dependent variation in energy needs should, in principle, be reflected in appetite. Brobeck (1948) claims that "everyone knows . . . that appetite fails in hot weather."

The inverse relation of appetite to environmental temperature may be examined in a number of different ways. Clearly, one might manipulate (or exploit naturally occurring variations in) ambient temperature and examine indices of appetite. One might manipulate (or exploit naturally occurring variations in) body temperature independent of environmental temperature—as in fever—and determine whether this form of hyperthermia suppresses appetite. Alternatively, one might manipulate the need to acquire or dissipate energy more indirectly, through exercise; exercise, by providing a short-term boost in internal heat, ought to reduce the need for further energy—in short, appetite should be suppressed. In the long-term, by depleting short-term energy stores, exercise should increase the cumulative demand for energy repletion.

A final research strategy involves examining the influence of eating itself. Food intake itself creates heat, in addition to providing stored energy for future use. The heat attendant on eating and digestion (the thermic effect of food) as well as the heat produced through the processes of postprandial thermogenesis, which is experienced when humans perspire or become flushed after overeating, ought to reduce appetite acutely. Eating-induced thermogenesis presumably combines with environmental heat, so that appetite will be more suppressed after a given mean in a hot environment than in a cold environment, all things being equal.

An inferential caution: Considerable research has been devoted to the effects of cold environments on physiology and behavior, including appetite. If cold exposure increases appetite compared to appetite under normal conditions, one might be tempted to conclude that heat exposure above normal levels should have the opposite effect. For example, if people eat more than normal when the ambient temperature drops from 70° to 55°F, one might be inclined to infer that appetite would be reduced below normal if the temperature were raised to 85°F. This temptation might be justified by the data, but in the absence of specific research on heat exposure, one should be cautious about extrapolating from research on cold exposure. Does unusual heat have the opposite effect from unusual cold? That is an empirical question.

Another inferential caution: The immediately foregoing analysis assumes that body temperature is regulated and that the heat generated by eating represents a major element in the regulatory equation. But temperature may not be the only important regulated variable. It is now widely believed that body weight or body fat or some associated variable is also regulated (for a review see Mrosovsky, 1990). Moreover, there is reason to believe that the level at which body weight/fat (hereafter BW) is regulated may shift in response to various inputs, perhaps including environmental temperature. What if the set-point for BW drops in the heat? (This would be a reasonable adaptive strategy physiologically, because humans require less insulation when the environmental temperature is high in order to maintain a comfortable body temperature. Note that the supposition of a BW set-point is not an alternative to the supposition of thermoregulation, but rather a complementary assumption.) If it is assumed that BW set-point drops in the summer or in response to elevated temperature in general, then the explanation for the finding that humans eat less in the heat becomes slightly more complicated. The more complicated interpretation is that heat lowers BW set-point and that appetite subsides because the animal's current weight is now excessive relative to set-point. Hyperthermia following excessive eating may contribute to the decline in intake, but increased heat dissipation and decreased intake may both be understood as mechanisms in the service of attaining a lowered level of BW, which in turn may be a mechanism in the service of more efficient thermoregulation in the heat. These regulatory adaptations, then, would seem to operate in concert. Mapping these causes and effects in a simple linear way is difficult at best and may not do justice to the mutual accommodations of physiological and behavioral systems.

The elegance and apparent prevalence of such regulatory adaptations in nature should not lead to the assumption without question that any change observed is necessarily perfectly functional. It is eminently possible that adaptation to one sort of challenge may prove to be contraadaptive in some other sense (see Mrosovsky [1990], for numerous examples of regulatory conflict). In the present example, it is certainly possible that a decline in appetite in response to heat—should it occur—will not be mediated by a lowering of BW set-point; rather, the set-point may remain where it began, and lowered BW may represent a departure from the regulated value. The consequence would be that people who eat less and lose weight or fat in a hot climate will become underweight relative to set-point. This relative underweight may apply even to obese individuals, whose BW set-point and/ or thermoregulatory set-point may be inordinately high (Wilson and Sinha, 1985). The consequences may be stressful, both physiologically and psychologically. Animals and people who maintain a BW below set-point show aberrant eating patterns, hyperemotionality (including irritability), distractibility, and a reduced sex drive (Nisbett, 1972). If heat does indeed drive appetite and BW downward, it would be important to know whether it does so in conjunction with a shift in BW set-point or in defiance of a stable set-point. It has been argued (Pénicaud et al., 1986) that temperature control has primacy over food intake control, albeit perhaps only in the short term. As long as such primacy is evident, it should not be surprising to discover disorder in the feeding system and perhaps further disorders at the psychological (emotional) and behavioral (performance) level.

Because analyzing the effects of heat on appetite presupposes an appreciation of the effects of appetite on thermoregulation, the latter question will be addressed first. Having gained a sense of the effects of appetite on heat, readers may then be in a better position to comprehend the effects of heat on appetite.

EFFECTS OF EATING ON THERMOREGULATION

Owing to the thermic effect of eating and metabolism, eating should be expected to provide warmth. This is certainly the case. "Food has a marked effect on body temperature; the temperature difference between a fed animal and an unfed one in the same cage, in the same room, at the same time can vary as much as one full degree F. This difference is due to the specific dynamic action of food" (Beller, 1977). This effect extends fully to humans; for example, Dallosso and James (1984) found that a 50 percent increase in caloric intake by the addition of fat to the diet produced a 47 percent increase in the thermic effects of eating. Eating ground beefsteak and stewed tomatoes to satiety raised skin temperature an average of 2°C about 1 hour after the meal (Booth and Strang, 1936).

Experimental demonstrations of increased metabolic rate, oxygen consumption, and thermogenesis are now so well established that research focuses mainly on subtleties of the response. For instance, LeBlanc and Cabanac (1989) recently demonstrated that the postprandial thermogenic effect has both a cephalic and a gastrointestinal phase; remarkably, the cephalic effect—which was evident in subjects who did not even swallow the food but who merely chewed and spit it out—was even stronger than was the subsequent gastrointestinal effect in subjects who consumed the food. In dogs, a large thermic effect was obtained when the animals were exposed only to the sight and smell of food for 3 minutes (LeBlanc and Diamond, 1986). Thus, eating produces heat, as was known all along; and even sensory exposure to food may produce conditioned or anticipatory thermogenesis or both. One possibly remote implication of this research is that in order to prevent thermogenetic increases in body heat, one may be required to avoid not only eating but all the sensory trappings of food.

Hypothalamic disturbances that produce substantial weight gain may do so at least partially by suppressing the heat dissipation by brown adipose tissue (BAT) that normally follows a meal (Hogan et al., 1986), although medially lesioned rats continue to show BAT activation during cold exposure (Hogan et al., 1982). This finding suggests that the lesioned rat, in defending an artificially higher BW set-point, will store whatever additional calories it can but not if its thermoregulation is threatened. Numerous studies (for example, Booth and Strang, 1936; Segal et al., 1987) have found a blunted thermogenic response to eating in obese humans.

If the suppression of appetite observed during heat exposure drives BW levels below set-point, this heat-induced appetite suppression might be expected to be accompanied by greater metabolic efficiency. A reduced intake, accordingly, should not be cause for concern. And if heat-induced appetite suppression is accompanied or caused by a lowering of the BW set-point, then there is all the more reason to avoid forced feeding, because such hyperphagia would probably lead to hyperthermia. (At 40°C, rats will stop feeding altogether, and if force fed by intubation, they suffer heat stress and occasionally die [Hamilton, 1967].) Either way, reduced intake in the heat would seem to be adaptive. The only issue concerns activity, which, if intensified, ought to place extra demands on energy stores. The prudent recommendation for heat exposure would seem to be to allow for reduced intake but to avoid, as much as possible, strenuous activity, which not only requires more energy but also generates more undesirable heat, and which also puts fluid balance in jeopardy. Reduced activity is a natural response to heat exposure. If bursts of activity are unavoidable, care should be taken to allow, as much as possible, for longer than normal metabolic recovery periods.

Although eating causes thermogenesis, it does not follow automatically that all thermogenesis will feed back as a regulator of eating. Glick et al. (1989) abolished the thermogenic response of brown adipose tissue during and after feeding in rats but found no indication that meal size was augmented, as would be expected under, say, Brobeck's (1948) theory, if heat provided a satiety signal. It remains true that "increases in body and brain temperature do not coincide exactly with the cessation of feeding" (Balagura, 1973). Of course, the apparent unimportance of BAT thermogenesis in the control of appetite does not mean that endogenous heat in general is irrelevant to the regulatory control of appetite. Rampone and Reynolds (1991) have recently outlined a proposal—a "fine-tuning" of Brobeck's (1948) proposal—in which diet-induced thermogenesis feeds back to activate temperature-sensitive neurons in the rostral hypothalamus, which in turn activate the ventromedial hypothalamus to induce satiety. They explain hyperphagia and weight gain as the result of inadequate diet-induced thermogenesis and consequent inadequate satiety, with the result that the animal takes in more energy than it expends. Consistent with this notion is the finding that animals with rostral lesions both overeat and become hyperthermic (Hamilton and Brobeck, 1964).

It should be noted that even if the abolition of all thermogenesis failed to affect satiety or the duration and/or size of a meal, it would not follow logically that thermogenesis is unimportant in the control of appetite. Conceivably, feeding might be responsive to the lack of energy/heat in the "system." Meal-induced thermogenesis might not act as a satiety signal, but still serve to delay the onset of a drop in heat below some threshold that serves as a hunger signal. In other words, the focus in this chapter on heat as a satiety signal fails to address the initiation of eating. Perhaps energy depletions as hunger signals ought to be considered, in which case heat might well remain an important determinant of feeding but more at the onset end than at the offset end. The unwarranted but prevalent assumption that the same types of signals control both meal termination and meal initiation—as in Rampone and Reynolds' (1991) hypothesis that heat induces satiety and cold induces hunger—adds to the confusion in this area. In general, more attention should be paid to whether the effect of heat on appetite suppression is expressed in terms of smaller meals (presumptive satiety effects) or less frequent meals (presumptive hunger effects); of course, these alternatives are not perfectly independent of one another. The frustratingly speculative nature of the foregoing discussion, in fact, is a reflection of the fact that "in most cases the measurement of postprandial heat [has been] undertaken with a totally different objective than that of assessing its effects on food intake" (Rampone and Reynolds, 1991). Thus, the call for more research may be extended to all aspects of endogenous heat production as a moderator of appetite.

Lack of adequate food induces cold. Keys et al. (1950) found that their semistarved volunteers complained of the cold even in warm summer weather. One might be tempted to suggest underfeeding troops in hot climates in order to minimize their problems with heat. Although a somewhat reduced intake is probably desirable and inevitable, given the various regulatory pressures that are activated automatically, deliberate food restriction below what the troops naturally desire would probably not be desirable, owing to all the negative effects of maintaining a suboptimal body weight. Metabolism is, if anything, speeded up in the heat and intake is reduced; the net effect is likely to be significant weight loss, and if that weight loss occurs in the absence of a resetting of the BW set-point, the result is likely to be a substantial energy deficit.

Most humans are not built to operate optimally in extremes of temperature. If faced with severe heat, people may reduce their intake and rely on metabolic processes to dissipate as much heat as possible, but this ultimately represents a loss of energy that might well interfere with other demands placed on them (for example, demands for intense activity). The solution, it would seem, is to avoid severe heat and function in a climate where thermoregulation is not a difficult challenge. Hot environments by definition provide such a challenge, but the best solution may be to find ways to keep cool, or at least thermoneutral, other than—or in addition to—reducing intake.

Climatic Adaptation

Physique

The ability to dissipate heat depends on various factors, not the least of which is physique. Bergmann's rule states that a bulkier shape minimizes heat loss, because the bulkier animal has a relatively smaller ratio of skin surface to metabolically active bulk, and skin surface determines heat dissipation (Beller, 1977). Allen's corollary to Bergmann's rule gives a heat-dissipating advantage to those with longer appendages. Accordingly, people with rounded physiques (endomorphs) should have more difficulty with heat dissipation than will those with linear physiques (ectomorphs). Presumably, a given meal will produce greater thermic overload for the endomorph, who ought to learn, eventually, to eat less in the interests of thermoregulatory comfort.

There is substantial evidence that people adapt to a hot climate. Of course, eating less may be construed as an adaptation par excellence; but other related adaptations have been proposed. It is suggested above that heat can drive one's set-point for BW downward. Physical anthropologists (see Beller, 1977 for a fascinating review) have long noted a correspondence between physique and climate (Bergmann's rule, noted above). That linear physiques generally do better in the heat may be seen as an evolutionary selection principle, with races adapting to hot environments by altering their physique in an ectomorphic direction. One strong implication of this adaptational point of view is that certain people will do better in a hot environment than will others. Presumably, an individual who is genetically preadapted to a hot climate will have less trouble adapting to such a climate; such a displacement ought to disrupt his or her eating patterns less.

More pertinent to this discussion, perhaps, is the question of individual rather than evolutionary adaptation. Does, or can, an individual's set-point shift in response to heat exposure? If so, then the individual should feel uncomfortably overweight on initial exposure and cut back on eating; with a reduced set-point, the individual would eventually maintain a lower BW, and show a continued suppression of appetite appropriate for his or her more svelte physique.

Adaptation to Heat or Cold?

Interestingly, the endomorphy of a population is not correlated with mean annual temperature so much as with mean January temperature in northern latitudes (Beller, 1977). This finding has a number of implications, foremost among which is that normative BW depends more on extremes of cold than on heat. As an adaptation, this makes sense, because in these northern or temperate latitudes—and even in some tropical latitudes where the temperature occasionally plummets—the risk of insufficient fat/energy is greater than the risk of an excess of fat/energy. When one focuses on adaptation to hot climates, the implications are confusing. The main threat facing an individual in the hot climate would seem to be a failure of thermoregulation: heat dissipation is the main concern. Yet if the nighttime temperature drops precipitously, as may happen in the desert, then heat adaptation during the day may be more than cancelled out by cold adaptation at night. Conceivably, cold desert nights could lead to a continuing high BW set-point, with dire implications for heat dissipation during the day. Even excessive use of air-conditioning might make heat adaptation and successful thermoregulation difficult.

It's Not the Heat, It's the Humidity

We think of high humidity as impairing our ability to perspire; humidity ought to impair heat dissipation and render the "functional temperature" even higher (for an overview see Burse, 1979). Heat combined with humidity should have a greater suppressive effect on appetite than dry heat. The anthropological evidence is confusing on this point. In Africa, humidity tends to be associated with a shorter, fatter physique in the native people, whereas in more northern climates (for example, Scandinavia), the wetter west coast breeds taller, thinner people than does the drier interior (Beller, 1977).

Gender Differences

There is reason to believe that men may be less heat tolerant than women. Beller (1977) notes that men have more, and a higher proportion of, metabolically active tissue than do women, who have a higher proportion of fat, and suggests that women's relative metabolic inactivity buffers them from heat stress. Beller goes even further and argues that women's extra fat tissue literally buffers them, by insulating them, from the external heat. It makes sense that a layer of fat might insulate one's internal core temperature from external heat sources; but such insulation should also make it more difficult to dissipate whatever heat is generated internally, through metabolism. Beller's conclusion is disputed, although not cited, by Burse (1979), who enumerates the physiological disadvantages of women working in the heat and urges that extreme caution be taken to prevent heat exhaustion in unacclimatized women.

Stress

Under acute stress, body temperature may rise. For example, boxers before a bout have a higher body temperature than they do before a routine practice. Mrosovsky (1990) refers to this temperature shift as *psychogenic hyperthermia* and attributes to it an enhancement of muscular activity. "The psychogenic contribution to such warming up may be to shift the thermoregulatory set-point" upward (Mrosovsky, 1990). To the extent that stress elevates the thermoregulatory set-point—or simply adds metabolic heat even without raising the thermoregulatory set-point—it should exacerbate whatever heat dissipation threats are encountered in hot climates. On balance, stress should further suppress appetite. Previous research concurs with this expectation, in that normal eaters in both laboratory and field settings have responded to stress by decreasing their food intake (Herman and Vaccarino, 1992). The major exception to this rule is provided by dieters, who often overeat in response to distress; presumably most military personnel would not fall into this category. Military personnel, however, are quite likely to experience stress independent of heat, and the suppressive effect on appetite must be taken into account. Such stress may have debilitating effects on its own, to which may be added whatever stress stems from long-term hunger, such as may occur if stress suppresses appetite without a corresponding suppression of BW set-point.

Activity

One effective short-term technique for achieving thermoregulation is activity, because strenuous activity has a thermogenic effect (Bellward and Dauncey, 1988). Animals who are energy-deficient (either cold or hungry) become more likely to move around; such activity both provides endogenous heat directly and makes it more likely that exogenous energy sources may be encountered. Eventually, this strategy may backfire, if the extra expenditure of energy is not repleted; but in the short-term, the animal will be closer to a thermal optimum. Lassitude in the heat, conversely, probably serves a useful physiological purpose and should not be countermanded as assiduously as it might be in a temperate climate.

Food Temperature

If food contains energy, and its thermic effect depends on the amount of that energy plus the assimilative cost of consuming and digesting it, then it should follow that adding energy to the food by heating it ought to have a relatively straightforward additive effect on the food's thermic value. Conversely, cold food ought to minimize the thermic effect of eating. Indeed, one gets the impression that if the food is served at a temperature significantly below body temperature it will have a cooling effect; this cooling effect should be more reinforcing for people who are hyperthermic.

Eating tends to add energy in the form of heat to the body; if the heat-exposed individual must eat, he or she should presumably prefer a cool version of a food to a hot version, on thermic grounds. But the hot version may in general be perceived as more palatable, insofar as warming brings out the presumably pleasant flavor of the food (Trant and Pangborn, 1983). Cabanac (1971) might argue that the enhanced palatability of warmed food might be a conditional preference, based on the thermic effect of the food. Negative alliesthesia effects (that is, decreased acceptability) might be expected for warm food as the internal environment heats up. In other words, warm food may not be intrinsically more palatable; rather, its palatability may depend directly on the state of the organism (in this case, whether the organism is hypo- or hyperthermic). For Cabanac, it is not that the hot food is rejected by the heat-exposed individual despite its greater palatability but because heat exposure detracts from the food's palatability.

That heat exposure might shift one's preferences away from hot food and toward cool food is understandable. But another question arises: Should heat exposure increase one's attraction to cool foods rather than to no food at all? Cooling food produces a peculiar condition: the food still contains latent calories and is likely on those grounds to raise body temperature; but the cool physical state of the food is likely to have an immediately cooling effect in the mouth and perhaps even further down the alimentary canal. From a thermoregulatory point of view, is the hyperthermic individual better off consuming a cool food or none at all?

Type of Food

It is widely accepted that "the amount of . . . added heat, of course, varies with the type . . . of food consumed" (Rampone and Reynolds, 1991). Yet there appears to be only a small variation in the thermic effect of food depending on the type of food ingested. "Eating proteins, which are somewhat more complicated to break down inside the body than carbohydrates or fats are, tends to raise body temperature very slightly more than these other two basic food components do" (Beller, 1977). Beller goes on to note (pages 157 to 158) that "this difference has probably received more attention than it deserves in the popular literature about nutrition," an allusion to the allegedly weight-reducing properties of a high-protein diet. Balagura (1973), in discussing this issue, notes that in general, animals prefer carbohydrate diets and especially prefer fat diets over protein diets, so the fact that eating terminates sooner on protein diets may be more a function of the diets' limited palatability than of their greater thermic effect. Of course, in nonhumans, palatability is often difficult to disentangle from eating itself; but in humans, the expressed preference for fats and sweets is well known (Drewnowski et al., 1989), so that if less of a high protein diet is consumed, it may well be due to taste and texture factors rather than to thermal satiety feedback. Whether in making diet prescriptions we ought to consider the thermic effect of macronutrients—or confine ourselves to a consideration of basic nutritional balance—is difficult to assess at present.

EFFECTS OF HEAT ON APPETITE

Effects of Environmental Temperature Variations on Amount Eaten

Acute Variations

Humans One of the earliest systematic reports of the effect of heat on appetite was Johnson and Kark's (1947) summary of ad lib intakes by soldiers in various geographic areas ranging from the mobile force "Musk Ox," stationed in the Canadian Arctic, to infantry troops on Luzon in the Philippines. Troops stationed in the tropics ate on average 3100 calories, whereas arctic troops ate 4900 calories; in both cases, troops were allegedly offered as much food as they wanted, although the skeptical reader might be able to imagine some interpretive confoundings in these results. Whether the size of the heat effect on appetite is as profound as suggested by Johnson and Kark is debatable, but the direction of the effect has not been disputed. Edholm et al. (1964) confirmed this pattern, observing a 25 percent decrease in food intake by soldiers in Aden compared to the United Kingdom (see also Collins and Weiner, 1968). More parochially, one Toronto restaurateur (unpublished data from consumer survey, 1991) conceded that "sales plunge during a heat wave . . . . People do not have the appetite for a large heavy meal when it is hot." Beller (1977) neatly summarized the effect of heat on appetite, explaining it on the basis of the thermic effect of food:

> The ability to raise body temperature through feeding is one that is shared by all warm-blooded animals. Cattle, swine, rats, goats, and U.S. Army men all eat more when the temperature is low than when it is high, and the reverse is equally true: at environmental temperatures of 90°F feeding begins to slow down in all these animals, and by the time rectal temperatures reach 104° (which is not an unheard-of reading, incidentally, for a man doing strenuous exercise for more than a few minutes at a time) virtually all species stop feeding entirely. This state of affairs is true not only for man and other homeotherms but for such disparate creatures as toads, single-celled paramecia, and honeybees (although the critical temperature maximum for a honeybee may not be quite the same as it is for a toad—or, of course, a man).

Logue (1986) makes the same point more colloquially: "An easy way to quell appetites at a summer dinner party is to turn off the air-conditioning." These generalizations suggest that acute temperature variations have a strong effect on appetite: specifically, heat impairs appetite. (And note that the implication of the turned-off air-conditioning scenario is that had the air-conditioning stayed on, appetite would have remained unquelled, despite it being summer. This suggests that acute temperature variations may have a significant effect over and above seasonal variations. The consumer survey (unpublished, 1991) yielded a strong consensus about the effect of air-conditioning on customer behavior. In the summer, "air-conditioning attracts customers and after sitting in the restaurant, many order 'normally'. . . . If we have an air-conditioning breakdown, sales drop dramatically." The summer peak in ice cream sales is much more noticeable in street outlets than in mall outlets, although it is unclear whether this is because the malls are air-conditioned in the summer or because they are heated in the winter. One ice cream chain blamed the increasing prevalence of air-conditioning for its slower gain in sales in recent years. It is worth noting here that there is some lingering confusion about whether the effect of air-conditioning on appetite (countering heat-induced appetite changes) depends on acute effects (that is, air-conditioning at the eating site) or more chronic effects (that is, exposure to air-conditioning through much of the day). Presumably the answer to this question depends on whether chronic exposure to air-conditioning counteracts a heat-induced drop in BW setpoint.

It is not clear what happens in an environment that is naturally hot much of the time but which cools off dramatically at other times. Such dramatic cooling may occur naturally at nighttime, or even during the day, with the advent of air-conditioning. How responsive is appetite to abrupt shifts in environmental temperature? Does one's appetite pick up when leaving the broiling heat to enter an air-conditioned dining room? Or does the pressure to dissipate heat carry over even in the air-conditioned environment? The same questions can be asked when substituting "cool nights" for "air-conditioning." One study, albeit on rats, speaks at least indirectly to this question. Refinetti (1988) examined feeding in rats that were housed in normal (29°C) or cold (19°C) conditions and fed in a separate chamber that was either normal temperature or cold. Both housing and feeding environment temperatures additively affected appetite; thus, the temperature that obtains when eating occurs does affect eating, but there is also some carryover from the external environment. One possibly significant finding in this study is that animals who went to a cold environment to feed gained much more weight than did animals who remained in a warm environment to feed. The finding suggests that if one spends most of one's time in the heat but eats in an artificially cooled environment, one might end up eating more than needed, with potential problems for heat dissipation when one returns to the hot environment.

Nonhumans Research on the effects of variations in environmental temperature on feeding was stimulated by Brobeck's (1948) hypothesis. He found that rats' food intake dropped precipitously as the environmental temperature rose from 18° to 36°C; these rats, acclimated to a temperature of 28° to 29°C, began to lose weight when the environmental temperature during feeding rose above 32°C. Numerous other investigators have found equivalent results with rats (Fletcher, 1986; Hamilton and Brobeck, 1964; Jakubczak, 1976; Leon and Woodside, 1983) and with other species, such as goats (Appleman and Delouche, 1959) that eat less and hoard less (Fantino and Cabanac, 1984) and frequently lose weight in hotter ambient temperatures. Kraly and Blass (1976) found that rats will work harder for food and consume more unpalatable food in the cold. Mice eat 43 percent less in an ambient temperature of 33°C than at 17°C (Thurlby, 1979; see also Donhoffer and Vonotzky, 1947), and pigs that were maintained at 32° to 35°C ate only half as much as pigs maintained at 10° to 12°C (Heath, 1980; Macari et al., 1986). Note that Swiergiel and Ingram (1986) found that piglets maintained at 35°C gained more weight than did piglets maintained at 10°C, but the intake levels appeared to have been controlled in this study; the higher BW of the 35°C piglets may have represented their attempt to store energy rather than burn it. Cafeteria-fed rats maintained at 29°C ate less, but if anything gained more weight than did those maintained at 24°C, presumably because in the hotter environment the rats became much more energy efficient, storing their excess calories rather than burning them and risking hyperthermia (Rothwell and Stock, 1986). Presumably in severe heat, thermogenic disposal of calories would pose enough of a threat so that the animal would quickly learn to cut back on its intake.

More proximal heating (that is, in the preoptic and anterior hypothalamic regions) serves to inhibit feeding in much the same way as does distal heating (that is, in the external environment) (Andersson and Larsson, 1961). This simply indicates that the effects of environmental heat must be registered somewhere in the central nervous system if they are to affect feeding; the hypothalamic tracts remain the prime candidates for the coordination of heat-and-feeding regulation. Other loci, such as the liver (DiBella et al., 1981) and even the skin (Booth and Strang, 1936), have also been nominated as crucial in producing regulatory thermal feedback in the control of eating.

In general, "reduced intake in warm environments [has] been shown in several endothermic animals" (Refinetti, 1988). One exception to the rule that animals eat less when it is hot is contained in a study by Bellward and Dauncey (1988); in this study, mice ate more at above-normal temperatures than at below-normal temperatures. The explanation for this contrary effect supports the general approach here: mice had to choose between heat (exposure to a heat lamp) and food. When it was cold, they tended to choose heat, at the expense of food. Presumably if they had been allowed access to food but not the heat lamp, they would have eaten less as the temperature rose.

One mechanism possibly contributing to increased intake in animals exposed to the cold is faster gastric emptying (Logue, 1986). Logue notes that rats exposed to the cold initiate more meals but do not eat more at a given meal. Presumably, gastric emptying rate does not affect the initial repletion rate of the stomach, and consequently the size of the meal, but does affect the length of time until the stomach again "demands" repletion, and consequently the frequency of meals. The faster the stomach empties, the sooner the next meal must begin. To extrapolate to the presumably reduced gastric emptying rate in animals exposed to the heat, one might speculate that the slowing of the digestive process is a means of muting the thermic effect of food.

Seasonal Effects

Casual inquiry yields a broad consensus that BW declines in the summer and rises in the winter. This seasonal variation is sometimes thought to be accompanied by a corresponding variation in appetite, although interestingly, people appear to be less cognizant of how much they eat than of how much they weigh. The thermoregulatory viewpoint considered above would seem to predict a decline in appetite in the summer heat as a means of ensuring that endogenous heat does not threaten one's thermoregulatory capacity. What remains uncertain—even if the appetitive shift occurs—is whether the shift in body weight is regulated or not. That is, does BW setpoint shift downward in the hot months, dragging appetite with it? Or does appetite decline on its own, as a thermoregulatory tactic, while BW setpoint remains high?

The need for less internal heat in the summer seems to be an adequate physiological rationale for lowered summer appetite. Other reasons may be suggested, however—notably, that people wear less clothing in the summer for thermoregulatory reasons and therefore become more concerned with their physical appearance. A bathing suit demands a slim physique, and perusal of popular magazines suggests that much of the springtime is devoted to shaping up for summer.

Among those who are exposed to summer heat involuntarily, reduced appetite would be expected. Solid evidence in support of this expectation is not abundant, if only because it has not been systematically collected. We know that the farmed polecat reduces its intake and weight during the summer months (Korhonen and Harri, 1986).

The most salient outcome of this literature search—other than consensual agreement with the general proposition that heat impairs appetite—is the dearth of actual experimental research on human consummatory response to variations in heat. It is somewhat reassuring, then, to note that retailers corroborate the consensual impression, often with hard data (sales figures). A number of restaurant chains in the Toronto area report decreased sales during the summer—not only fewer customers, as might be expected because of vacations, but also a decline in the average purchase per customer (range of decrease: 2 to 20 percent). The only exceptions to this rule were a chain of restaurants specializing in salads and two chains specializing in ice cream desserts.

Fever

Fever, of course, is not an exogenous source of heat, but it may be considered as a means of inducing heat in the internal environment. Fever is usually associated with decreased appetite, which follows from most analyses of feeding in which thermoregulation is a consideration. Raising the internal temperature ought to trigger compensatory decreases in feeding if feeding threatens to raise the internal temperature even further. This conclusion is premised on the notion that fever represents a state of hyperthermia relative to some internal optimum. Note that it does not follow that if hyperthermia suppresses voluntary appetite, then voluntary appetite suppression necessarily indicates hyperthermia. Appetite suppression and indications of hypothermia coexist, for instance, in anorexia nervosa (Garfinkel and Garner, 1982).

The possibility remains, of course, that fever might not represent true hyperthermia but rather a resetting of the thermoregulatory set-point at a higher level (Mrosovsky, 1990); in this case, the body might "want" to maintain a higher temperature, and a decline in feeding would not be expected. Intraperitoneal injection of interleukin-1, normally released in the presence of pathogens, raises body temperature and ordinarily is associated with appetite suppression; but when injected intracerebroventricularly, interleukin-1 raises body temperature in rats without affecting intake (McCarthy et al., 1986). This suggests that fever-induced anorexia may not be mediated by thermic mechanisms. Conversely, injecting endotoxin substantially lowers intake even when temperature elevation is prevented by administration of sodium salicylate (Baile et al., 1981; McCarthy et al., 1984), although the suppression may be less than when fever is not prevented (Baile et al., 1981). Another study, in which rats' body weights were lowered before the administration of interleukin-1, found that despite elevated body temperature, the animals were initially hyperphagic in defense of an albeit subnormal body weight (Mrosovsky et al., 1989); in other words, it may be that pathogens—or the interleukin-1 stimulated by them—produce a lowered BW set-point, pulling appetite down, independent of heat compensation (see also O'Reilly et al., 1989). There are plausible adaptive reasons why maintaining a lowered BW might help to fight or "starve" pathogens (Murray and Murray, 1977).

Food Temperature

One consensual belief, at least among nonscientists, is that hot foods have a greater thermogenic effect. Accordingly, people seek hot foods when they are cold, and cold foods, if any, when they are hot. Turning this prescription around, the conclusion emerges that hot foods ought to have a greater suppressive effect on appetite than cold foods.

Humans Because warming a food tends to enhance its flavor and aroma (Trant and Pangborn, 1983), one might expect that hotter, more palatable food will generate increased intake initially, with perhaps a subsequent caloric compensation—or perhaps not, depending on the strength of compensatory pressures. Actually, one should be careful about assuming that accentuating the flavor will make the food more palatable; some things—notably beverages such as water—are more palatable when cool (Szlyk et al., 1989). And if the food is unpalatable to begin with, warming it may make it taste worse! Holding intake constant, one might expect hot food to suppress appetite by suppressing gastric emptying rate, just as exposure to cold environments speeds gastric emptying, as shown above. Or hot food might suppress appetite by raising body temperature and inducing satiety.

No significant effect on subsequent intake of cheese sandwiches or on sensations of hunger or fullness was observed when experimental subjects were given a fixed portion of V8 juice served at 1°C or 60° to 62°C (Rolls et al., 1990). The cold juice, while not affecting intake, did reduce reported desire to eat, in male subjects only, and reduced thirst as well. No clear explanation is available for the ambiguously suppressive effect of a cold beverage on mens' appetites.

Notwithstanding these sparse and nondefinitive data, there is a strong consensus among retailers and their customers that cold foods are preferred when the ambient temperature is high (unpublished data from consumer survey, 1991). The summer sales peak for ice cream would seem to depend more on the "ice" than on the "cream." In the words of one restaurateur, "cold menu items make them [the customers] feel even cooler." Soup and bakery item sales are slow in the summer.

Nonhumans The effect of food temperature on eating in humans may be powerful, if as yet undemonstrated; in other species, it appears to be negligible. Rats who were served cold (12°C), normal (29°C), or hot (48°C) pellets showed only a weak and insignificant tendency to eat more of the hotter food. As with humans, one is entitled to wonder whether hotter food might smell or taste better, enhancing appetite, while also providing more energy and suppressing appetite. Intriguing studies in ruminants (Bhattacharya and Warner, 1968; Gengler et al., 1970) indicate that if the rumen is heated by the addition of warm water or by heating coils, intake may decline by as much as 45 percent. One is tempted to imagine studies in humans where the effect of heating on flavor is separated from its direct thermic effect. Heating a basically unpalatable food would presumably suppress intake substantially if it brought out the aversive flavor as well as added unwanted heat to the system. Presumably a study in which the animal or person was offered a choice between hot and cold versions of the same food might help to disambiguate these results.

Effects of Light on Appetite

Although there is obviously not an invariant connection between environmental heat and environmental light, some of the hottest environments, especially desert areas, are notable for the intensity of the light. This fact becomes relevant, perhaps, in conjunction with recent work on seasonal affective disorder (SAD), a variant of clinical depression that is seasonal in nature and, more specifically, responsive to "light therapy" (for example, exposure for a period of hours to a bright [2500 lux] full-spectrum fluorescent light). The connection between SAD and appetitive disorders has been remarked on repeatedly (for example, Rosenthal et al., 1986; Wurtman, 1988). Specifically, the depressive phase is associated with overeating, carbohydrate craving, and weight gain. Periodic exposure to bright light produced weight loss in SAD patients, although this effect was accompanied by a decrease in their surprisingly high resting metabolic rate (Gaist et al., 1990). It is tantalizing to imagine that bright sunlight might contribute to the appetite suppression observed in hot environments; however, there is essentially no evidence that normal control subjects' appetites are affected by light exposure. Rats show a transient decline in appetite when exposed to constant light (Dark et al., 1980); but rats are nocturnal feeders, so the extended presence of light would be expected to disrupt feeding briefly, independent of profound physiological changes. The relevance to humans of studies of rats' reactions to extra light is probably negligible.

Effects of Environmental Temperature on Food Preferences

Acute Variations

The discussion above regarding thermic effects of different macronutrients suggests that, in the heat, there should be a relative suppression of the already relatively suppressed (Drewnowski et al., 1989) protein preference/intake. Johnson and Kark (1947), in their survey of wartime military nutrition, found that "regardless of environment, the percentage of proteins voluntarily chosen from the rations was practically constant." Edholm et al. (1964) concur. In mice exposed to hot and cold environments, the only substantial variation was in carbohydrate (starch) intake, which was strongly elevated by cold and suppressed by heat, but not below the level for casein- and lard-supplemented diets (Donhoffer and Vonotzky, 1947). Two restaurant chains reported a decided shift away from sandwiches toward salads in the summer (unpublished data from consumer survey, 1991). Ice cream consumption, which peaks in the summer (unpublished data from consumer survey, 1991), seems to be an exception to the rule of heat-suppressed carbohydrate consumption; however, most observers regard the summer appeal of ice cream to reside in its coldness more than its sweetness. In fact, one ice cream chain reported that while ice cream sales tended to rise with increases in environmental temperature from 72° to 82°F, above 82°F customers switch to more thirst-quenching products (for example, ices and "light" ice creams).

Rothwell and Stock's (1986) casual observations suggested that food selection of rats offered a cafeteria diet was unaffected by variations (from 24° to 29°C) in environmental temperature. As already shown, however, the ability of protein to differentially suppress appetite has probably been overstated; accordingly, it should not be surprising if heat has little observable effect on macronutrient preferences. Ashworth and Harrower (1967) reported that proportional nitrogen loss from sweating is lower than normal in acclimatized tropical workers, again suggesting no need for supplemental protein in the diet, a conclusion seconded by Collins et al. (1971) and Weiner et al. (1972). Still, it would seem a reasonable precaution to maintain protein intake at or slightly above a nutritionally desirable minimum in hot environments, especially before full acclimatization has been achieved.

Seasonal Effects

Donhoffer and Vonotzky (1947) cite well-known seasonal changes in thyroid activity as a possible mediator of the heat-induced differential suppression of carbohydrate intake. How thyroid activity might control qualitative aspects of appetite and whether humans are susceptible to such seasonal variations remain obscure.

The consumer survey yielded fairly strong data regarding shifts in food preference in the summer. As noted above, the restaurant chain specializing in salads had its sales peak during the summer. Not surprisingly, so did the ice cream parlors. Seasonal shifts in consumer preferences, however, may not be driven entirely by physiology. A number of retailers indicated that intense promotional activity of different types of foods occurs on a seasonal basis; conceivably, some of the seasonal shift in preferences actually represents conformity with expectations or financial and social pressures. One hamburger chain claimed that "consumption patterns are marketing driven";

that is, people eat what they are told by advertisers or induced by incentives to eat.

CONCLUSIONS AND RECOMMENDATIONS

Research Recommendations

Almost any systematic research on the effects of heat on appetite would be welcome. Beyond the general and vague conclusion that heat suppresses appetite—and possibly renders cooler foods more palatable—researchers are forced to surmise where they would prefer to know. Studies of the following sort would be most desirable, although the list is somewhat arbitrary and certainly not exhaustive:

• Straightforward studies that examine food intake in environments in which the temperature has been artificially elevated, in comparison with food intake in normal or cooled environments. Such studies should examine (a) quantity consumed, (b) preference shifts among macronutrients and/or basic food groups, and (c) preference shifts for heated versus cooled versions of the same foods.

• Similar studies conducted in thermoneutral, heated, and cooled environments during summer versus winter. Whether living in an air-conditioned environment mitigates the effects of environmental heat should be investigated.

• Variations on the foregoing studies in which adaptation periods are varied: (a) short-term adaptations over the course of minutes or hours (as when one acclimates to an air-conditioned room) and (b) long-term adaptation (for example, at the beginning of a heat wave versus after a week or two of a heat wave).

• Studies on the effects on appetite of humidity manipulations in conjunction with heat manipulations.

• Studies of the effects of heat on appetite in situations where the subjects' ad lib consumption is monitored with a specific view to determining whether appetite suppression occurs because meal size decreases and meal frequency remains constant, or because meal frequency decreases and meal size stays constant. These studies should address whether heat enhances satiety or impairs hunger.

• Studies of the thermic effect of different diets. Do different macronutrients have different thermic effects? Enough to bother about?

• Studies of the thermic effects of food at different temperatures.

• Studies of the palatability of foods at different temperatures while manipulating environmental temperature and, if possible, body temperature.

• Alliesthesia studies like that of Cabanac (1971) to determine whether heat suppression of appetite occurs in conjunction with a lowered BW set-point—in which case preference for sweets following a glucose load should decline—or whether heat suppression of appetite occurs in defiance of an unchanged BW set-point—in which case preference for sweet after a glucose load should remain high.

Practical Recommendations for Working in Hot Environments

In general, work in a hot environment demands close attention to factors that might threaten either thermoregulation or BW regulation. In the absence of knowledge about whether these regulatory mechanisms act in conflict or in concert in hot environments, it is probably safest to focus on thermoregulation, which poses the most immediate physiological challenge.

• Allow for reduced intake. Unless BW falls to dangerously low levels, if heat suppresses appetite, it should be recognized that this as an adaptive strategy in the best interest of the individual's thermoregulatory well-being.

• Allow for some shifts in food preferences, to be determined empirically. There may be a shift in the preferred macronutrient balance; more likely, there will be a shift in the preferred temperature, toward cooler foods and, especially, beverages.

• Ensure that protein intake is maintained at a healthy level. This is not likely to require much if any intervention.

• Encourage adaptation to the heat through regular, graded exposure to the hot environment. During the first few days in a hot environment, exposure should be gradually increased, with care taken to provide opportunities to cool off between exposures. Excessive cooling is not advised, because it will probably interfere with heat adaptation and may conceivably interfere with the adaptive resetting of regulatory set-points.

• Minimize activity, especially during the first few days of heat exposure. Strenuous exercise provides an additional heat challenge and may disrupt appetite in such a way as to interfere with normal regulatory adaptations. As with heat exposure, exercise may be increased gradually.

• Women may have more difficulty than men adapting to heat, so the foregoing recommendations should be observed especially closely for women.

REFERENCES

Andersson, B., and B. Larsson
    1961   Influence of local temperature changes in the preoptic area and rostral hypothalamus on the regulation of food and water intake. Acta Physiol. Scand. 52:75-89.
Appleman, R.D., and J.C. Delouche
    1959   Behavioral, physiological and biochemical responses of goats to temperature 0° to 40°C. J. Anim. Sci. 17:326-335.

Ashworth, A., and A.D.B. Harrower
    1967   Protein requirements in tropical countries: Nitrogen losses in sweat and their rela-
            tion to nitrogen balance. Br. J. Nutri. 21:833-843.
Baile, C.A., J. Naylor, C.L. McLaughlin, and C.A. Catanzano
    1981   Endotoxin elicited fever and anorexia and elfazepam-stimulated feeding in sheep.
            Physiol. Behav. 27:271-277.
Balagura, S.
    1973   Hunger: A Biopsychological Analysis. New York: Basic Books.
Beller, A.S.
    1977   Fat and Thin: A Natural History of Obesity. New York: Farrar Straus, & Giroux.
Bellward, K., and M.J. Dauncey
    1988   Behavioural energy regulation in lean and genetically obese (ob/ob) mice. Physiol.
            Behav. 42:433-438.
Bhattacharya, A.N., and R.G. Warner
    1968   Influence of varying rumen temperature on central cooling or warming and on
            regulation of voluntary feed intake in dairy cattle. J. Dairy Sci. 51:1481-1489.
Booth, G., and J.M. Strang
    1936   Changes in temperature of the skin following the ingestion of food. Arch. Int.
            Med. 57:533-543.
Brobeck, J.R.
    1948   Food intake as a mechanism of temperature regulation. Yale J. Biol. Med. 20:545-
            552.
Burse, R.L.
    1979   Sex differences in human thermoregulatory response to heat and cold stress. Hum.
            Factors 21:687-699.
Cabanac, M.
    1971   Physiological role of pleasure. Science 17:1103-1107.
Collins, K.J., and J.S. Weiner
    1968   Endocrinological aspects of exposure to high environmental temperature. Physiol.
            Rev. 48:785-839.
Collins, K.J., T.P. Eddy, A. Hibbs, A.L. Stock, and E.F. Wheeler
    1971   Nutritional and environmental studies on an ocean-going oil tanker. 2. Heat accli-
            matization and nutrient balance. Br. J. Indu. Med. 28:246-258.
Dallosso, H.M., and W.P.T. James
    1984   Whole-body calorimetry studies in adult men. 2. The interaction of exercise and
            over-feeding on the thermic effect of a meal. Br. J. Nutr. 52:65-72.
Dark, J., L.L. Rayha, I. Clark-Lane, and V. Kimler
    1980   Melatonin and lighting condition: Absence of long-term effects on food intake and
            body weight regulation in the albino rat. Physiol. Behav. 25:855-857.
DiBella, L., G. Tarozzi, M.T. Rossi, and G. Scalera
    1981   Effect of liver temperature increase on food intake. Physiol. Behav. 26:45-51.
Donhoffer, S., and J. Vonotzky
    1947   The effect of environmental temperature on food selection. Am. J. Physiol. 150:329-
            333.
Drewnowski, A., E.E. Shrager, C. Lipsky, E. Stellar, and M.R.C. Greenwood
    1989   Sugar and fat: Sensory and hedonic evaluation of liquid and solid foods. Physiol.
            Behav. 45:177-184.
Edholm, O.G., R.H. Fox, R. Goldsmith, I.F.G. Hampton, C.R. Underwood, E.J. Ward,
            H.S. Wolf, J.M. Adam, and J.R. Allan
    1964   Report to the Medical Research Council, No. APRC64/65. London: Army Person-
            nel Research Committee.

Fantino, M., and M. Cabanac
1984   Effect of a cold ambient temperature on the rat's food hoarding behavior. Physiol.
        Behav. 32:183-190.
Fletcher, J.M.
1986   Effects on growth and endocrine status of maintaining obese and lean Zucker rats
        at 22°C and 30°C from weaning. Physiol. Behav. 37:597-602.
Gaist, P.A., E. Obarzanek, R.G. Skwerer, C.C. Duncan, P.M. Shultz, and N.E. Rosenthal
1990   Effects of bright light on resting metabolic rate in patients with seasonal affective
        disorder and control subjects. Biol. Psychiatry 28:989-996.
Garfinkel, P.E., and D.M. Garner
1982   Anorexia Nervosa: A Multidimensional Perspective. New York: Brunner-Mazel.
Gengler, W.R., F.A. Martz, H.D. Johnson, G.F. Krause, and L. Hahn
1970   Effect of temperature on food and water intake and rumen fermentation. J. Dairy
        Sci. 53:434-437.
Glick, Z., A. Uncyk, J. Lupien, and L. Schmidt
1989   Meal associated changes in brown fat thermogenesis and glycogen. Physiol. Behav.
        45:243-248.
Hamilton, C.L.
1967   Food and temperature. Pp. 303-317 in Handbook of Physiology: Section 6, vol. 1,
        C.F. Code, ed. Washington, D.C.: American Physiological Society.
Hamilton, C.L., and J.R. Brobeck
1964   Food intake and temperature regulation in rats with rostral hypothalamic lesions.
        Am. J. Physiol. 207:291-297.
Heath, M.E.
1980   Effects of rearing temperature on the thermoregulatory behavior of pigs. Behav.
        Neural. Biol. 28:193-202.
Herman, C.P., and F.J. Vaccarino
1992   Appetite. Pp. 79-86 in Encyclopedia of Food Science and Technology, Y.H. Hui,
        ed. New York: Wiley.
Hogan, S., D.V. Coscina, and J. Himms-Hagen
1982   Brown adipose tissue of rats with obesity-inducing ventromedial hypothalamic
        lesions. Am. J. Physiol. 243:E338-E344.
Hogan, S., J. Himms-Hagen, and D.V. Coscina
1986   Lack of diet-induced thermogenesis in brown adipose tissue of obese medial hypo-
        thalamic-lesioned rats. Physiol. Behav. 35:287-294.
Jakubczak, L.F.
1976   Food and water intakes of rats as a function of strain, age, temperature, and body
        weight. Physiol. Behav. 17:251-258.
Johnson, R.E., and R.M. Kark
1947   Environment and food intake in man. Science 105:378-379.
Keys, A., J. Brôzek, A. Henschel, O. Mickelson, and L.L. Taylor
1950   The Biology of Human Starvation. Minneapolis, Minn.: University of Minnesota
        Press.
Korhonen, H., and M. Harri
1986   Seasonal changes in energy economy of farmed polecat as evaluated by body
        weight, food intake and behavioral strategy. Physiol. Behav. 37:777-783.
Kraly, F.S., and E.M. Blass
1976   Increased feeding in rats in a low ambient temperature. Pp. 77-89 in Hunger: Basic
        Mechanisms and Clinical Implications, D. Novin, W. Wyrwicka and G.A. Bray,
        eds. New York: Raven Press.

LeBlanc, J., and M. Cabanac
  1989   Cephalic postprandial thermogenesis in human subjects. Physiol. Behav. 46:479-482.
LeBlanc, J., and P. Diamond
  1986   Effects of meal size and frequency on postprandial thermogenesis in dogs. Am. J. Physiol. 250:E144-E147.
Leon, M., and B. Woodside
  1983   Energetic limits on reproduction: Maternal food intake. Physiol. Behav. 30:945-957.
Logue, A.W.
  1986   The Psychology of Eating and Drinking. New York: W. H. Freeman.
Macari, M., S.M.F. Zuim, E.R. Secato, and J.R. Guerreiro
  1986   Effects of ambient temperature and thyroid hormones on food intake by pigs. Physiol. Behav. 36:1035-1039.
McCarthy, D.O., M.J. Kluger, and A.J. Vander
  1984   The role of fever in appetite suppression after endotoxin administration. Am. J. Clin. Nutr. 40:310-316.
  1986   Effect of centrally administered interleukin-1 and endotoxin on food intake of fasted rats. Physiol. Behav. 36:745-749.
Mrosovsky, N.
  1990   Rheostasis: The Physiology of Change. New York: Oxford.
Mrosovsky, N., L.A. Molony, C.A. Conn, and M.J. Kluger
  1989   Anorexic effects of interleukin 1 in the rat. Am. J. Physiol. 257:R1315-R1321.
Murray, M.J., and A.B. Murray
  1977   Starvation suppression and refeeding activation of infection. Lancet 1:123-125.
Nisbett, R.E.
  1972   Hunger, obesity, and the ventromedial hypothalamus. Psychol. Rev. 79:433-453.
O'Reilly, B., A.J. Vander, and M.J. Kluger
  1989   Effects of chronic infusion of liposaccharide on food intake and body temperature of the rat. Physiol. Behav. 42:287-291.
Pénicaud, L., D.A. Thompson, and J. Le Magnen
  1986   Effects of 2-deoxy-d-glucose on food and water intake and body temperature in rats. Physiol. Behav. 36:431-435.
Rampone, A.J., and P.J. Reynolds
  1991   Food intake regulation by diet induced thermogenesis. Med. Hypotheses. 34:7-12.
Refinetti, R.
  1988   Effects of food temperature and ambient temperature during a meal on food intake in the rat. Physiol. Behav. 43:245-247.
Rolls, B.J., I.C. Federoff, J.F. Guthrie, and L.J. Laster
  1990   Effects of temperature and mode of presentation of juice on hunger, thirst and food intake in humans. Appetite 15:199-208.
Rosenthal, N.E., M. Genhart, F.M. Jacobsen, R.G. Skwerer, and T.A. Wehr
  1986   Disturbances of appetite and weight regulation in seasonal affective disorder. Ann. N.Y. Acad. Sci. 499:216-230.
Rothwell, N.J., and M.J. Stock
  1986   Influence of environmental temperature on energy balance, diet-induced thermogenesis and brown fat activity in "cafeteria"-fed rats. Br. J. Nutr. 56:123-129.
Segal, K.R., B. Gutin, J. Albu, and F.X. Pi-Sunyer
  1987   Thermic effect of food and exercise in lean and obese men of similar lean body mass. Am. J. Physiol. 252:E110-E117.

Strominger, J.L., and J.R. Brobeck
    1953   A mechanism of regulation of food intake. Yale J. Biol. Med. 25:383-390.
Swiergiel, A.H., and D.I. Ingram
    1986   Effect of diet and temperature acclimation on thermoregulatory behavior in pig-
            lets. Physiol. Behav. 36:637-642.
Szlyk, P., I.V. Sils, R.P. Francesconi, R.W. Hubbard, and L.E. Armstrong
    1989   Effects of water temperature and flavoring on voluntary dehydration in man. Physiol.
            Behav. 45:639-647.
Thurlby, P.L.
    1979   Ph.D. dissertation. Studies on thermoregulatory thermogenesis in relation to en-
            ergy balance in genetically obese (ob/ob) mice. D35261/79 AX: Cambridge Uni-
            versity.
Trant, A.S., and R.M. Pangborn
    1983   Discrimination, intensity, and hedonic responses to color, aroma, viscosity, and
            sweetness of beverages. Lebens. Wissen. Technol. 16:147-152.
Weiner, J.S., J.O.C. Willson, H. El-Neil, and E.F. Wheeler
    1972   The effect of work level and dietary intake on sweat nitrogen losses in a hot
            climate. Br. J. Nutr. 27:543-552.
Wilson, L.M., and H.L. Sinha
    1985   Thermal preference behavior of genetically obese (ob/ob) and genetically lean (+/
            ?) mice. Physiol. Behav. 35:545-548.
Wurtman, J.J.
    1988   Carbohydrate craving, mood changes, and obesity. J. Clin. Psychiatry 49:37-39.

DISCUSSION

DR. NESHEIM: Any questions?

PARTICIPANT: Mike Sawka mentioned yesterday that discomfort is closely related to skin temperature. I wonder if you think that a feeling of discomfort in the heat would also affect appetite, and if that might be part of the appetite suppression mechanism—as opposed to solely internal body temperature?

DR. HERMAN: Certainly. I know that if you manipulate skin temperature directly, at least in nonhuman animals, that you will get a suppression of appetite. Of course we don't have subjective discomfort ratings in that situation, but I can't help but think heat discomfort would be very much a factor.

PARTICIPANT: Do you know of any studies that have tried to pinpoint whether it was blood temperature, skin temperature, a certain anatomical section, or physiological section that might be impacting on that sensation of heat discomfort?

DR. HERMAN: No, the manipulation was too crude and the measurement was just done at the skin surface. We also don't know whether there were cascading effects to the internal environment.

We know that heating deep core organs like the hypothalamus in animals will have the same effect. So my guess would be that almost anywhere along the chain that you apply heat, it is likely to have a suppressive effect on appetite.

Nutritional Needs in Hot Environments
Pp. 215–243. Washington, D.C.
National Academy Press

11

Situational Influences on Food Intake

Edward S. Hirsch[1] and F. Matthew Kramer

INTRODUCTION

If one were asked to describe a situation where eating was not likely to occur, the description would probably contain many elements of the battlefield. It is striking that the thorough nutritional surveys taken during World War II were virtually unanimous in reporting the absence of nutritional disease among troops when food supplies were adequate (Bean, 1946; Johnson and Kark, 1946; Youmans, 1955). These surveys also frequently found weight loss (Youmans, 1955). Consistent with these observations, surveys of troops during World War II found that 54 to 73 percent reported that they were hungry during combat (Webster and Johnson, 1945). More recent observations in the Falkland islands (McCaig and Gooderson, 1986) and a retrospective survey of U.S. Marines who had served in World War II, Korea, and Vietnam (Popper et al., 1989) indicated that during combat, troops reported eating considerably less than usual. The picture that emerges is that under combat conditions troops consume sufficient food to avoid frank nutritional disease but do not consume enough food to meet their energy needs, and some weight loss occurs.

THE UNDERCONSUMPTION PROBLEM

During the past 10 years, the full range of current military rations has been rigorously tested under various field and climatic conditions by the

---

[1] Edward S. Hirsch, U.S. Army Natick Labs, Mail Stop STRNC/YBF, Natick, MA 01760

U.S. Army Natick Research Development and Engineering Center and the U.S. Army Research Institute of Environmental Medicine. With one instructive exception, these studies have uniformly found that energy intake in the field is not sufficient, and weight loss occurs.

Of the various military rations, the meal, ready-to-eat (MRE), a general purpose ration designed to be eaten when hot food is not available, has undergone the most thorough testing in the widest variety of circumstances. Table 11-1 shows the composition of the menus in an early version of this ration, the MRE IV. Newer improved versions are similar in configuration, with each meal consisting of an entree, a dessert, a beverage, crackers and a spread, and a starch in some instances. Hot sauce, fruit-flavored beverages, and new or reformulated items as well as larger entrees have replaced many of the items in Table 11-1. MRE IV provided 3669 calories in three meals whereas MRE VIII provides over 3900 calories in three meals.

Table 11-2 shows the results of nine studies conducted with various versions of the MRE fed as the sole source of subsistence for periods ranging from 5 to 34 days, in environments as different as Hawaii and Alaska, and with troops that were relatively inexperienced compared to the highly trained and disciplined U.S. Army Special Forces. Caloric intake and body weight loss varied with the nature of the environment, duration of the test, experience of the participating troops, and version of the MRE tested. However, because of nonsystematic variations across tests, it is impossible to attribute differences in intake and weight loss to these factors independently. What is clear from this table is that energy intake is not sufficient and that weight loss occurs when this ration is fed as the sole source of food. The trend is likely to be even more pronounced in the high heat environment of the desert where the MRE has yet to be tested.

PROBLEM DEFINITION

The question arises whether these observations are an immutable fact of military feeding in the field, which those responsible for the health and well-being of troops will have to acknowledge and plan for, or whether their source can be uncovered and the situation can be remedied. What factors are responsible for the underconsumption of operational rations?

WHY IS RATION INTAKE INSUFFICIENT?

Most troops and their leaders would probably explain the inadequate consumption of rations in terms of the nature and quality of the food. However, this is probably not the complete answer for several reasons. First, the various field tests of the MRE have generally shown that troops report the MRE to be acceptable on a 9-point hedonic scale. For example, in a 34-day

TABLE 11-1   Menus in the Meal, Ready-To-Eat (MRE) IV Ration

Menu No.	Entree	Other Components
1	Pork sausage patty, freeze-dehydrated; catsup, dehydrated; applesauce; crackers	Cheese spread; cookies, chocolate-covered; cocoa beverage powder
2	Ham/chicken loaf; strawberries, freeze-dehydrated; crackers	Peanut butter; pineapple nut cake
3	Beef patty, freeze-dehydrated; soup and gravy base; beans with tomato sauce; crackers	Cheese spread; brownies, chocolate-covered; candy
4	Beef slices with barbecue sauce; crackers; peanut butter; cookie, chocolate-covered	Peaches, freeze-dehydrated; candy
5	Beef stew; crackers; peanut butter; fruit, mixed, freeze-dehydrated	Cherry nut cake; cocoa beverage powder
6	Frankfurters; catsup, dehydrated; beans with tomato sauce; crackers	Jelly; candy; cocoa beverage powder
7	Turkey, diced with gravy; potato patty, freeze-dehydrated; beans with tomato sauce; crackers	Maple nut cake; candy
8	Beef, diced with gravy; beans with tomato sauce; crackers	Cheese spread; brownie, chocolate-covered
9	Cooked beef or chicken à la king; catsup, dehydrated; crackers; cheese spread	Fruitcake; cocoa beverage powder
10	Meatballs with barbecue sauce; potato patty, freeze-dehydrated; crackers	Jelly; chocolate nut cake; cocoa beverage powder
11	Ham slices; crackers; cheese spread; peaches, freeze-dehydrated	Orange nut roll; cocoa beverage powder
12	Chicken loaf or ground beef with spiced sauce; crackers; peanut butter; strawberries, freeze-dehydrated	Cookies, chocolate-covered; candy

NOTE: All menus include instant coffee; dry, nondairy cream substitute; granulated sugar; salt; and candy-coated chewing gum. Nonfood components are spoon, matches, and toilet paper.

test, the average acceptability rating of all items in the ration was 7.05, which corresponds to the description *like moderately* on the acceptability scale, and there was no indication that food acceptability decreased over time despite an almost 30 percent reduction in food intake from the first week of the test to the last (Fox et al., 1989; Hirsch et al., 1985). These observations clearly suggest that the nature of the food is not the sole or perhaps not even a critical factor in limiting consumption of the MRE in field tests.

TABLE 11-2 Caloric Intake and Body Weight Loss in Troops Fed Only MRE (Meal, Ready-to-Eat) Meals

Ration	Environment	Eating Conditions	Caloric Intake (Kcal)	Body Weight Loss (%)	Reference
MRE IV	Temperate, 6000 feet, Hawaii	Three MREs per day for 34 days. Issued three per day, no special provisions for heating, training exercise.	2189	5.8	Hirsch et al., 1985
MRE IV	Temperate, 7200 feet, Hawaii	Three MREs per day for 12 days, ran strenuous cross-country course for 2 hours per day for 7 days.	2282	3.0	Askew et al., 1986
MRE IV MRE VII Improved MRE	Temperate, 6000 feet, 35° to 80°F, Hawaii	Three MREs per day for 11 days, no provisions for heating food.	2517 2517 2842	2.98 3.20 2.28	Popper et al., 1987
MRE VI	Temperate, cool, 40° to 51°F, Vermont	Thirty days, Special Forces, surveillance, reconnaissance, no foraging permitted.	2782; no trends over time	2.2	Askew et al., 1987
MRE V	Cold, 4° to 35°F, White Mt. National Forest	Four MREs per day for 10 days, outside all the time.	2733	4	Engell et al., 1987
Improved MRE VIII	Cold, Mountain Warfare Training Center	Four MREs per day; days 1-5 in field, 6-7 in garrison, 8-11 in field; leadership course; high activity.	3217	3.3	Morgan et al., 1988
MRE VIII	Cold, 14° to 43°F, Wisconsin	Four MREs per day for 3 days, three different heating methods,* ate outside.	2250 (canteen cup stand) 2289 (ration heater pad) 2206 (control)	1.7 2.1 2.5	Lester et al., 1990

Four MRE VI	Cold, −40° to +35°F, Alaska	Ten days, some days high activity other days defensive position, meals eaten in tents.	2009	2.8	Edwards et al., 1989
Four MRE VIII			2802	2.0	
Three MRE VI and supplement			2830	1.9	
Three MRE VIII and supplement			3553	1.7	
Three MRE VIII and supplement	Cold, −55° to +26°F, Alaska	Air assault and defensive positions, meals eaten in warm tents.	2729	1.6	Edwards et al., 1990

*Three groups of U.S. Marines were provided with different heating methods. One group was given a canteen cup stand and a more-than-sufficient supply of heat tabs. A second group was given ration heater pads and the third group, the control, was given the Optimus Hiker Stove, which is standard issue by the Marine Corps.

A much stronger argument against the notion that low intakes of rations in the field are due to the nature of the food derives from a series of studies conducted where the identical ration was fed either in the field or in a dining room environment.

LABORATORY AND FIELD DIFFERENCES

The impetus for the initial laboratory study of the MRE arose because this ration had never been tested as the sole source of food for extended periods of time. Military planners and logisticians would like to be able to provide only packaged operational rations to troops for prolonged time periods. This type of subsistence plan would obviously save on equipment, personnel, and money if it could be accomplished without compromising troop morale and performance. In addition, information was needed to set policy on how long the MRE could be fed as the sole source of food without affecting health and nutritional status. It seemed prudent to determine if intake was adequate under controlled conditions prior to field testing, where serious nutritional and health problems might develop, at which time they would be more difficult to treat.

In response to these concerns, a laboratory study was conducted with paid student volunteers at the Massachusetts Institute of Technology (E. Hirsch and F. M. Kramer, unpublished data). One group of 17 healthy, normal-weight male students was fed the MRE IV as their sole source of food for 6 weeks. A second group of 16 subjects was fed freshly prepared food that provided 3600 calories per day and closely matched the MRE in macronutrient composition. The control diet was fed in a 12-day menu cycle and consisted of high-preference food items offered in traditional meals. Both groups ate in a small, pleasant dining room with meals available at traditional times for a 2-hour period. Subjects eating the MRE were free to exchange items with each other as is typical of the field. Uneaten MRE components were noted and were available for later consumption by members of the MRE group. The control group could also consume extra food if, at the end of a meal, there were leftovers in the kitchen. Thus, it was possible for some subjects to consume more than the 3600 calories provided in a day's allotment. The MRE was provided at ambient temperature, but components could be heated in a nearby microwave oven. Similarly, hot and cold water was available for mixing beverages or rehydrating ration components. Dinner plates, silverware, bowls, glasses, and cups were available to the MRE group for consuming their food and beverages. The general eating environment can best be described as pleasant, clean, and social.

Figure 11-1 shows that during the first two weeks of the experiment the two dietary groups had comparable levels of energy intake. During later weeks, although intake remained relatively constant in the control group it

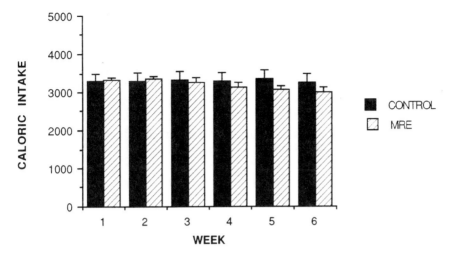

FIGURE 11-1 Mean daily caloric intake for student volunteers fed three MREs per day or freshly prepared food (control) for 6 weeks. SOURCE: Kramer et al. (1992); used with permission.

declined in the MRE group to a value of 3017 calories per day in the final week of the study. Mean caloric intake averaged 3465 calories per day in the control group and 3149 in the MRE group over the course of the experiment. The group differences in caloric intake and the decline in intake over time by the MRE group were statistically reliable (p's < 0.01). At these levels of food intake the control group showed a slightly positive energy balance and gained 0.68 kg over the six weeks of the study whereas the MRE group showed a slightly negative energy balance and lost 0.69 kg. The group differences in energy intake are not readily accounted for by differences in food acceptability, as measure by hedonic ratings. In this study the ration was as highly rated as the freshly prepared food and the reduction in consumption that developed over time in the ration group was not accompanied by changes in food acceptability ratings. At this juncture an explanation of why caloric intake dropped in the MRE group awaits additional research.

These findings contrast sharply with data from the field. When troops were fed MRE IV as their sole source of food for 34 days, their average energy intake was only 2190 calories per day (Hirsch et al., 1985; Wenkam et al., 1989). Thus, in the field, intake of the identical ration was almost 1000 calories lower than it was in a dining room environment.

Differences in food intake that were observed in the preceding studies suggest that the nature of the feeding environment can dramatically affect daily energy intake. However, it is also possible that this difference is due to comparing a student population to infantry troops. These populations differ in many dimensions that could affect intake such as, fitness, experience with military food, perceptions of the military and military rations, ethnic and racial composition and food habits. Accordingly, a second study of this type was conducted where troops were fed an improved version of the ration (MRE VIII) either in a field setting or in a garrison dining room (E. Hirsch and F. M. Kramer, unpublished data) for 5 days.

The troops in the field were engaged in small-unit training and were provided with three MRE VIIIs, which provide approximately 3900 calories per day. The garrison group ate all meals for a 5-day period at fixed times in a dining room. Meals were prepared and served, restaurant style, on individual trays with plates, bowls, cups, and utensils. Serving sizes were identical to those provided in the ration packages with the exception that cold beverages were served in 200-ml rather than 355-ml portions. Additional portions were available, and subjects could also request ration items for between-meal snacks. Thus, garrison subjects were able to consume more than 3900 calories per day. The field group received one freshly prepared meal on the first and fifth day of the study. For this reason intake on only the middle 3 days, when they were consuming only operational rations, was analyzed.

Troops who received rations in the dining room consumed 3848 calories per day compared to the field group, which consumed 2870 calories per day. Level of intake in the field was similar to the level previously observed in a field test with a prototype version of the MRE that was very similar to MRE VIII in a temperate environment (Popper et al., 1987). The large difference in food intake when the MRE VIII was fed to troops in the field compared to troops in a garrison dining hall replicates our earlier finding of about a 1000 calorie difference in intake when the MRE IV was fed to students in a dining room relative to troops in the field. The same finding with more similar subjects in the two eating environments (field versus garrison) strengthens the view that situational factors, such as the nature of the feeding environment, play a critical role in controlling human food intake.

To identify specific aspects of the feeding environment that promote this higher food intake in the dining room setting, levels of intake of various classes of food in the ration were examined. Figure 11-2 shows that consumption of desserts and cold beverages was almost 100 percent higher in the dining room than the field, while intake of the other ration components was similar. Higher intake of these items was due to dining room consumption rather than to between-meal snacks. Why these two ration components were consumed at such markedly higher levels remains an open question.

A final example of field-dining room differences in energy intake pro-

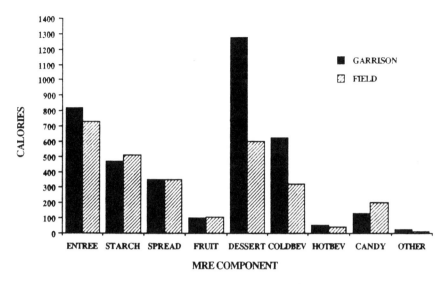

FIGURE 11-2   Mean daily caloric intake from each food class of the MRE (meal, ready-to-eat) for troops in garrison or in the field.

vides additional support for the notion that the nature of the feeding situation has a substantial influence on food intake. Over the past several years, the U.S. Army Research Institute of Environmental Medicine has been assessing the impact of the Army's initiatives to improve the healthfulness of the diet eaten by troops in garrison dining facilities. As part of this effort researchers have examined the nutrient intakes of troops in garrison over 7-day periods. Table 11-3 shows the level of caloric intake they have observed in five studies of this type where troops were provided with three A-ration meals per day. In contrast to operational rations, such as the MRE, which are designed to be eaten hot or cold from shelf-stable, packaged components, A-ration meals consist of fresh foods, prepared and cooked in the field. A remarkably narrow range of caloric intakes (2978 to 3199) was measured in troops that ranged from new recruits in basic training (Fort Jackson) to those attending a leadership course (Fort Riley) and in facilities that were operated by either the military or contractors as illustrated in the first five studies in the table. The final entry in this table is from a field study where, due to unusual circumstances, an artillery unit was engaged in sustained operations for an 8-day period; where sleep was limited and fragmented; and where three A-ration meals per day were provided. The hot meals were brought to the troops in the field, ample time for eating was allowed, and seconds were available. Under these conditions, troops in the field consumed an average of 3713 calories per day and gained 0.8 kg over

TABLE 11-3 Energy Intake by Troops Fed A-Rations in the Garrison or Field for Three Meals per Day

Population	Location	Energy Intake in Calories (Standard Deviation)	Reference
43 Male students attending primary leadership development course; attended all meals	Fort Riley	3112 (758)	Carlson et al., 1987
31 Male soldiers stationed at Ft. Lewis; most meals in dining facility	Fort Lewis	3173 (616)	Szeto et al., 1987
54 Male soldiers stationed at Ft. Devens who habitually ate at dining hall	Fort Devens I	2978 (527)	Szeto et al., 1988
52 Male soldiers stationed at Ft. Devens who habitually ate at dining hall	Fort Devens II	3165 (511)	Szeto et al., 1989
41 Male and 40 female basic trainees; limited meal time; socializing discouraged	Fort Jackson	3199 (736), men 2467 (560), women	Rose et al., 1989
31 Male artillery soldiers engaged in 8 days of sustained operations; food brought to them, and ample time allowed to eat	Fort Sill	3713 (785) gained 0.8 kg in 8 days	Rose and Carlson, 1987

the 8 days. The male soldiers in the field study consumed an average of 588 calories per day more than the men in the combined garrison studies. Perhaps the higher A-ration intake in the field occurred because in these unusual circumstances feeding was in some sense easier and more convenient than even in the garrison dining facility. The observed weight gain in a field setting with A-rations is also in marked contrast to the typical weight loss of 1-2 kg in an MRE field trial of comparable duration.

SITUATIONAL INFLUENCES

The question arises why such large differences in food intake are observed when the identical ration is provided in garrison dining facilities or in a field setting. This laboratory has begun to study how aspects of the eating situation other than food affect food acceptability and consumption both in single meals and over longer periods of time. The dimensions of the eating situation being studied fall into the general areas of constraints on food intake, social influences, and time of day.

Constraints on Food Intake

For most organisms, food and water rarely are freely available. Time and effort must be expended to obtain these commodities. Animal research has demonstrated clear relationships between patterns of ingestion and food choice and the cost-benefit structure of an animal's niche and current habitat (for example, Collier, 1989). Although the conceptual leap from animal models of optimal foraging to human feeding behavior is substantial, these authors believe that a comprehensive model of human ingestive behavior must ultimately embrace this class of variables. Further, a consideration of these variables probably will provide insight into the factors that influence the initiation, continuation, and termination of feeding by troops in the field and in combat.

Reflecting on the events involved in preparing, consuming, and cleaning up from a meal of operational rations in the field indicates that a series of time-consuming and effortful actions may be required. Potential actions to be carried out include finding a safe or protected location, finding water, rendering it potable, cleaning oneself, opening ration packages, rehydrating foods and beverages that require it, choosing a heating method, actually heating those items one wants hot, and finally eating food items contained in as many as five different packages. If the entire meal is to be eaten in one setting, a place to eat that is relatively flat and dry must be found or prepared. Throughout this entire sequence, orders to move on or perform another task may be issued. Cleaning up may involve burying or burning trash and cleaning a canteen cup if it was used to heat food or prepare beverages. These events become more difficult in a cold, dark, or muddy environment. These constraints on feeding appear to play a major role in limiting the intake of operational rations under field conditions. A corollary of this conjecture is that whatever makes eating easier, less time consuming, and free from situational limitations will lead to higher levels of food intake. The scene just described is obviously complex, with many factors that are difficult to operationalize or to quantify. Studies that vary the effort or cost, of obtaining food may provide an appropriate model for a better understanding of eating behavior in this environment.

The literature is limited on the effects of either cost or effort, broadly defined to include physical cost, monetary cost, physiological cost, or cost in a cost-benefit sense on human ingestion. Most of the initial studies were conducted in the context of testing Schachter's (1971) hypothesis that the obese differ from normal-weight individuals in that their feeding behavior is more responsive to external food-related cues than to internal physiological signals related to hunger and satiety. Within this framework, Schachter and Friedman (1974) placed either shelled or unshelled almonds in front of obese and normal subjects while they were filling out a questionnaire. More obese subjects ate almonds when the shells were removed than did normal subjects, and fewer ate almonds when the shells were left on. Singh and Sikes (1974) reported a similar pattern when cashew nuts were wrapped in aluminum foil or left unwrapped. Although the obese and normal subjects differed in the degree of their responsiveness, this simple manipulation showed that even apparently trivial increases in effort had a substantial impact on the intake of these snack items. Two observational studies conducted in a cafeteria context also showed that seemingly minor changes in the accessibility of high-calorie desserts (Meyers et al., 1980) or ice cream (Levitz, 1975) affected food selection in both normal-weight and obese subjects. Both groups reduced their selection of these items when they were made less accessible.

Studies that have directly manipulated response cost or effort (Lappalainen and Epstein, 1990) or monetary cost (Durrant and Garrow, 1982) have shown that food choices in a short test session (Lappalainen and Epstein, 1990) or over 24 hours (Durrant and Garrow, 1982) are sensitive to the cost aspects of food availability. When the response cost or effort associated with obtaining a preferred food was increased relative to a less preferred food, responding for the preferred food dropped to zero. In the Durrant and Garrow (1982) study, baseline food choices from a dispenser by obese subjects were obtained. Subjects were then given sufficient money to maintain their baseline intake only if they chose from the less preferred items (preferred foods were relatively costly). Under this regimen, subjects showed a 20 percent reduction in energy intake but a 65 percent reduction in intake of preferred foods. Thus, subjects were willing to sacrifice intake of more desirable foods to maintain overall intake but not to the extent of completely eliminating the preferred items.

Water intake is also sensitive to the effort associated with obtaining it during a luncheon meal (Engell and Hirsch, 1991). Subjects were randomly assigned to one of three conditions of water availability: (1) a pitcher within reach on the dining table, (2) an immovable dispenser approximately 20 feet from the dining table, and (3) an immovable dispenser in another room approximately 40 feet from the dining table. In the last condition, subjects were told that the water was in the other room for a taste test being conducted there. Figure 11-3 shows that under these conditions of water availability, more than twice as much water was consumed when it was located on the dining room table relative to the two other conditions. Figure 11-4 shows that premeal thirst ratings did not differ in the three groups, but the group that had water on the table was the only one to report a reduction in postmeal levels of thirst.

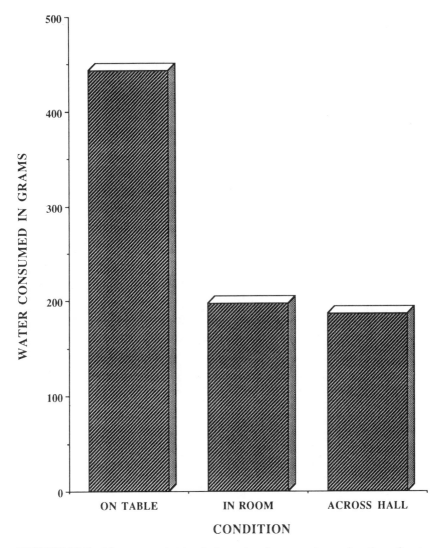

FIGURE 11-3 Mean water intake during a luncheon meal as a function of water accessibility.

Encouraged by these laboratory observations and reports that troops frequently do not heat operational rations in the field (Popper et al., 1987), Lester and Kramer (1991) reasoned that if troops were provided with a convenient way to heat their rations, acceptability and consumption should improve. They tested this idea in a 5-day field study in a cold environment. Three groups of U.S. Marines fed MRE VIII were provided with different heating methods. One group was given a canteen cup stand and a more-

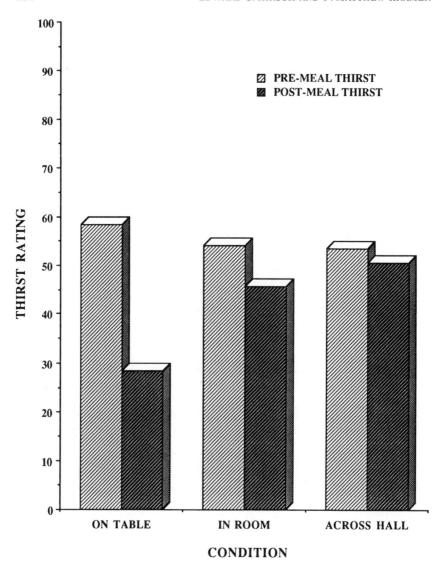

FIGURE 11-4 Mean thirst ratings on a 100-mm visual analogue scale prior to and after a luncheon meal as a function of water accessibility.

than-sufficient supply of heat tabs. With this method, a canteen cup containing water and an MRE package is placed on top of the stand and the heat tab is lit. A second group was given ration heater pads—an alloy/polymer composite that reacts with water to produce heat—to heat both food items and water. The third group was given an Optimus Hiker Stove, which is issued by the Marine Corps as the standard cold weather gear for heating rations. One stove was available for approximately every five subjects. A final questionnaire revealed that the two individual heating methods were viewed as more convenient than the group method, but the two individual methods differed with respect to their effectiveness and ease of heating food or water. The canteen cup stand was viewed as more effective for water, and the ration heater pad was best for entrees. Group differences in energy intake and food acceptability were consistent with these questionnaire ratings. In general, convenience in heating and increased frequency of using the heating devices were associated with increased acceptance and consumption of the heated items and the ration as a whole.

This brief overview reveals that data on the effects of effort and cost on human food intake are limited but remarkably consistent. Increases in the cost or effort associated with obtaining, preparing, or consuming food or water lead to a reduction in intake. The limited nature of the database urges caution, but the pronounced effects of what appear to be minor changes in these dimensions also encourage the speculation that whatever can be done to make eating easier and less constrained in the field (doctrine, command emphasis, food packaging, heating methods, and so on) will enhance consumption.

Social Influences

The marketing and advertising budgets of the food industry provide ample testimony to the perceived power of social forces on eating behavior, yet this aspect of the feeding environment has been largely ignored by research. In domains other than eating, social influences on behavior and attitudes have been intensively researched and found to exert powerful effects. Studies by Asch (1956) on group conformity and by Milgram (1973) on obedience to authority have dramatically illustrated the power of social forces on the behavior and expressed attitudes of individuals. Studies by Zimbardo and colleagues (Haney et al., 1973) of a mock prison system similarly provide a powerful example of how the social context can alter behavior of a group. Two aspects of social influence seem especially pertinent. First, social influence may occur within the soldier's peer group (for example, soldiers grumbling about the food) or through the chain of command. NCOs (noncommissioned officers; that is, sergeants) have the greatest day-to-day influence, but opinions and thereby influence can filter down from higher levels as well. Second, social facilitation of eating can either have a direct impact on eating or be a vehicle for transmission of peer and leadership behaviors and attitudes.

Although the practical application of social forces to the shaping of eating behavior is limited at this time, evidence exists for its importance in food consumption and acceptance in both humans (de Castro and de Castro, 1989) and animals (Galef, 1986). Indeed, sociocultural factors are a primary influence in food intake and acceptance (Axelson, 1986; Rozin and Vollmecke, 1986). Similarly, societal norms for beauty and body weight play a major role in eating disorders (Polivy and Herman, 1985; Striegel-Moore et al., 1986). Finally, food and mealtimes have immense symbolic value in the cultural and interpersonal domain (Messer, 1984).

What then is the evidence for social influence on feeding behavior? A number of recent publications have confirmed that meal size is larger when people eat together than when they eat alone (Edelman et al., 1986; Klesges et al., 1984). The most systematic work in this area has been reported by de Castro (de Castro, 1990; de Castro and de Castro, 1989; de Castro et al., 1990). As part of his ongoing investigation of factors influencing meal size, he has concluded that the number of people present at a meal is the single most important predictor of amount eaten (de Castro and de Castro, 1989). Caloric intake in meals eaten with others averaged 44 percent more than meals eaten alone (de Castro and de Castro, 1989). He also found that social facilitation of eating is apparent not only in comparing eating alone to eating with others but also in comparing groups of different sizes (de Castro and de Castro, 1989). The upper limit for this effect and its variability from situation to situation remain to be determined.

De Castro has also examined how social facilitation affects eating in the context of other potential influences (for example, hunger, prior meal size). Social facilitation appears to have an additive effect to these variables (de Castro, 1990; de Castro and de Castro, 1989). Social facilitation also appears to take place regardless of time of day, place, or whether one eats a meal or a snack (de Castro et al., 1990). The results do not appear to be explained by either increased hunger under social conditions, generalized increases in arousal, or level of deprivation. Social facilitation may have a disruptive effect on satiety in that the amount eaten in a given social occasion does not have any clear influence on eating later in the day.

The meal characteristic most linked to group size is meal duration. As group size increases so does meal length. Regression analyses indicate that both number of people and meal length, although correlated, have independent effects on meal size (de Castro, 1990). De Castro (1990) raises a number of possible explanations for his results. Under more social conditions, people may linger over their meal longer and as a result eat more. Likewise, larger meals will tend to increase meal duration. Social factors might also diminish or distract people from psychological or physiological constraints on eating. Social facilitation of eating appears to be robust, but its mechanism cannot be well explained at this time.

Social facilitation in a group context is illustrated by data collected during a field evaluation of the T-ration, a group feeding method in which the main components of the meal are in large cans (Salter et al., 1991). Intake was collected over a 2-week period, at the end of which soldiers completed a questionnaire that, among other information, asked about the social context of meals. Figure 11-5 shows average daily intake as a function of number of meals eaten socially. Social eating was defined as eating with a small group, and nonsocial eating was defined as eating alone or as part of an undifferentiated large group of 50 to 70 people. As can be seen, caloric intake increased linearly as the number of social meals increased. The increase is modest (about 150 calories per day), but given its consistency with prior research and the limitations of the approach, these results suggest that more controlled investigation is warranted.

Social influence on food intake and acceptance may also take place through the behavior and stated opinions of other people in the environment. It is clear that modeling can have a potent effect on food acceptance and consumption. Polivy et al. (1979) recruited subjects to eat a meal with

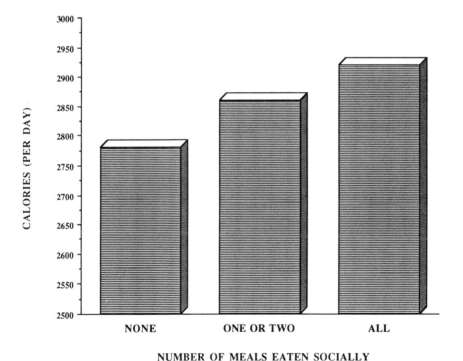

FIGURE 11-5 Mean daily caloric intake as a function of the number of daily meals eaten in a social group in troops fed T-rations.

one other person who was actually a confederate. The confederate ate either two or eight sandwich quarters and either identified herself as a dieter or did not. Both amount eaten by the confederate and identification as a dieter had an impact on subjects' eating. Subjects ate more when the confederate had eight sandwich quarters than when she had two and ate less when the confederate identified herself as a dieter. An example from research in this laboratory illustrates the phenomenon (Engell et al., 1990). Two groups of soldiers along with their longstanding NCO were recruited to eat two lunch meals of military rations. Unbeknownst to the soldiers, the NCO acted as a confederate. Each soldier was given a meal tray and instructed to taste and rate each item before eating freely. After these initial ratings, the NCO made a brief positive or negative comment about the food, such as "this food is a lot better than I thought it would be" and ate appropriately (most of the food versus approximately 65 percent of the food served). Soldiers then ate as much or as little as they wished and were given repeated opportunities to have additional servings. Once the meal was finished, the subjects again rated all of the items. As seen in Figure 11-6, soldiers ate approximately 11 percent more when the NCO was positive than when he was negative. Similarly, food acceptance from before to after the meal showed a significant decline in the negative condition and a nonsignificant increase in the positive group (Figure 11-7). Military food is traditionally described in a negative manner, but as demonstrated here, a simple verbal statement and appropriate modeling had a noticeable impact on both ration consumption and acceptance.

What remains to be determined is whether such modeling can (and under which conditions) have an effect on extended consumption of operational rations. In addition, a potentially important distinction exists between social influences on public versus private attitudes and behavior. Studies using Asch's (Asch, 1956) classic method have consistently found a marked effect of social pressure on behavior in a group but little evidence to suggest that private attitudes or behavior are changed. This distinction between the impact of social influences on food attitudes versus eating behavior is provided by Smith (1961) in which different methods were used in an attempt to persuade soldiers to eat fried grasshoppers. In one condition, a rationale for eating grasshoppers under extreme conditions was presented by an NCO who concluded his talk by eating a grasshopper. The author assessed both change in the acceptance rating from before to after the manipulation and number of grasshoppers consumed. Soldiers in the group with the NCO showed little change in attitude about eating grasshoppers, but nearly 90 percent ate one or more grasshoppers. In contrast, subjects who were told they would be paid $.50 for each grasshopper eaten following a presentation by a cool, formal experimenter showed a substantial and positive change in attitude, but over 50 percent refused to eat any grasshoppers.

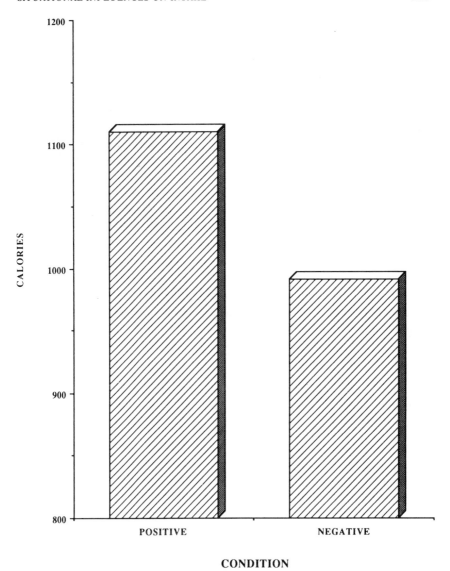

FIGURE 11-6   Mean caloric intake in a luncheon meal following negative or positive comments at the start of the meal.

Time of Day

Time of day plays a large role in setting peoples' daily routines. Sociocultural conventions guide these decisions, and like other behavior, eating often is determined by time of day (Schachter and Gross, 1968). For example, although some foods are considered suitable for any meal, most

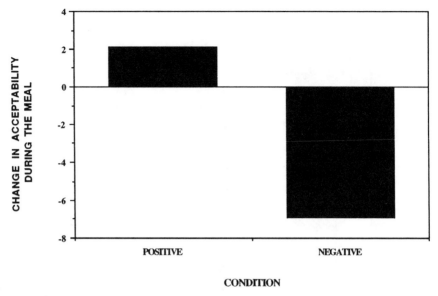

FIGURE 11-7 Mean change in acceptability on a 100-mm visual analogue scale of food consumed in a lunch meal following negative or positive comments at the start of the meal.

foods are considered appropriate for only selected meals. In particular, a distinction exists between morning meals and meals later in the day. Although many breakfast foods are eaten later in the day, few people would consider roast beef, vegetables, or ice cream as appropriate for breakfast. Operational military rations have been especially noted for lacking sufficient numbers of acceptable breakfast meals. Soldiers comment that they would like to have more breakfast meals and better ones than those presently available. Furthermore, when MREs are the sole source of food, soldiers eat less and rate the food as less acceptable at morning meals (Hirsch et al., 1985; Lester et al., 1990). One study found effects of time of day on hedonic ratings (Birch et al., 1984), but recent reports also show that even under normal day-to-day conditions, breakfast is typically the smallest meal of the day (Chao and Vanderkooy, 1989; Fricker et al., 1990). Thus, whether time of day is affecting overall intake requires further exploration.

To better determine the relevance of time of day, this laboratory conducted a study in which subjects ate four meals (Kramer et al., 1991). Two meals were served at 8:00 a.m. and two at 12:00 noon. One meal at each time consisted of lunch-type foods such as a turkey sandwich, and one consisted of breakfast foods such as bacon and eggs. Subjects were given a serving of each item with additional servings available on request. Contrary to what was expected, no clear effect of meal "appropriateness" was found. Mean caloric intake at each meal is shown in Figure 11-8. Both the time when the meal was eaten and the type of food served affected consumption. Subjects ate more at noon than at 8:00 a.m., and subjects ate more when offered a lunch menu than a breakfast menu. The hypothesized statistical interaction between menu type and serving time did not approach significance. Hedonic ratings were also not affected by time of day. These results suggest that the best strategy to improve consumption is to focus primarily on developing the most acceptable and nutritious meals possible without regard to their time-of-day appropriateness. Interestingly, subjects' hunger ratings after the meal gave some indication that appropriateness is a salient feature. Although changes in hunger from immediately before to after the meal did not differ across the meal, hunger did recover more rapidly following inappropriate meals than following appropriate meals. Given that intake and acceptance were not affected by time of day, the importance of this finding remains to be determined.

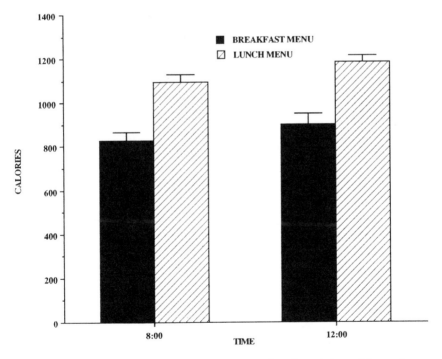

FIGURE 11-8 Mean caloric intake in meals as a function of time of day and type of food.

The results suggest that when subjects do not have a choice about type of food, the appropriateness of those foods for that time of day will have little impact on intake or hedonic ratings. However, as noted earlier, soldiers engaged in field training typically eat less and rate the foods lower for morning meals than for meals at other times of day. Whether this finding merely reflects that morning meals tend to be smaller or is more closely linked to a lack of appropriate breakfast foods cannot be determined with current data.

CONCLUSIONS AND RECOMMENDATIONS

Three major themes are developed in this review. First, a consistent pattern of underconsumption relative to maintenance needs is apparent when troops subsist on operational rations in combat or training environments. Second, the dining room-laboratory environment embodied features that support substantially higher levels of food intake than a field environment. Third, seemingly minor changes in the feeding situation can have marked effects on food acceptance, food choice, and food intake. It is possible to translate these themes into recommendations that are relevant to troops living and working in hot weather environments, with the caveat that there is limited information concerning the specific effects of situational factors on human food intake to strongly support particular conclusions.

The general conceptual model posited here says that whatever makes eating in the field easier and less constrained will enhance consumption. This approach could be accomplished through military doctrine, command emphasis, ration design and configuration, or materials used in food preparation and disposal. Similarly, social factors could be exploited in a direct fashion, such as by encouraging scheduled group feeding or through leadership influence and example. These authors believe the latter in tandem with marketing and training offers particular promise. Although instituting a policy of eating with one's buddies at every meal is not possible, officers can be given a basis for describing, and encouraged to describe, rations in a positive way.

REFERENCES

Asch, S.
   1956   Studies of independence and conformity: A minority of one against a unanimous majority. Psychol. Monogr. 70:No. 9, Whole No. 416.
Askew, E.W., J.R. Claybaugh, S.A. Cucinell, A.J. Young, and E.G. Szeto
   1986   Nutrient intakes and work performance of soldiers during seven days of exercise at 7,200 ft altitude consuming the meal, ready-to-eat ration. Technical Report T3-87. U.S. Army Research Institute of Environmental Medicine, Natick, Mass.

Askew, E.W., I. Munro, M.A. Sharp, S. Siegel, R. Popper, M.S. Rose, R.W. Hoyt, J.W. Martin, K. Reynolds, H.R. Lieberman, D.B. Engell, and C.P. Shaw.
1987   Nutritional status and physical and mental performance of special operations soldiers consuming the ration, lightweight or the meal, ready-to-eat military field ration during a 30-day field training exercise. Technical Report T7-87. U.S. Army Research Institute of Environmental Medicine, Natick, Mass.

Axelson, M.L.
1986   The impact of culture on food related behavior. Ann. Review Nutr. 6:345-363.

Bean, W.B.
1946   Nutrition survey of American troops in the Pacific. Nutr. Rev. 4:257-259.

Birch, L.L., J. Billman, and S.S. Richards
1984   Time of day influences food acceptability. Appetite 5:109-116.

Carlson, D., T. Dugan, J. Buchbinder, J. Allegretto and D. Schnakenberg
1987   Nutritional assessment of the Ft. Riley Non-Commissioned Officer Academy Dining Facility. Technical Report 14-87. U.S. Army Institute of Environmental Medicine, Natick, Mass.

Chao, E.S.M, and P.S. Vanderkooy
1989   An oversview of breakfast nutrition. J. Can. Diet. Assoc. 50:225-228.

Collier, G.
1989   The economics of hunger, thirst, satiety and regulation. Ann. N.Y. Acad. Sci. 575:136-154.

de Castro, J.M.
1988   Physiological, environmental, and subjective determinants of food intake in humans: A meal pattern analysis. Physiol. Behav. 44:651-659.
1990   Social facilitation of duration and size but not rate of the spontaneous meal intake of humans. Physiol. Behav. 47:1129-1135.

de Castro, J.M., and E.S. de Castro
1989   Spontaneous meal patterns of humans: Influence of the presence of other people. Am. J. of Clin. Nutr. 50:237-247.

de Castro, J.M., E.M. Brewer, D.K. Elmore, and S. Orozco
1990   Social facilitation of the spontaneous meal size of humans occurs regardless of time, place, alcohol or snacks. Appetite 15:89-101.

Durrant, M.L., and J.S. Garrow
1982   The effect of increasing the relative cost of palatable food with respect to ordinary food on total-energy intake of eight obese inpatients. Int. J. Obes. 6:153-164.

Edelman, B., D. Engell, P. Bronstein, and E. Hirsch
1986   Environmental effects on the intake of overweight and normal-weight men. Appetite 7:71-83.

Edwards, J.S.A., D.E. Roberts, T.E. Morgan, and L.S. Lester
1989   An evaluation of the nutritional intake and acceptability of the meal, ready-to-eat consumed with and without a supplemental pack in a cold environment. Technical Report T18-89. U.S. Army Research Institute of Environmental Medicine, Natick, Mass.

Edwards, J.S.A., D.E. Roberts, S.H. Mutter, and R.J. Moore
1990   A comparison of the meal, ready-to-eat VIII with supplemental pack and the ration cold weather consumed in an arctic environment. Technical Report T21-90. U.S. Army Research Institute of Environmental Medicine, Natick, Mass.

Engell, D., and E. Hirsch
1991   Environmental and sensory modulation of fluid intake in humans. Pp. 382-390 in Thirst: Physiological and Psychological Aspects, D.J. Ramsey and D. Booth, eds. London, U.K.: Springer-Verlag.

Engell, D.B., D.E. Roberts, E.W. Askew, M.S. Rose, J. Buchbinder, and M.A. Sharpe
  1987   Evaluation of the ration cold weather during a 10-day cold weather field training
          exercise. Natick Technical Report TR-87/030. U.S. Army Natick Research, Devel-
          opment and Engineering Center, Natick, Mass.
Engell, D., F.M. Kramer, S. Luther, and S.O. Adams
  1990   The effect of social influences on food intake. Presented at the Society for Nutri-
          tion Education 1990 Annual Meeting, Anaheim, Calif.
Fox, M., N. Wenham, and E. Hirsch
  1989   Acceptability studies of military ration: Meal, ready-to-eat. J. Foodserv. Systems
          5:189-197.
Fricker, J., S. Giroux, F. Fumeron, and M. Apfelbaum
  1990   Circadian rhythms of energy intake and corpulence status in adults. Int. J. Obes.
          14:387-393.
Galef, B.G.
  1986   Social interaction modifies learned aversions, salt appetite, and both palatability
          and handling-induced dietary preference in rats (*Rattus norvegicus*). J. Comp.
          Psychol. 100:432-439.
Haney, C., W.C. Banks, and P. Zimbardo
  1973   Interpersonal dynamics in a simulated prison. Int. J. Criminol. Penol. 1:69-97.
Hirsch, E., H.L. Meiselman, R.D. Popper, G. Smits, B. Jezior, I. Lichton, N. Wenkam, J. Burt,
          M. Fox, S. McNutt, M.N. Thiele, and O. Direge
  1985   The effects of prolonged feeding meal, ready-to-eat (MRE) operational rations.
          Technical Report Natick TR-85/035. U.S. Army Natick Research, Development
          and Engineering Center, Natick, Mass.
Johnson, R.E., and R.M. Kark
  1946   Feeding problems in man as related to environment. An analysis of United States
          and Canadian army ration trials and surveys, 1941-1946, Chicago, Quartermaster
          Food and Container Institute for the Armed Forces, Research and Development
          Branch, Office of the Quartermaster General.
Klesges, R.C., D. Bartsch, J.D. Norwood, D. Kautzman, and S. Haugrud
  1984   The effects of selected social and environmental variables on the eating behavior
          of adults in the natural environment. Int. J. Eating Disord. 3:35-41.
Kramer, F.M., K. Rock, and D. Engell
  1992   Effects of time of day and appropriateness on food intake and hedonic ratings of
          morning and midday. Appetite 14:1.13.
Lappalainen, R., and L.W. Epstein
  1990   A behavioral economics analysis of food choice in humans. Appetite 14:81-93.
Lester, L.S., and F.M. Kramer
  1991   The effects of heating on food acceptability and consumption. J. Foodserv. Sys-
          tems.
Lester L.S., F.M. Kramer, J. Edinberg, S. Mutter, and D.B. Engell
  1990   Evaluation of the canteen cup stand and ration heater pad: Effects on acceptability
          and consumption of the meal, ready-to-eat in a cold weather environment. Techni-
          cal Report Natick TR-90/008L. U.S. Army Natick Research, Development and
          Engineering Center, Natick, Mass.
Levitz, L.
  1975   The susceptibility of feeding to external control. Pp. 53-60 in Obesity in Perspec-
          tive, G. A. Bray, ed. Department of Health, Education, and Welfare Publication
          No. NIH 75-708. Washington, D.C.: U.S. Government Printing Office.
Lichton, I.J., J.B. Miyamura, and S.W. McNutt
  1988   Nutritional evaluation of soldiers subsisting on meal, ready-to-eat operational ra-

tions for an extended period: Body measurements, hydration, and blood nutrients. Am. J. Clin. Nutr. 48:30-37.

McCaig, R.H., and C.Y. Gooderson
1986   Ergonomic and physiological aspects of military operations in a cold wet climate. Ergonomics 29:849-857.

Messer, E.
1984   Anthropological perspectives on diet. Annu. Rev. Anthropol. 13:205-249.

Meyers, A.W., A.J. Stunkard, and M. Coll
1980   Food accessibility and food choice. Arch. Gen. Psychiatry 37:1133-1135.

Milgram, S.
1973   Obedience to Authority. New York: Harper and Row.

Morgan, T.E., L.A. Hodgess, D. Schilling, R.W. Hoyt, E.J. Iwanyk, G. McAninch, T.C. Wells, and E.W. Askew
1988   A comparison of the meal, ready-to-eat, ration, cold weather, and ration, light-weight nutrient intakes during moderate altitude cold weather field training operations. Technical Report T5-89. U.S. Army Research Institute of Environmental Medicine, Natick, Mass.

Polivy, J., and C.P. Herman
1985   Dieting and binging: A causal analysis. Am. Psychol. 40:193-201.

Polivy, J., C.P. Herman, J.C. Younger, and B. Erskine
1979   Effects of a model on eating behavior: The induction of a restrained eating style. J. Pers. 47:100-117.

Popper, R., E. Hirsch, L. Lesher, D. Engell, B. Jezior, B. Bell, and W.T. Matthew
1987   Field evaluation of Improved MRE, MRE VII, and MRE IV. Technical Report Natick TR-87/027. U.S. Army Natick Research, Development and Engineering Center, Natick, Mass.

Popper, R., G. Smits, H.L. Meiselman, and E. Hirsch
1989   Eating in combat: A survey of U.S. Marines. Milit. Med. 154:619-623.

Rose, M.S., and D.E. Carlson
1987   Effect of A-ration meals on body weight during sustained field operations. Technical Report T2-87. U.S. Army Research Institute of Environmental Medicine, Natick, Mass.

Rose, R.W., C. Baker, C. Salter, W. Wisnaskas, J.S.A. Edwards, and M.S. Rose
1989   Dietary assessment of U.S. Army basic trainees at Fort Jackson, SC. Technical Report T6-89. U.S. Army Research Institute of Environmental Medicine, Natick, Mass.

Rozin, P., and T.A. Vollmecke
1986   Food likes and dislikes. Ann. Rev. Nutr. 6:433-456.

Salter, C.A., D. Engell, F.M. Kramer, L.S. Lester, J.J. Kalick, L.L. Lester, S.L. Dewey, and D. Caretti
1991   The relative acceptability and consumption of the current and proposed versions of the T Ration. Technical Report 91/031. U.S. Army Natick Research, Development and Engineering Center, Natick, Mass.

Schachter, S.
1971   Some extraordinary facts about obese humans and rats. Am. Psychol. 26:129-144.

Schachter, S., and L.N. Friedman
1974   The effects of work and cue prominence on eating behavior. Pp. 11-14 in Obese Humans and Rats, S. Schachter and J. Rodin, eds. Potomac, Md.: Earlbaum Associates.

Schachter, S., and L. Gross
1968   Manipulated time and eating behavior. J. Personal. Soc. Psychol. 10:98-106.

Singh, D., and S. Sikes
   1974   Role of past experience on food-motivated behavior of obese humans. J. Comp.
             Physiol. Psychol. 86:503-508.
Smith, E.E.
   1961   The power of dissonance techniques to change attitudes. Public Opin. Q. 25:626-
             639.
Striegel-Moore, R.H., L.R. Silberstein, and J. Rodin
   1986   Toward an understanding of risk factors for bulimia. Am. Psychol. 41:246-263.
Szeto, E.G., D.E. Carlson, T.B. Dugan, and J.C. Buchbinder
   1987   A comparison of nutrient intakes between a Ft. Riley contractor-operated and a Ft.
             Lewis military-operated garrison dining facility. Technical Report T2-88. U.S.
             Army Research Institute of Environmental Medicine, Natick, Mass.
Szeto, E.G., T.B. Dugan, and J.A. Gallo
   1988   Nutrient intakes of habitual diners in a military-operated garrison dining facility—
             Ft. Devens I. Technical Report T3-89. U.S. Army Research Institute of Environ-
             mental Medicine, Natick, Mass.
Szeto, E., J.A. Gallo, and K.W. Samonds
   1989   Passive nutrition intervention in military-operated garrison dining facility—Ft. Devens
             II. Technical Report T7-89. U.S. Army Research Institute of Environmental Medi-
             cine, Natick, Mass.
Webster, E.C., and F.H. Johnson
   1945   Questionnaire of wounded soldiers. Part II. Data on rations in combat and behind
             the lines. Report No. C6162 to the Associate Committee Army Medical Research,
             National Research Council Canada.
Wenkam, N.S., M. Fox, M.N. Thiele, and I.J. Lichton
   1989   Energy and nutrient intakes of soldiers consuming MRE operational rations: Physiological
             correlates. J. Am. Diet. Assoc. 89:407-409.
Youmans, J.B.
   1955   Malnutrition and deficiency diseases. Pp. 159-170 in Preventive Medicine in World
             War II, J.B. Coates, Jr., and E.C. Hoff, eds. Washington, D.C.: Office of the
             Surgeon General, Department of the Army.

DISCUSSION

DR. NESHEIM: Any questions?

PARTICIPANT: A couple of comments. One of them is about getting up in the morning—the attendance being low for the breakfast items in the field kitchens—when you talk about the notion about how much work is involved, breakfast is a good case. Going to breakfast is a little bit more trouble, often, than it is to go to eat at lunchtime when you are already up.

But the other thing that I think needs to be emphasized is that as the Army goes more and more to continuous operations which go around the clock, it is really very difficult to say what time of day is breakfast.

So the notion of the meal that is served early in the morning being everybody's breakfast, I think, needs to be reevaluated because for many of the troops, particularly the light infantry, who do most of their raids at night, the meal that they eat early in the morning is the meal they are eating before they go to bed.

So the whole notion of what is breakfast becomes very confused and that needs to be given some consideration.

PARTICIPANT: One of the things that we heard yesterday from most speakers and you mentioned also, is the availability of time and eating on the run. I have noticed that that is one of the variables that you didn't have any data on, people who had more access to time.

DR. HIRSCH: I think it is critical. Since the first MRE test, we have been trying to line up a field study where troop commanders would allow us to schedule meals and provide ample time for eating.

Even during a training exercise, troop commanders don't want to relinquish that kind of control and impose that lack of flexibility on themselves. It is a real problem and I think particularly in the heat, which we were fortunate to escape this time around.

PARTICIPANT: One other question related to that, we heard about the number of packets that they have to deal with. Would it make sense to consider greater proportions of calories in something that could be consumed between meals, on-the-go type of things.

DR. HIRSCH: I think we will probably move in that direction. On-the-go food items are one of the items that troops were asking for.

PARTICIPANT: I just want to address the question about putting lunch and dinner type items in breakfast menus and this is in the early 1980s. We only had really about five entrees but they told us that we will eat anything you give us for breakfast. So we went to that concept of putting what we felt were mildly flavored lunch and dinner items at breakfast.

The comments that came back, even though they told us to do this, were abominable. They didn't want to see another beef stew or peppers or lasagna or whatever we put—I don't remember.

We had excesses that we had to use up for years in the 1984, 1985 and 1986 time frame. I am not saying that in the 1990s now that people are used to it and we have been to work, that that might not work, but we did try that and that was—we lost so much credibility with the agency that was doing menus at the time that I would be reluctant to do that again, and we were listening to the troops.

DR. HIRSCH: Yes, but I think at that point in time you were dealing with such a limited range of entrees that were available, that what you were giving them for breakfast they were also seeing for lunch and dinner. No wonder they were upset with you.

PARTICIPANT: I was just curious about the breakfast items. Were they significantly worse?

DR. HIRSCH: I invite you to join us for a tray pack breakfast when you are up in Boston.

PARTICIPANT: I can tell you that a breakfast tray pack doesn't look very good.

PARTICIPANT: Even in a civilian setting, the breakfast meal is usually the one where people are willing to put forth the least effort. They want a breakfast cereal or something you could pour milk on, something that is fast.

I would guess that in a military setting, you have the additional effort of having to get up earlier and you have to go to the effort of heating water and rehydrating something. The whole environment would argue against their eating it.

It seems like it is almost a set-up to almost ensure that you are going to have minimal consumption. I would think the effort would have to be directed to greater ease of preparation, something that could be eaten cold perhaps.

DR. HIRSCH: Well, they are certainly moving in that direction with the breakfast cereals which are very popular.

PARTICIPANT: A comment on that, one of the things that people ask for from home to kind of fill that is things like pop tarts and granola bars which they would often eat for breakfast.

PARTICIPANT: I notice that now. Kids eat poptarts now without putting them in the toaster. They eat them cold out of the package.

DR. HIRSCH: My own guess is that as the American culture moves more and more toward packaged eat-on-the-run foods, it will be much easier for the soldier to find that part of his military ration and be very comfortable with it.

In the past, when we have tried to feed people unconventional foods that they have never seen before or had a strange name or a strange sight, they really resist it.

Over the past several years there have been some, senior generals had very strong opinions about the rations and let it be known to their troops and you could just see that attitude in working with the troops.

As a matter of fact, in testing one of the new versions of the MRE, we were kind of told that before we went to the field with it, we had to test it with his troops, and until his troops told him it was okay, he was going to fight it.

And fortunately, the product was good enough that with this version of the MRE, his troops endorsed it and he went along. But the senior leadership effect is very dramatic. I can't quantify it but I certainly see it every time I am out with troops.

PARTICIPANT: To what extent have cold instant breakfasts consumed as beverages been tried?

DR. HIRSCH: I can't think of any.

PARTICIPANT: Just an editorial comment on whether the leadership has any impact, but one thing that is real obvious in the field is many of the senior NCOs that were in Vietnam had the C rations, whether they like it or not, in their mind it was better.

And routinely you will have 18-, 19-year-old soldiers who wouldn't know one if a palette-full dropped on them, will tell you, C rations were much better than MREs. People they trust say it is, so it must be so.

DR. NESHEIM: Thank you very much.

PART III

U.S. Army Presentations: A Reevaluation of Sodium Requirements for Work in the Heat

OVERVIEW

PART III CONSISTS OF THREE CHAPTERS that present different aspects of a team research project undertaken by the Army at the U.S. Army Research Institute of Environmental Medicine. This project focused on the important issue of the level of dietary sodium needed for work during heat acclimation. The study was conducted with volunteers in the temperature controlled environmental chambers in Natick, Massachusetts. Similar to the participants whose papers form Part II, all authors of papers in Part III were asked to provide copies of at least three background articles related to their portion of the project to the Committee on Military Nutrition Research prior to the workshop. There was a recorded question and answer period at the end of each presentation. Selected questions directed toward the speakers and their responses are included at the end of each chapter. After the workshop, all authors were given the opportunity to revise or add to their papers based on committee questions. The papers were then submitted in writing and used by the committee in the development of Part I. All recommended background articles and selected references from the chapters in Part III are included in the Selected Bibliography on Nutritional Needs in Hot Environments in Appendix B. The research reported in these chapters has relevance to all individuals who are concerned about their diets and exercise in the hot environments whether outdoors or in more climatically controlled settings such as indoor tracks, gymnasiums, and racket courts.

Nutritional Needs in Hot Environments
Pp. 247–258. Washington, D.C.
National Academy Press

12

Responses of Soldiers to 4-gram and 8-gram NaCl Diets During 10 Days of Heat Acclimation

Lawrence E. Armstrong,[1] Roger W. Hubbard, Eldon W. Askew, and Ralph P. Francesconi

INTRODUCTION

The reported dietary sodium (Na^+) intake of adults in the United States ranges from 1800 to 5000 mg (78 to 218 mEq Na^+) per day, depending on the method of assessment (National Research Council, 1989a,b). Empirical studies have demonstrated that this intake is greater than the levels consumed by the inhabitants of several tropical countries (Conn, 1963; Dahl, 1958; Hubbard et al., 1986) and that the basal biologic human requirement for Na^+ ranges from only 50 to 175 mg (2 to 8 mEq Na^+) per day (Dahl, 1958). These facts, and previous studies that related dietary sodium chloride (NaCl) to hypertension (Tobian, 1989), led to a recent dietary recommendation of 2400 mg (104 mEq) of Na^+ per day (National Research Council, 1989a) for U.S. residents living in temperate climates.

However, observations made in hot environments (National Research Council, 1989b) suggest that this dietary recommendation may be inadequate because of increased daily Na^+ losses during exercise in the heat. For example, Denton (1982) reported losses of up to 24 g NaCl per day (408 mEq Na^+ per day) in the sweat of unacclimatized humans in hot climates. Several laboratory studies concluded that humans who eat low Na^+ diets and perform strenuous exercise in the heat have an increased risk (Armstrong et al., 1987; Hubbard and Armstrong, 1988) or incidence of

---

[1] Lawrence E. Armstrong, The Human Performance Laboratory, The University of Connecticut, Sports Center, Room 223, U-110, 2095 Hillside Road, Storrs, CT 06269-110

heat exhaustion (Taylor et al., 1944) or heat syncope (Bean and Eichna, 1943). Other experts (Consolazio, 1966; Ladell et al., 1954; Strauss et al., 1958) used field observations to derive Na^+ recommendations for soldiers of 13,000 to 48,000 mg NaCl (221 to 816 mEq Na^+) per day.

In contrast to those findings, laboratory studies of human heat acclimation (HA) (Armstrong et al., 1985; Conn, 1963) and dietary Na^+ intake (Dahl, 1958; National Research Council, 1989b) have suggested that humans function well when consuming relatively low Na^+ diets ranging from 1930 to 6000 mg NaCl per day (33 to 103 mEq Na^+ per day). Unfortunately, those human studies often did not involve prolonged exercise-heat exposure on many successive days or allow ample time for dietary Na^+ stabilization prior to HA. Therefore, the purpose of the current investigation was to evaluate the effects of moderate Na^+ diets ([8g NaCl] 137 mEq Na^+; abbreviated MNA) and low Na^+ diets ([4 g NaCl] 68 mEq Na^+; abbreviated LNA) on thermoregulatory, cardiovascular, hematologic, and fluid-electrolyte variables during 10 consecutive days of prolonged intermittent exercise (8 hours per day) in a simulated desert environment. This experiment was relevant to military populations because the caloric and Na^+ intakes typically decrease during the initial days of deployment in a hot environment, and because the maintenance of intravascular and intracellular fluid-electrolyte balance is essential to prolonged exercise in heat.

METHODS

The subjects of this investigation were 17 males who were not acclimated to heat; who gave their informed, voluntary consent to participate in the current investigation; and who underwent a medical examination. Selected physical characteristics for both treatment groups appear in Table 12-1.

During this 17.5-day study, subjects were housed 24 hours each day in a research building that contained sleeping, dining, and environmentally controlled chamber facilities. A proctor was present at all times to ensure that no subject left and that no food entered the research building. During the initial 7-day dietary equilibration period (days 1 to 7), all 17 subjects consumed MNA and were housed in an ambient temperature of 21°C. During the subsequent 10-day HA period (days 8 to 17), nine subjects continued to consume MNA and eight subjects began to consume LNA. On days 8 to 17, breakfast and dinner were consumed in the dormitory kitchen (21°C) while lunch was eaten in the tropical chamber (41°C) during the fifth rest period. Three primary meals and two snacks provided subjects with 55 percent carbohydrate, 13 percent protein, 32 percent fat, and 3600 kcal per day, in both LNA and MNA. Subjects drank assorted beverages ad libitum, when not involved in HA trials.

Upon awakening each morning (days 1 to 18), the following measures

TABLE 12-1 Day 1 Mean (±SE) Characteristics of Subjects Consuming Low Na$^+$ Diets (LNA) (n = 8) and Moderate Na$^+$ Diets (MNA) (n = 9)

Variable (unit)	Diet		Statistical Significance
	LNA[*]	MNA[†]	
n	8	9	—
Age (years)	20 ± 1	20 ± 1	NS[‡]
Height (cm)	180.1 ± 2.3	178.7 ± 2.3	NS
Mass (kg)	79.80 ± 3.18	77.86 ± 3.80	NS
Estimated body fat (%)[§]	14 ± 1	14 ± 1	NS
$\dot{V}_{O_2}$ peak (ml per kg per minute)	45.73 ± 1.69	47.09 ± 1.54	NS
HR (heart rate) peak	207 ± 9	211 ± 7	NS

[*]4 g NaCl, 68 mEq Na$^+$.
[†]8 g NaCl, 137 mEq Na$^+$.
[‡]NS, not significantly different (p > .05).
[§]Calculation from Jackson and Pollock (1978).

were taken: nude body weight (±50 g), first void urine specific gravity (refractometer), and first void urine Na$^+$ and potassium (K$^+$) concentrations (flame photometer). Blood samples also were collected prior to exercise on days 8, 11, 15, and 17. Subjects entered the 41°C environment and stood quietly for 20 minutes before the sample was drawn. Daily HA trials were conducted in ambient conditions of 41°C, 21 percent relative humidity (rh), and 1.2 m per second air speed (8.5 hours per day); during the remainder of each day (15.5 hours per day), subjects lived at an ambient temperature of 21°C in an effort to simulate a 24-hour desert temperature cycle. Exercise involved 8 periods of alternating rest (30 minutes per hour) and moderate (5.6 km per hour, 5 percent grade) treadmill exercise (30 minutes per hour) while wearing shorts, socks, and sneakers. Exercise was terminated (and subjects rested in the heat for the remainder of the trial) if heart rate (HR) exceeded 180 beats per minute, if rectal temperature (T_{re}) exceeded 39.5°C, or if T_{re} rose 0.6°C during any 5-minute period. Subjects drank pure or flavored water (<1 mEq Na$^+$ per liter, 10° to 15°C) ad libitum from canteens during treadmill walking and rest periods. Body weight was maintained each hour by requiring that subjects drink a volume of pure water, at the end of each rest period, that matched the amount of body mass not replaced by ad libitum drinking.

Statistical significance was tested by using a repeated measures analysis of variance (ANOVA) with Tukey's post hoc analysis (Zar, 1974). The two factors in this design were diet (LNA and MNA) and days (days 1 to 17; days 8 to 17; days 8, 11, 15, 17). The null hypotheses were rejected at the p = .05 confidence level. All data were expressed as mean ± standard error.

RESULTS

Morning Body Mass and Urinalysis

There were no between-diet differences in mean morning body mass values for LNA and MNA (days 1 to 18, $p > .05$, NS). Between-day differences ($p < .001$) were observed in the body mass of LNA, in that days 10 to 15 were significantly lower ($p < .001$) than day 8 (the initial day of heat exposure). The day-to-day body mass fluctuations in LNA and MNA may have involved changes in body fat, fat-free mass, or total body water. However, estimates of percent body fat showed no significant diet or day effects: day 1, 14 ± 1 percent (LNA), 14 ± 1 percent (MNA); day 8, 13 ± 1 percent (LNA), 14 ± 2 percent (MNA); day 17, 14 ± 1 percent (LNA), 15 ± 1 percent (MNA).

The mean morning urine specific gravity values for LNA and MNA (days 1 to 18) showed no between-diet differences ($p > .05$, NS). All mean urine specific gravity values (range: 1.016 to 1.023) indicated normal hydration status for both LNA and MNA on all days.

Figure 12-1 presents the concentrations of Na^+ and K^+ (mEq per liter) in the initial morning urine samples. The extremely low mean Na^+ concentration on days 9 to 15 indicated that LNA adhered to the salt-restricted dietary regimen. The significant between-diet (LNA versus MNA) differences ($p < .05$ to .001) in Na^+ and K^+ are represented by asterisks. The differences in urinary Na^+ were attributed to differential Na^+ consumption and conservation, while differences in urinary K^+ were of unknown origin and may have involved type I statistical errors of null hypothesis testing. Significant day-to-day differences in urinary Na^+ (not shown in Figure 12-1) were identified for LNA between day 1 and days 3 to 18 ($p < .05$ to .001), as well as between day 8 and days 9 to 17 ($p < .05$ to .001). Significant day-to-day differences were observed for urine Na^+ in group MNA between day 1 and days 2 to 18 ($p < .01$ to .001).

Preexercise Blood Measurements

Mean values for hematologic variables in Table 12-2 represent preexercise samples drawn at 7:30 a.m. on days 8, 11, 15, and 17. A noteworthy between-diet difference in percent change in plasma volume (PV) occurred on days 11 and 15. Although the LNA group exhibited a significantly smaller ($p < .05$) expansion of PV than MNA on days 11 and 15, both treatment groups manifested a similar percent change in PV by day 17 (+12.3 percent versus +12.4 percent). Similar, significant between-day decreases (Table 12-2) were identified for total plasma protein in LNA and MNA (day 8 versus days 11, 15, 17; $p < .01$), even though PV expansion exhibited

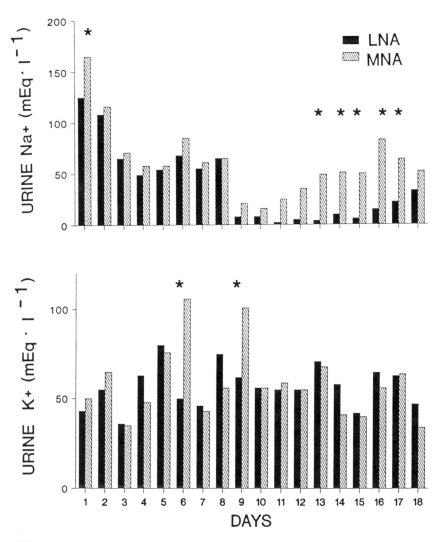

FIGURE 12-1 Mean Na$^+$ and K$^+$ concentrations (mEq per liter) of urine samples collected from low Na$^+$ diets (4 g NaCl, 68 mEq Na$^+$) (LNA) and moderate Na$^+$ diets (8 g NaCl, 137 mEq Na$^+$) (MNA) after awakening each morning. The significant between-diet (LNA versus MNA) differences ($p < .05$ to $.001$) in Na$^+$ and K$^+$ are represented by asterisks.

significant between-group differences (LNA versus MNA, $p < .05$) on days 11 and 15.

Responses During Heat Acclimation Trials

Although no cases of heat exhaustion, heat syncope, heat cramps, or heatstroke (Hubbard and Armstrong, 1988) occurred, the prolonged exercise resulted in numerous foot blisters and minor orthopedic injuries, which allowed only four subjects to complete all 80 of the 30-minute exercise bouts. The total distances walked by LNA and MNA, respectively, were 168.7 ± 18.9 and 185.4 ± 10.1 km per 10 days; these distances were not different ($p > .05$, NS) and were not significantly correlated with $\dot{V}_{O_2}$ peak ($p > .05$, NS).

There were no between-diet (LNA versus MNA) differences in heart rate (HR), on any day. Both MNA and LNA resulted in similar day 8 versus day 17 decreases in HR (for example, 140 beats per minute on day 8 versus 121 beats per minute on day 17), at the end of all exercise periods. Similarly, there were no between-diet differences (LNA versus MNA) in T_{re}, on any day. Both MNA and LNA resulted in similar day 8 versus day 17 decreases in T_{re} (for example, 38.3°C on day 8 versus 37.8°C on day 17), at the end of all exercise periods.

Sweat rate measurements during heat exposure were analyzed each day, for all subjects who completed eight exercise periods. These values ranged from 2850 to 3000 g per m^2 per 8 hours for LNA and from 2900 to 3050 g per m^2 per 8 hours for MNA on days 8 to 17 (the total volume of sweat approximated 6 kg per 8 hours). There were no between-diet differences and no between-day differences ($p > .05$, NS).

DISCUSSION

An evaluation of physical characteristics (Table 12-1), morning body mass, and morning urine specific gravity indicated no LNA versus MNA differences. With respect to HA trials, there were no between-diet differences in total distance walked, in HR, in T_{re}, in sweat rate, or in six out of seven blood variables (Table 12-2). The absence of heat cramps, heat syncope, or heat exhaustion in both LNA and MNA supported these data. It was concluded that dietary Na$^+$ restriction (LNA) resulted in HA responses that were similar to those exhibited during moderate Na$^+$ intake (MNA). In fact, only three variables showed LNA versus MNA differences: urine Na$^+$ (days 13 to 17), urine K$^+$ (days 6 and 9), and percent change in PV (days 11 and 15; see Table 12-2 and Armstrong et al. [1987]). Although an increase in sweat rate often occurs during human HA, it is not invariably present (Armstrong et al., 1985). A review of this topic (Henane, 1980) noted that

TABLE 12-2 Blood Variables of Low Na$^+$ Diets (LNA) ($n = 8$) and Moderate Na$^+$ Diets (MNA) ($n = 9$) at the Beginning of Heat Acclimation Trials on Days 8, 11, 15, and 17

Measurement (unit)	Diet	Day 8	11	15	17
Serum Na$^+$ (mEq per liter)	LNA*	137 ± 2	138 ± 2	140 ± 3†	137 ± 2‡
	MNA§	140 ± 1	140 ± 1	140 ± 1	139 ± 2
Serum K$^+$ (mEq per liter)	LNA	4.5 ± 0.2	4.5 ± 0.3	4.5 ± 0.2	4.4 ± 0.1
	MNA	4.2 ± 0.2	4.3 ± 0.2	4.3 ± 0.2	4.3 ± 0.2
Plasma osmolality (mOsmol per kg)	LNA	287 ± 1	285 ± 3	286 ± 3	287 ± 4
	MNA	287 ± 2	287 ± 2	288 ± 4	289 ± 2
Percent change in PV	LNA	—	+2.0 ± 1.8	+6.6 ± 2.0¶	+12.3 ± 1.7¶
	MNA	—	+11.5# ± 2.8	+12.8# ± 2.2	+12.4 ± 1.7
MCHC (g per 100 ml rbc)	LNA	33.90 ± 0.94	33.76 ± 1.13	34.40 ± 1.18	33.79 ± 0.68
	MNA	34.00 ± 0.90	34.34 ± 0.78	34.65 ± 1.01	33.87 ± 0.79
Total plasma protein (g per 100 ml)	LNA	8.8 ± 0.5	7.5 ± 0.3†	7.1 ± 0.4†	7.2 ± 0.3†
	MNA	8.6 ± 0.9	7.4 ± 0.4†	7.1 ± 0.3†	7.3 ± 0.3†
COP (mm Hg)	LNA	27.4 ± 1.3	28.6 ± 1.9	27.0 ± 1.4	26.3 ± 1.7
	MNA	29.7 ± 2.5**	28.0 ± 2.3**	28.2 ± 1.8	29.3 ± 2.2

NOTE: PV = plasma volume; MCHC = mean corpuscular hemoglobin concentration; rbc = red blood cells; COP = colloid osmotic pressure.

*4 g NaCl, 68 mEq Na$^+$.
†Significantly different ($p < .05, .01$) from day 8.
‡Significantly different ($p < .05$) from day 15.
§8 g NaCl, 137 mEq Na$^+$.
¶Significantly different ($p < .05, .01$) from day 11.
#Significant difference ($p < .05$) between LNA and MNA.
**Significant interaction effect ($p < .05, .01$) from day 8 to 11, and from day 11 to 15.

36 percent of HA studies ($n = 55$) showed no changes in sweat rate during HA and that sweat rate remained unchanged in hot-dry environments, such as this investigation, but increased markedly in humid environments. In addition, the day-to-day decline in T_{re} during exercise reduced the central drive for sweat production.

Plasma Volume Expansion

Table 12-2 demonstrates that the LNA group exhibited a significantly smaller ($p < .05$) expansion of PV than MNA on days 11 and 15, and that both treatment groups experienced a similar percent change in PV by day 17 (+12.3 percent versus +12.4 percent). A similarly delayed PV expansion was previously reported (Armstrong et al., 1987) for subjects consuming a low Na^+ diet (98 mEq Na^+ per day), when compared to a high Na^+ diet (399 mEq Na^+ per day), during an HA regimen involving 90 minutes of continuous daily exercise. It was suggested that such a delay in PV expansion might increase the risk of circulatory inadequacy or heat exhaustion on days 3 to 6 of HA because several between-diet differences (for example, HR, T_{re}, percent change in PV, sweat Na^+, and plasma Na^+) were observed (Armstrong et al., 1987). However, the absence of any form of heat illness (for example, heat exhaustion) in the current study strongly suggests that LNA does not elicit an increased risk of circulatory incompetence or heat exhaustion. The effects of high-intensity exercise or concurrent illness (for example, diarrhea) in the heat, while consuming LNA, are unknown and could have significant effects on fluid-electrolyte balance and physical performance (Ladell, 1957).

Na$^+$ Balance During Heat Acclimation

It is relevant to ask if there is a minimal or optimal range of daily salt consumption that optimally supports the acquisition and sustainment of HA. Because HA is intimately linked with adrenocortical regulation of urine/ sweat Na^+ losses and because NaCl losses may be large during exercise-heat exposure (Denton, 1982), several authors have concluded that a high salt diet is advisable prior to and during exercise in the heat (Consolazio, 1966; Ladell et al., 1954; Strauss et al., 1958) and that excess Na^+ simply would be excreted in urine without harm to health. However, an excess of whole body Na^+ will typically repress plasma aldosterone levels (Conn, 1963; Ladell, 1957). This is exactly opposite the hormonal status desired, especially if secondary challenges (that is, decreased food consumption, increased work requirements) are presented, and it could lead to an increased incidence of heat illness (Hubbard and Armstrong, 1988; Hubbard et al., 1986).

Morning urine samples from both LNA (day 16) and MNA (day 11) demonstrated that mean morning urine Na^+ concentrations increased late in the course of HA (MNA, day 11; LNA, day 16; see Figure 12-1). This result demonstrated renal escape from the effects of aldosterone (Conn, 1963) and suggests that retention of Na^+ at the kidney (and probably the sweat glands, see Armstrong et al., 1985; Conn, 1963) eventually resulted in Na^+ balance in both LNA and MNA, which agrees with previous research (Armstrong et al., 1985; Conn, 1963). Strauss et al. (1958) demonstrated that such increases in urinary Na^+ would not have occurred if a balance of the daily Na^+ turnover had not been achieved by day 17.

CONCLUSIONS

A diet typical of normal garrison Na^+ consumption (8-gram NaCl diet) adequately stimulated HA and maintained human performance during 10 days of prolonged (8.5 hours per day), intermittent exercise in the heat. Moreover, if Na^+ consumption was reduced by 50 percent (4-gram NaCl diet), HA was still effected, and performance was maintained. The requirement to replace sweat and urine losses with water, during each hour of HA, was believed to be an important factor in the abilities of groups LNA and MNA to walk an average of 16.9 and 18.5 km per day ($p > .05$, NS), respectively, in the 41°C environment.

This investigation reduced concerns about the occurrence of salt depletion heat exhaustion (McCance, 1936) and increased risk of heat illness (Armstrong et al., 1987; Bean and Eichna, 1943; Hubbard and Armstrong, 1988; Taylor et al., 1944) among humans consuming LNA and MNA. Although each subject lost approximately 60 liters of sweat during the 10-day course of HA, no subject exhibited the symptoms of salt-depletion heat exhaustion (vertigo, hypotension, tachycardia, and vomiting; see Hubbard and Armstrong, 1988), heat cramps, or heat syncope during the 10 days of HA.

These observations, in agreement with the results of Johnson et al. (1988), indicate that a well-balanced diet and a regimen of required water consumption will adequately maintain performance and result in normal fluid-electrolyte measurements during strenuous physical activity (8 hours per day) in a hot environment for 10 consecutive days.

ACKNOWLEDGMENTS

The authors gratefully acknowledge the many hours of dedicated assistance provided by Jane P. De Luca, Catherine O'Brien, Angela Pasqualicchio, Robert J. Moore, Natalie Leva, Patricia C. Szlyk, Ingrid V. Sils, Richard F. Johnson, William J. Tharion, Glenn J. Thomas, and Simone Adams.

REFERENCES

Armstrong, L.E., D.L. Costill, W.J. Fink, M. Hargreaves, I. Nishibata, D. Bassett, and D.S. King
1985   Effects of dietary sodium intake on body and muscle potassium content in unacclimatized men during successive days of work in the heat. Eur. J. Appl. Physiol. 54:391-397.

Armstrong, L.E., D.L. Costill, and W.J. Fink
1987   Changes in body water and electrolytes during heat acclimation: Effects of dietary sodium. Aviat. Space Environ. Med. 58:143-148.

Bean, W.B., and L.W. Eichna
1943   Performance in relation to environmental temperature. Reactions of normal young men to a simulated desert environment. Fed. Proc. 2:144-158.

Conn, J.W.
1963   Aldosteronism in man: Some clinical and climatological aspects. Part 1. J. Am. Med. Assoc. 183:775-781.

Consolazio, C.F.
1966   Nutrient requirements of troops in extreme environments. Army Res. Dev. Mag. 11:24-27.

Dahl, L.K.
1958   Salt intake and salt need. New Engl. J. Med. 258:1152-1157.

Denton, D.
1982   The Hunger for Salt. New York: Springer-Verlag.

Henane, R.
1980   Acclimatization to heat in man: Giant or windmill, a critical reappraisal. Pp. 275-284 in Pecs: Proceedings of the 28th International Congress of Physiological Science, F. Obal and G. Benedek, eds. New York:Pergamon Press.

Hubbard, R.W., and L.E. Armstrong
1988   The heat illnesses: Biochemical, ultrastructural, and fluid-electrolyte considerations. Pp. 305-360 in Human Performance Physiology and Environmental Medicine at Terrestrial Extremes, K.B. Pandolf, M.N. Sawka, and R.R. Gonzalez, eds. Indianapolis, Ind.:Benchmark Press.

Hubbard, R.W., L.E. Armstrong, P.K. Evans, and J.P. De Luca
1986   Long-term water and salt deficits—A military perspective. Pp. 29-48 in Predicting Decrements in Military Performance Due to Inadequate Nutrition. Committee on Military Nutrition, Food and Nutrition Board. Washington, D.C.: National Academy Press.

Jackson, A.S., and M.L. Pollock
1978   Generalized equations for predicting body density of men. Br. J. Nutr. 40:497-504.

Johnson, H.L., R.A. Nelson, and C.F. Consolazio
1988   Effects of electrolyte and nutrient solutions on performance and metabolic balance. Med. Sci. Sports Exerc. 20:26-33.

Ladell, W.S.S.
1957   Disorders due to heat. Trans. R. Soc. Trop. Med. Hyg. 51:189-216.

Ladell, W.S.S., J.C. Waterlow, and M.F. Hudson
1954   Desert climate: Physiological and clinical observations. Lancet 2:491-497.

McCance, R.A.
1936   Experimental sodium chloride deficiency in man. Proc. R. Soc. Lond. [Biol] 119:245-268.

National Research Council
1989a   Diet and Health: Implications for Reducing Chronic Disease Risk. Report of the

Committee on Diet and Health, Food and Nutrition Board. Washington, D.C.: National Academy Press.

1989b   Recommended Dietary Allowances, 10th ed. Report of the Subcommittee on the Tenth Edition of the RDAs, Food and Nutrition Board, Commission on Life Sciences. Washington, D.C.: National Academy Press.

Strauss, M.B., E. Lamdin, W.P. Smith, and D.J. Bleifer
1958   Surfeit and deficit of sodium. Arch. Int. Med. 102:527-536.

Taylor, H.L., A. Henschel, O. Mickelsen, and A. Keys
1944   The effect of sodium chloride intake on the work performance of man during exposure to dry heat and experimental heat exhaustion. Am. J. Physiol. 140:439-451.

Tobian, L.
1989   The relationship of salt to hypertension. Am. J. Clin. Nutr. 32:2739-2748.

Wyndham, C.H., A.J.A. Benade, C.G. Williams, N.B. Strydom, A. Golden, and A.J.A. Heynes
1968   Changes in central circulation and body fluid spaces during acclimatization to heat. J. Appl. Physiol. 25:586-593.

Zar, J.H.
1974   Biostatistical Analysis. Englewood Cliffs, New Jersey:Prentice Hall.

DISCUSSION

DR. NESHEIM: Questions for Dr. Armstrong?

PARTICIPANT: I wasn't sure how to read that one slide. Are you showing, then, on the 8-gram diet, a higher body weight? Is that what this shows?

DR. ARMSTRONG: You saw a decrease in body weight at the midpoint.

PARTICIPANT: So you were showing that—explain that slide again.

DR. ARMSTRONG: On the 8-gram diet yes, there was, on the average an increase in body weight.

PARTICIPANT: So the people on the moderate salt diet had a higher body weight.

DR. ARMSTRONG: Not statistically significant.

PARTICIPANT: But you could argue, since the tonicity was the same, that they may have had a slightly increased extracellular food volume.

DR. ARMSTRONG: Yes.

PARTICIPANT: What happened in the urine tests? You showed urine sodium. What happened to urine potassium?

DR. ARMSTRONG: There were two spikes that were significantly different. I am only looking at the a.m. value, however, and that may have been due to drinking fruit juice, for example, the night before or to some other source of potassium. Captain Moore can probably speak more to the 24-

hour balance. Other than that, there were no between-diet or between-day differences.

The two spikes came, interestingly, the day before heat acclimation and day after heat acclimation began.

DR. NESHEIM: Maybe we should go through all these presentations and then we can have a discussion about that then.

PARTICIPANT: That excretion then was expressed per liter.

DR. ARMSTRONG: Yes.

Nutritional Needs in Hot Environments
Pp. 259–275. Washington, D.C.
National Academy Press

13

Endocrinological Responses to Dietary Salt Restriction During Heat Acclimation

*Ralph P. Francesconi,[1] Lawrence E. Armstrong, Natalie M. Leva,
Robert J. Moore, Patricia C. Szlyk, William T. Matthew,
William C. Curtis, Jr., Roger W. Hubbard, and Eldon W. Askew*

INTRODUCTION

There are many, albeit sometimes inconsistent, reports related to the salt (NaCl) requirements of people working in hot environments. Dill (1938) recommended that 10 to 15 g per day of NaCl would be adequate to maintain electrolyte equilibrium despite the increased salt loss of men working in the heat. Later, Taylor et al. (1944) and Consolazio (1966) suggested an optimal intake of 13 to 17 g per day and 15 to 20 g per day, respectively. At about the same time, other investigators argued that, in heat-acclimatized men, salt deficits could be avoided by consuming only 5 g per day (Ladell, 1957) or 6 g per day of NaCl (Conn, 1949). Of course, the latter view is supported by the considerable populations that flourish in extremely hot global environments despite dietary NaCl intakes of from 2 to 6 g per day (Ladell, 1957; Orr and Gilks, 1931). A recent review from this laboratory (Hubbard et al., 1986) has pointed out that some of these early studies were uncontrolled with respect to heat acclimation, exercise level, and the period of dietary stabilization.

It has been well established that the acquisition of heat acclimation or natural acclimatization reduces significantly the amount of salt lost in the sweat (Allan and Wilson, 1971; Kirby and Convertino, 1986) and urine (Bonner et al., 1976; Costill et al., 1975; Finberg and Berlyne, 1977; Francesconi

[1] Ralph P. Francesconi, Comparative Physiology Division, U.S. Army Research Institute of Environmental Medicine, Natick, MA 01760-5007

et al., 1977). However, it is unknown whether these adaptive responses are sufficient to acquire and sustain acclimation during unaccustomed restriction of dietary salt intake. For example, there have been no comprehensive studies on the minimal daily consumption of salt necessary to acquire and sustain heat acclimation in individuals who ordinarily ingest 8 to 15 g per day of NaCl. This question is particularly important to military planners. When troops are rapidly deployed from garrison to field conditions, their normal salt intake in many cases drops precipitously due to the altered salt content of the issued field rations and the generally reduced total ration consumption, especially during the first several days of the deployment. If the mobilization destination is a desert or jungle environment, the problem is compounded by enhanced salt losses in sweat, especially during the early stages of heat acclimation.

It has been extensively documented, however, that reduced consumption of salt in the human diet results in hormonal adaptations designed to reduce urinary and sweat losses of sodium (Na^+). Initially, reductions in Na^+ content of the glomerular filtrate are perceived by cells of the distal tubules, thus stimulating the biosynthesis of renin (Rowell, 1986). Elevations in plasma renin activity (PRA) are followed rapidly by an increased biosynthesis and release of aldosterone (ALD), which promotes reabsorption of Na^+ by the distal tubules, with obligatory retention and return of water to the extracellular space. Thus, PRA and ALD, in conjunction with arginine-vasopressin (antidiuretic hormone, AVP), are the humoral factors most instrumental in the regulation of fluids and electrolytes, especially under conditions of reduced availability of either.

The responses of these hormones have been extensively studied during passive heat exposure (Adlerkreutz et al., 1977; Kosunen et al., 1976), during exercise in the heat (Francesconi et al., 1983, 1985), and during periods when these stressors have been combined with restricted or supplemented sodium intake (Brandenberger et al., 1986; Davies et al., 1981). Armstrong et al. (1987) reported that during heat acclimation subjects who consumed a diet providing 5.7 g per day of NaCl had higher heart rates and rectal temperatures, as well as attenuated increments in plasma volume, than when the same group repeated the acclimation while ingesting 23 g per day of NaCl. Endocrinological responses were not described.

The current study offered a unique opportunity to assess and quantitate the endocrinological responses during, and perhaps integral to, the acquisition of heat acclimation and prolonged periods of work in a desert environment (Costill et al., 1976). Further, consumption of a low-salt diet during the acclimation period was expected to amplify these hormonal adaptations (Follenius et al., 1979) and provide important information on their role in the individual's response to recurrent and prolonged exercise in the heat. A prior dietary stabilization period in which all test subjects consumed the same daily moderate level of Na^+ provided for a relatively homogeneous range of initial levels of ALD, PRA, and AVP, thus stabilizing the usual lability of these variables in young adult men. Finally, the opportunity to evaluate hormonal responses across a 10-day acclimation period permitted the addition of confirmational data to earlier findings on the effects of acclimation on the responses of these hormones to exercise in the heat (Francesconi et al., 1983, 1984).

METHODS

Subjects

Seventeen young adult males (mean age 19.8 ± 0.6 years) participated in this study after providing their written voluntary consent. Average height was 179.4 ± 1.6 cm, average weight was 78.5 ± 2.4 kg, and body surface area was 1.97 ± 0.03 m^2. Subjects were briefed orally on the procedures, risks, and benefits of the study, as well as on their right to withdraw at any time for any reason without penalty. Prior to their participation, all subjects were medically screened and examined and found to be in good health; the mean maximal oxygen consumption for these subjects was 46.5 ± 1.1 ml per minute per kg.

Design

The study was divided into two time intervals: (a) a 7-day dietary stabilization period under dormitory conditions and a temperature of 21°C and (b) a 10-day heat acclimation period, each day of which simulated an "average" 8-hour workday in a desert environment. During the complete 17-day interval, test volunteers were dedicated to the study and supervised 24 hours per day by test investigators who had total dietary control. During the 7-day dietary stabilization period, all volunteers consumed approximately 4000 kcal per day, which was adequate to sustain initial weights; the NaCl content of the diet was constant at 8 g per day for all subjects during this control interval. On day 8 of the study (day 1 of heat acclimation and work in the heat), subjects were randomly divided into two dietary groups, one of which continued to consume the moderate NaCl diet (8 g per day) and served as the control, while the second was placed on a low-salt diet (4 g per day) for the remainder of the test. Appropriate caloric consumption was sustained during the 10-day heat acclimation period for both groups as evidenced by minimal reductions in body weight over the experimental interval with no effects of diet on body weight.

Heat Acclimation and Work in the Heat

To ensure that both the duration of heat exposure and the amount of work done in the heat were adequate to elicit effects of the low-salt diet, subjects remained in the hot environment for approximately 8.5 hours per day. They entered a large environmental chamber (41°C dry bulb, 21 percent relative humidity, 1.1 to 1.2 meters per second wind speed) at approximately 7:30 a.m. on each of the 10 heat acclimation days and remained standing for at least 20 minutes to stabilize body fluid compartments prior to blood sampling (Hagan et al., 1978). At approximately 8:00 a.m. on each day of acclimation (days 8 to 17), subjects began exercise (treadmill, 5 percent grade, 5.6 km per hour) in this hot environment. They then walked for 30 minutes and rested for 30 minutes each hour for the next 8 hours with water available (temperature of water, 10° to 15°C). Fluid consumption and body weight were monitored at 30-minute intervals, and subjects were instructed to maintain euhydration levels by consuming the full complement (based on body weight measures) that was allowed during each 30-minute interval. Lunch was presented at approximately 12:30 p.m. (fifth rest period), and subjects were allowed to exit the chamber shortly after the eighth walk upon completing other physiological and behavioral measures (approximately 4:00 p.m.). If a person was unable to complete all of the work cycles on a particular day, he remained in the chamber and participated in all other aspects of the protocol (for example, diet, drinking, other tests). Thus, the continuity of the heat exposure component of the acclimation process was uninterrupted. After completing the daily chamber exposure, subjects returned to their dormitory setting until the regimen was repeated the next morning.

Blood Sampling

During the dietary stabilization period, on days 1, 4, and 7 a 6-ml sample of blood was removed by venipuncture from a superficial arm vein by a trained phlebotomist using aseptic techniques. This sample was removed at approximately 7:45 a.m. after subjects had been standing for 20 minutes; room temperature was $21° \pm 1°C$ during the entire stabilization period. During the heat-work period (days 8 to 17) three samples were taken on each of experimental days 8, 11, 15, and 17, which corresponded to days 1, 4, 8, and 10 of heat acclimation. Because of the requirement for repeated blood sampling on these days, a catheter was aseptically inserted into each subject's superficial arm vein. The first blood sample of the day (T_1) was taken after subjects had stood in the heat for 20 minutes, prior to exercise, at approximately 7:45 a.m. to correspond with the time of blood sampling during the dietary stabilization period. The second blood sample

(T_2) was removed immediately after the fourth work bout (approximately 11:30 a.m.). The final blood sample (T_3) was withdrawn after the final walk (approximately 3:30 p.m.). Collecting tubes were immediately placed into ice and transported to the laboratory for centrifugation (4°C, 10,000 rpm); EDTA plasma or serum was removed and stored (–20°C) for subsequent analysis.

Radioimmunoassays

Aldosterone was quantitated in serum using commercially available kits purchased from the Diagnostic Products Corporation (Los Angeles, California) and following techniques described in their technical bulletin (Aldosterone, No Extraction, Coat-A-Count[R]). This technique provides an approximate detection limit of 16 picograms (pg) per ml and is extremely specific for aldosterone; the range for this hormone is usually 4 to 31 nanograms (ng) per deciliter in salt-replete, standing adults (Aldosterone, No Extraction, Coat-A-Count[R]). Plasma renin activity was estimated by the quantitation of angiotensin I in EDTA plasma. Commercially available test kits (RIANEN Angiotensin I [^{125}I] RIA Kit) were purchased from DuPont NEN Products (Boston, Massachusetts), and the assay was performed according to techniques outlined in their technical manual (RIANEN Assay System, Angiotensin I, Instruction Manual). When endogenous converting enzyme and angiotensinases of human plasma are appropriately inhibited, then angiotensin I formation quantitatively reflects PRA. Control values in adult men ordinarily range from 1 to 4.1 ng angiotensin I formed per ml per hour (Young, 1987).

Arginine-vasopressin was quantitated in EDTA plasma according to the techniques outlined by LaRose et al. (1985). One ml of EDTA plasma was treated with 10 µl per ml of 50 percent trifluoroacetic acid to acidify the sample to a pH of 4.0 to 4.5. Rabbit antibody to arg[8]-vasopressin was purchased from the Calbiochem Corporation (San Diego, California), and ^{125}I-AVP was purchased from the DuPont NEN Corporation. Prepared standards were purchased from the Incstar Corporation (Stillwater, Minnesota). The range of circulating AVP in healthy adult males has been reported to be non-detectable to 4.7 pg per ml (Incstar, Vasopressin ^{125}I RIA Kit).

Statistical Analysis

Repeated measures analysis of variance was performed using statistical package BMDP4V (BMDP Statistical Software, Los Angeles, California). Tukey's mean critical difference test was applied post hoc to determine significant differences of appropriate mean values. The null hypothesis was rejected at $p < .05$.

RESULTS

Due to the chronicity of the heat acclimation regimen and the need to complete eight work-rest cycles on a given day, all subjects were unable to complete the 80 treadmill walks (224 km). The main reasons for not completing all trials included foot blisters, inner thigh skin chafing, heat rash, and leg muscle pain. However, there was no significant difference in the proportion of the maximal possible walks completed between the two groups (control = 82.7 percent, low-salt = 75.4 percent). Further, as noted previously, if subjects could do only a portion of the total walks on a given day, they remained in the chamber and maintained the same rigorous nutritional, hydrational, and psychological testing requirements of the study as their walking counterparts. For these reasons the endocrinological data of subjects who did not walk the full complement of trials on all days were included in the mean values reported as well as the statistical analyses.

Figure 13-1 illustrates the effects of the low-salt diet and recurrent exercise in the heat on plasma levels of aldosterone. During the dietary stabilization period (days 1, 4, and 7) there were no significant differences ($p > .05$) noted between the control and low-salt groups on any of the days; in fact, the two groups displayed remarkably consistent between-group values in this sometimes labile variable. The slight elevation in levels of both groups on day 4 may have been in response to the dietary stabilization intake of NaCl (8 g), which probably represented a decrement in salt intake for most of these young adult men in comparison to their normal garrison consumption (approximately 11 to 15 g per day; Szeto et al., 1987). This increment nearly achieved statistical significance (for example, on day 1, low-salt, mean = 18.3 ng per dl; on day 4, low-salt, mean = 33.2 ng per dl, minimal critical difference of the means necessary for significance = 15.1 ng per dl, $p > .05$).

On the first day of both heat acclimation and dietary manipulation (eighth experimental day) plasma ALD levels at T_1, T_2, and T_3 were not significantly different between groups ($p > .05$). However, the effects of exercise in the hot environment are noted in the elevated plasma ALD levels in both groups at T_2, which achieved statistical significance by T_3 in both the control and the low-salt groups ($p < .05$). By day 11, the marked effects of the low-salt diet on circulating ALD were manifested in significant ($p < .01$) increments at all sampling times when compared to the control levels. In the low-salt group, the increment observed between T_1 and T_2 narrowly failed to achieve significance (difference of means = 45.73, minimal difference for significance = 46.46 ng per dl).

A strikingly similar pattern emerged on day 15. Thus, at each of the sampling times, plasma ALD in the low-salt group was significantly elevated ($p < .01$) when compared to the respective mean of the control

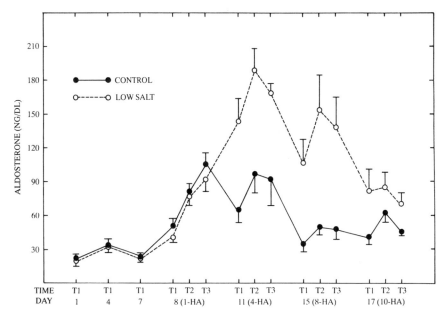

FIGURE 13-1 The effects of consuming a low-salt diet (4 g per day) or a moderate-salt diet (8 g per day) and of work in the heat (41°C; 21 percent relative humidity, treadmill, 5 percent grade, 5.6 km per hour, 30 minutes per hour, 8 hours per day) on plasma levels of aldosterone. During the dietary stabilization period (days 1 to 7), blood samples were taken at approximately 7:45 a.m. on days 1, 4, and 7; during the heat acclimation (HA) period (days 8 to 17), the first blood sample (T_1) was removed after each subject remained upright in the heat chamber for at least 20 minutes, also at about 7:45 a.m. The second (T_2) and third (T_3) samples were removed after the fourth and eighth walks, respectively, on days 8, 11, 15, and 17. Mean values ± standard errors of the mean are depicted for all values.

group. Likewise, the apparent increment in circulating ALD in the low-salt group between T_1 and T_2 once again barely failed to achieve statistical significance (difference of means = 46.13, minimal difference for significance = 46.46 ng per dl). However, by day 17 (corresponding to day 10 of both dietary and heat-work manipulations), the effects of the low-salt diet were minimized, and there were no significant effects of either NaCl consumption or exercise in the heat on circulating levels of ALD. There were no between-diet effects on circulating Na^+ concentrations, and these levels remained within the range of normal (135.6 to 140.8 mEq per liter) throughout the experimental period. As anticipated, urinary Na^+ in the low-salt group fell precipitously (to less than 10 mEq per liter) during the 10 days of low-salt-exercise in the heat.

The responses of ALD to the low-salt-heat-work regimen were nearly mirrored in the effects of these parameters on PRA (Figure 13-2). In examining first the PRA of both groups during the dietary stabilization period, there were no significant differences in plasma levels between groups on day 1. In progressing from day 1 to day 4, a trend occurred toward elevations in PRA in both groups, but neither achieved statistical significance. However, in the low-salt group, the sharp decrement between day 4 and day 7 resulted in a significant difference ($p < .05$) in mean levels. On the first heat acclimation day, although there were no significant intergroup effects, exercise in the heat elicited a significant elevation ($p < .01$) in PRA in the low-salt group (T_1 versus T_3); other trends toward increased activity on day 8 failed to achieve statistical significance. On day 11 (fourth day of heat acclimation), there was a significant elevation ($p < .05$) of PRA in the low-salt group at T_1. However, because of the slight decrements in activity in

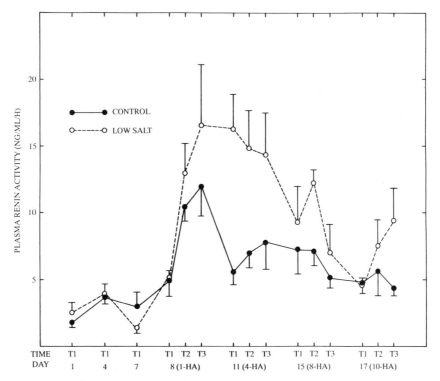

FIGURE 13-2 The effects of consuming a low-salt or moderate-salt diet and of recurrent exercise in the heat on levels of plasma renin activity. All conditions, times, and parameters are as noted in Figure 13-1. HA = days of heat acclimation period and T_1, T_2, and T_3 are the first, second, and third blood samples, respectively.

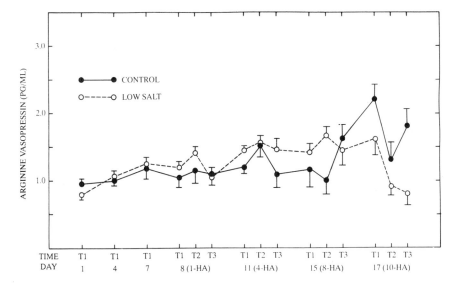

FIGURE 13-3   The effects of consuming a low-salt or moderate-salt diet and of recurrent exercise in the heat on circulating levels of arginine-vasopressin. All conditions are as noted in Figure 13-1. HA = days of heat acclimation period and T_1, T_2, and T_3 are the first, second, and third blood samples, respectively.

the low-salt group and the concomitant minor increments in PRA in the controls, no further significant differences were noted in any of the other time intervals. Moreover, as the chronicity of heat acclimation increased (days 15 and 17), all effects of the low-salt diet as well as exercise in the heat were negated, and no further intergroup or between-time differences were observed.

During the dietary stabilization period, there were no significant intergroup or across-time differences in levels of AVP (Figure 13-3). Further, even after dietary manipulation and consecutive days of exercise in the heat, the data indicated that throughout the period of heat acclimation there were no significant effects on AVP of either the dietary manipulation or the recurrent exercise in the hot environment.

DISCUSSION

Because the endocrinological variables under consideration in the current experiments are significantly affected by dietary salt consumption (McDougall, 1987), hydration state (Convertino et al., 1981), exercise and training (Geyssant et al., 1981), and thermal exposure (Kosunen et al., 1976), it was considered important that all test subjects undergo an adequate stabilization period prior to salt restriction and recurrent exercise in the heat. Thus, during the first 7 days of the experiment all subjects remained under the 24-hour control of test investigators with obligations only to the study (as was the case throughout the experiment). During this interval, subjects consumed the same test diets—which delivered 8 g of NaCl daily for each volunteer—and adhered to a structured and consistent schedule of activity that included completion of questionnaires (for example, environmental symptoms, thermal comfort), simulated target acquisition and firing, a maximal oxygen uptake test on day 4, and at least 4 hours per day of light recreational activity that included reading, videos, and games. All of this activity took place after blood sampling on all days.

During the stabilization period, circulating levels of all three hormones were generally consistent between groups, with some minor variation over time. All values were well within the normal range for young adult males, except for ALD levels on day 4, which were approximately 4 ng per dl above the upper limit of the normal range. This increment was probably due to the reduced NaCl content of the stabilization diet (8 g per day) as compared to the normal salt content of military dining hall rations, which is usually 11 to 15 g per day (Szeto et al., 1987). By day 7, mean ALD levels had returned to within the normal range.

Francesconi et al. (1983, 1985) and others (Finberg and Berlyne, 1977; Finberg et al., 1974) have reported—and current results confirm—that the acquisition of acclimation attenuates the response to exercise in the heat of both PRA and ALD. In the current experiments, the effects of acclimation were manifested in mean daily ALD levels of 79 and 84.9 ng per dl on days 8 and 11 (days 1 and 4 of heat acclimation), respectively, which were reduced by days 15 and 17 (days 8 and 10 of heat acclimation) to 44.3 and 51.3 ng per dl, respectively, in the control group. Even in the low-salt group, the mean plasma ALD concentration on day 11 was a markedly elevated 167.3 ng per dl, which was reduced to 133.5 and 78.7 ng per dl on days 15 and 17, respectively. By day 17 there were no significant differences in plasma ALD either between the control and low-salt groups at any of the individual sampling times or between the T_1, T_2, and T_3 values for either group. These results suggest that the chronicity of both the heat acclimation regimen and the low-salt diet engender temporally related endocrinological accommodations to these experimental manipulations. Thus, the attenuated hormonal responses over time may be related to the following: increased plasma volume of heat acclimation (Bonner et al., 1976), generally reduced adrenocorticotrophic activity with decreased physiological strain (that is, a reduced stress response to the experimental conditions) (Francesconi et al., 1984), decreased sensitivity to adrenocorticotrophic hormone (McDougall, 1987), increased renal sensitivity to ALD-induced sodium reabsorption mechanisms (Smiles and Robinson, 1971), and a general improvement of the Na^+

balance due to improved Na^+ conservation at the level of the kidney and sweat gland (Allan and Wilson, 1971).

Similar arguments and rationale can be made for the pattern of PRA levels observed in the current experiments. For example, in the control group, mean PRA peaked on day 1 of heat acclimation (9.04 ng per ml per hour) followed by a declining trend (6.8, 6.6, and 5.3 ng per ml per hour) on days 4, 8, and 10, respectively, of heat acclimation. Moreover, in the low-salt group, by using the rationale developed above for ALD, maximal effects of the low-salt diet and exercise in the heat would be expected on day 4 of heat acclimation (15.2 ng per ml per hour) followed by moderation on day 8 (9.6 ng per ml per hour) with further reductions on day 10 (7.3 ng per ml per hour). The endocrinological adaptations that occur early in the acclimation process are necessary to maintain electrolyte balance and ultimately to expand extracellular fluid volume and may be closely related to the acquisition of full acclimation. Moreover, when the physiological strain of exercise in the heat has been reduced after full acclimation and expansion of plasma volume have been achieved, these hormonal responses are obviated.

In the current experiments, subjects on the low-salt diet gradually achieved the same state of acclimation as the control group over the 10-day acclimation period as suggested by significant reductions in heat- and exercise-induced heart rate, rectal temperature, urinary Na^+, and perceived exertion. Further, neither these variables nor the distance walked during the 10-day acclimation period differed significantly between the control and low-salt groups. The moderation of the endocrinological responses during the latter phase of the acclimation interval probably reflects, most importantly, the attendant plasma volume expansion and achievement of electrolyte balance. However, successful acclimation to recurrent and prolonged exercise in the heat on 4 g per day of NaCl was accomplished under the specific conditions of this study. It is unknown whether successful adaptation to this low-salt diet could have been accomplished if the exercise or environmental conditions were more intense.

It is generally agreed that AVP is most responsive to dehydration and increments in plasma osmolality (Von Ameln et al., 1985). Accordingly, Greenleaf et al. (1983) reported that when water intake was increased during an acclimation period from 450 ml per hour on day 1 to approximately 1000 ml per hour on days 5 to 8, there also occurred a significant decrement in plasma AVP. In the current experiments, subjects were weighed every 30 minutes during each of the 8-hour workdays, were encouraged to drink, and were provided fresh, cool water at 30-minute intervals. Thus, dehydration was not a significant observation in either group of subjects, and AVP levels remained generally consistent throughout both the stabilization and the heat acclimation intervals. In fact, the range of AVP for both groups over all sampling periods (0.80 to 2.21 pg per ml, mean values) is within the range of normal for young adult men with plasma osmolality less than 290 milliosmoles per kg.

CONCLUSIONS AND RECOMMENDATIONS

As shown from these studies, young adult men consuming a daily diet containing only 4 g of NaCl can work consecutive days in a desert environment and achieve full acclimation to this specific heat-work scenario. The endocrinological adaptations occurring especially during the first several days of the dietary-heat-work regimen may be important to the physiological adaptations and electrolyte equilibria needed for achieving acclimation. These hormonal responses moderated during the latter portions of the experimental regimen, which indicates a dietary and acclimation steady-state characterized by greatly reduced physiological strain to the test volunteers. These results imply that healthy young individuals can acclimate quite rapidly to work in desert environments despite relatively restricted salt intake.

ACKNOWLEDGMENTS

The authors gratefully acknowledge the technical, technological, and logistical support of many U.S. Army Research Institute of Environmental Medicine and U.S. Army Natick Research, Development, and Engineering Center personnel. A special thanks to the test volunteers who participated in this study. Without their cooperation, it could not have been executed.

REFERENCES

Adlerkreutz, H., K. Kosunen, K. Kuoppasalmi, A. Pakarinen, and S. Karonen
    1977   Plasma hormones during exposure to intense heat. Proc. Cong. Int. Med. 13:346-355.
Allan, J.R., and C.G. Wilson
    1971   Influence of acclimatization on sweat sodium concentration. J. Appl. Physiol. 30:708-712.
Armstrong, L.E., D.L. Costill, and W.J. Fink
    1987   Changes in body water and electrolytes during heat acclimation: Effects of dietary sodium. Aviat. Space Environ. Med. 58:143-148.
Bonner, R.M., M.H. Harrison, C.J. Hall, and R.J. Edwards
    1976   Effect of heat acclimatization on intravascular responses to acute heat stress in man. J. Appl. Physiol. 41:708-713.
Brandenberger, G., V. Candas, M. Follenius, J. Libert, and J. Kahn
    1986   Vascular fluid shifts and endocrine responses to exercise in the heat: Effects of rehydration. Eur. J. Appl. Physiol. 55:123-129.
Conn, J.W.
    1949   Acclimatization to heat. Adv. Int. Med. 3:337.

Consolazio, D.F.
1966   Nutrient requirements of troops in extreme environments. Army Res. Dev. Mag. Nov:24-27.

Convertino, V.A., L.C. Keil, E.M. Bernauer, and J.E. Greenleaf
1981   Plasma volume, osmolality, vasopressin, and renin activity during graded exercise in man. J. Appl. Physiol. 50:123-128.

Costill, D.L., R. Cote, E. Miller, T. Miller, and S. Wynder
1975   Water and electrolyte replacement during repeated days of work in the heat. Aviat. Space Environ. Med. 46:795-800.

Costill, D.L., G. Branam, W. Fink, and R. Nelson
1976   Exercise induced sodium conservation: Changes in plasma renin and aldosterone. Med. Sci. Sports 8:209-213.

Davies, J., M. Harrison, L. Cochrane, R. Edwards, and T. Gibson
1981   Effect of saline loading during heat acclimatization on adrenocortical hormones. J. Appl. Physiol. 50:605-612.

Dill, D.B.
1938   Life, Heat, and Altitude. Cambridge, Mass.: Harvard University Press.

Finberg, J.P.M., and G.M. Berlyne
1977   Modification of renin and aldosterone response to heat by acclimatization in man. J. Appl. Physiol. 42:554-558.

Finberg, J.P.M., M. Katz, H. Gazit, and G.M. Berlyne
1974   Plasma renin activity after acute heat exposure in nonacclimatized and naturally acclimatized man. J. Appl. Physiol. 36:519-523.

Follenius, M., G. Brandenberger, B. Reinhardt, and M. Simeoni
1979   Plasma aldosterone, renin activity, and cortisol responses to heat exposure in sodium depleted and repleted subjects. Eur. J. Appl. Physiol. 41:41-50.

Francesconi, R., J.T. Maher, G. Bynum, and J. Mason
1977   Recurrent heat exposure: Effects on plasma and urinary sodium and potassium in resting and exercising men. Aviat. Space Environ. Med. 48:399-404.

Francesconi, R.P., M.N. Sawka, and K.B. Pandolf
1983   Hypohydration and heat acclimation: Plasma renin and aldosterone during exercise. J. Appl. Physiol. 55:1790-1794.

1984   Hypohydration and acclimation: Effects on hormone responses to exercise/heat stress. Aviat. Space Environ. Med. 55:365-369.

Francesconi, R.P., M. Sawka, K. Pandolf, R. Hubbard, A. Young, and S. Muza
1985   Plasma hormonal responses at graded hypohydration levels during exercise/heat stress. J. Appl. Physiol. 59:1855-1860.

Geyssant, A., G. Geelen, C. Denis, A.M. Allevard, M. Vincent, E. Jarsaillon, C. A. Bizollon, J.R. Lacour, and C. Gharib
1981   Plasma vasopressin, renin activity, and aldosterone: Effect of exercise and training. Eur. J. Appl. Physiol. 46:21-30.

Greenleaf, J.E., P.J. Brock, L.C. Keil, and J.T. Morse
1983   Drinking and water balance during exercise and heat acclimation. J. Appl. Physiol. 54:414-419.

Hagan, R.D., F.J. Diaz, and S.M. Horvath
1978   Plasma volume changes with movement to supine and standing positions. J. Appl. Physiol. 45:414-418.

Hubbard, R.W., L.E. Armstrong, P.K. Evans, and J.P. DeLuca
1986   Long-term water and salt deficits: A military perspective. Pp. 29-48 in Predicting Deficits in Military Performance Due to Inadequate Nutrition. Washington, D.C.: National Academy Press.

Kirby, C.R., and V.A. Convertino
  1986   Plasma aldosterone and sweat sodium concentrations after exercise and heat accli-
          mation. J. Appl. Physiol. 61:967-970.
Kosunen, K. J., A.J. Pakarinen, K. Kuoppasalmi, and H. Adlerkreutz
  1976   Plasma renin activity, angiotensin II, and aldosterone during intense heat stress. J.
          Appl. Physiol. 41:323-327.
Ladell, W.S.S.
  1957   Disorders due to heat. Trans. R. Soc. Trop. Med. Hyg. 51:189-216.
LaRose, P., H. Ong, and P. DuSouich
  1985   Simple and rapid radioimmunoassay for the routine determination of vasopressin
          in plasma. Clin. Biochem. 18:357-361.
McDougall, J.G.
  1987   The physiology of aldosterone secretion. News Physiol. Sci. 2:126-128.
Orr, J.B., and J.L. Gilks
  1931   Studies of nutrition: The physique and health of two African tribes. Medical Re-
          search Council London, Special Reports, Series 155:82, His Majesty's Stationery
          Office, London.
Rowell, L.B.
  1986   Human Circulation: Regulation During Physical Stress. New York: Oxford Uni-
          versity Press.
Smiles, K.A., and S. Robinson
  1971   Sodium ion conservation during acclimatization of men to work in the heat. J.
          Appl. Physiol. 31:63-69.
Szeto, E.G., D.E. Carlson, T.B. Dugan, and J.C. Buchbinder
  1987   A comparison of nutrient intakes between a Ft. Riley contractor-operated and a Ft.
          Lewis military-operated garrison dining facility. U.S. Army Research Institute of
          Environmental Medicine Tech Rep. T2-88:1-65, Natick, Mass.: U.S. Army Re-
          search Institute of Environmental Medicine.
Taylor, H.L., A. Henschel, O. Mickelson, and A. Keys
  1944   The effect of sodium chloride intake on the work performance of man during
          exposure to dry heat and experimental heat exhaustion. Am. J. Physiol. 140:439-
          451.
Von Ameln, H., M. Laniado, L. Rocker, and K.A. Kirsch
  1985   Effects of dehydration on the vasopressin response to immersion. J. Appl. Physiol.
          58:114-120.
Young, D.S.
  1987   Implementation of SI units for clinical laboratory data. Ann. Int. Med. 106:114-
          129.

DISCUSSION

PARTICIPANT: What was driving the aldosterone and plasma renin activity responses? What was the relationship between those hormones and plasma volume, plasma osmolality, plasma sodium concentrations?

DR. FRANCESCONI: Well, the circulating sodium concentrations were actually not too different between groups, as Dr. Armstrong indicated. In addition to circulating sodium levels, circulating potassium levels, circulating protein levels, and osmolality were also not really significantly different.

Aldosterone biosynthesis is ordinarily stimulated by reduced dietary sodium, heat exposure, exercise, and usually by increases in plasma renin activity although we have seen conditions where the two have been separated.

So I can only conclude that increased sodium and fluid reabsorption in the face of reduced dietary salt intake was the driving factor for those endocrinological responses.

Increased plasma renin activity was probably due to diminished splanchnic blood flow, as Rowell (Rowell, 1986) has shown; decreased plasma volume or reduced renal blood flow ordinarily elicits a very immediate response in terms of renal tubular biosynthesis and release of plasma renin. These endocrinological responses thus stimulate very efficient electrolytes and, thus, fluids.

PARTICIPANT: I was going to ask somewhat of a similar question. I was trying to figure out the mechanisms, first, when you kept everything constant, the aldosterone and renin went up. I was fascinated that they went back down.

DR. FRANCESCONI: They did and that could be a result of just the achievement of new steady states after the full acquisition of acclimation and expansion of plasma volume. It could be an increased sensitivity of both the sweat glands and the kidney cells to the activity of the PRA and the aldosterone.

Nothing that we saw would indicate that any of the subjects were becoming either hyponatremic or hypokalemic in these studies.

PARTICIPANT: As acclimation progressed, the intensity of these endocrine responses was moderated. Is that just due to increased sensitivity to PRA and ALDO.

DR. FRANCESCONI: That is just one of the mechanisms proposed.

PARTICIPANT: But, the mechanisms remain very vague.

DR. FRANCESCONI: As an aside, I have had rats on low sodium diets for up to 70 or 80 days with no real significant effects on circulating sodium levels and almost nonexistent urinary or salivary sodium.

PARTICIPANT: I am not so sure that is a change in sensitivity because in one of those slides that you showed where you looked at preacclimatization and postacclimatization, if you looked at the two lines there was a difference between the two, but those two lines looked like they were parallel. They appeared to be rising at the same rate for PRA and ALDO.

It looked as if the sensitivity was the same but just the initial values were different.

DR. FRANCESCONI: Actually, on day 1 of heat acclimation the responses were quite similar, but, of course, on that day the volunteers in both groups were coming off the same stabilization diet and level of salt intake. By day 4 of heat acclimation, the T_1 values for PRA and ALD were remarkably different due to the low-salt diet.

And clearly, if acclimation increases plasma volume, which it has been reported to do up to 18 percent, there should indeed be a reduction in both the T_1 levels and the responses as acclimation progresses.

In fact, at one time we infused hyperoncotic albumin to test volunteers to increase plasma volume in a matter of hours versus the six or eight days that Dr. Armstrong showed were required here in this study.

And in that condition also we had repression of baseline levels of those hormones, not great, but statistically significant.

PARTICIPANT: Did you measure blood pressure during that period of time? Because that could change glomerular filtration rate and explain some of these differences.

DR. FRANCESCONI: There were actually some decreases in blood pressure during heat acclimation. In fact, I think Lt. Colonel William Curtis has much data on that which he is about to present at a different meeting. There were some decrements in blood pressure.

PARTICIPANT: I am trying to remember, from the military initiatives study, what was the sodium intake of soldiers in garrison? What were measured in some of those studies?

PARTICIPANT: At least 4500 mg of sodium per day.

PARTICIPANT: So that would be roughly 9 grams of salt, or 11 or 12. So maybe a little more.

Would you speculate that if you were to take soldiers coming right off the food that they would be consuming normally when they are on base and were dropped into Saudi Arabia and eating only MREs getting 4 grams of salt, that you would see the same kinds of results that you saw there?

DR. FRANCESCONI: I think I probably would. If they had responsive and well-functioning endocrinological systems, young, healthy adult males and if they were drinking well, yes.

DR. NESHEIM: Any other questions?

PARTICIPANT: Just point of clarification. Our current MRE is much higher in salt than the 4 grams.

DR. FRANCESCONI: Yes. That is true.

PARTICIPANT: Do you expect any differences in that level for women?

DR. FRANCESCONI: No, I don't. The hypohydration study which I have referenced actually had 12 women in that group of 24 test subjects and I saw no differences in hormonal responses and I don't think Dr. Sawka saw any differences in physiological responses in that study.

PARTICIPANT: My question is, do you anticipate that—this is a very small population you are looking at. There are some changes that are occurring here. Do you expect that there might be some people in a group of young men like this that might not respond the same way?

DR. FRANCESCONI: Clearly, we can only speak for the volunteers and the conditions in this study, at least at this time. However, the consistency of the responses indicated that such responses should generally occur, especially considering the numbers of papers in the literature describing the effects of heat and exercise on circulating levels of these hormones.

PARTICIPANT: It could represent a little caution in interpreting that everybody would respond that way.

PARTICIPANT: That is what I am worried about. If you look at the number of people who have heat stroke, it is a small number but they do occur.

PARTICIPANT: I just wanted to ask—Larry [ed. Dr Armstrong] mentioned that some people couldn't make it through this rigorous heat/exercise protocol for orthopedic reasons. How bad was the drop-out rate and maybe these people don't have the endocrinological response.

DR. FRANCESCONI: I didn't see any correlation. As Dr. Armstrong mentioned, the drop-outs were primarily for reasons that you would expect on this kind of a march—foot blisters primarily, ankle pain, intra-thigh chafing, especially for subjects that were a little heavier, all those kinds of things. In some instances the volunteers would miss one or two of the 30-minute marches and then rejoin the group. In other instances they may have missed a day that was not a blood-sampling day. However, they did remain in the heat all day on those days.

DR. JOHNSON: One note that might address your question: Even though people may have stopped walking on the treadmill, they stayed in the wind tunnel. They didn't leave the hot environment. They were still there.

Nutritional Needs in Hot Environments
Pp. 277–293. Washington, D.C.
National Academy Press

14

Subjective Reports of Heat Illness

Richard F. Johnson[1] and Donna J. Merullo

INTRODUCTION

During the first several days of rapid deployment of soldiers to the field, dietary salt consumption is often reduced due to the altered salt content of field rations and a general reduction in total ration consumption (USARIEM, 1990). If the deployment is to a hot environment, such as a jungle or a desert, decreased salt consumption becomes particularly problematic due to increased salt losses during sweating. To shed light on the minimum daily consumption of salt required to acquire and sustain heat acclimation during simulated desert living, a large study was conducted on the effects of salt intake on young soldiers during heat acclimation. A detailed description of the study is presented elsewhere in this volume (Chapter 12). Briefly, the study compared the effects of diets containing low-normal (8 g) and low (4 g) levels of daily dietary salt intake in 17 healthy soldiers. The soldiers underwent a 7-day dietary stabilization period (no heat exposure) followed by 10 days of heat acclimation (8 hours per day at 41°C, 20 percent relative humidity, walking at 5.6 km per hour for 30 minutes per hour). The physiological response data resulting from the study are presented by Armstrong et al. in Chapter 12. The focus of this chapter is on the influence of dietary salt intake on the soldiers' subjective reports of symptoms of heat illness during heat acclimation. Symptoms of heat illness,

---

[1] Richard F. Johnson, Military Performance and Neuroscience Division, U.S. Army Research Institute of Environmental Medicine, Natick, MA 01760-5007

as experienced by the individual soldier exercising in the heat, are important because they are the sole indications by which the soldier judges the onset of heat injury (Armstrong et al., 1987).

In a study of the signs and symptoms of one type of heat illness—heat exhaustion—Armstrong et al. (1987) exposed 14 healthy unacclimated men to 8 days of heat acclimation by intermittent treadmill running in an environmental chamber set at 41°C, 39 percent relative humidity. During the study, the subjects experienced nine different signs and symptoms: abdominal cramps, chills, dizziness, flushed skin with "heat sensations," elevated resting heart rate, hyperirritability, "rubbery" legs, piloerection, and vomiting and nausea. The incidence of these signs and symptoms decreased as the number of days of heat exposure increased. The signs and symptoms were gathered through careful clinical observations and the solicitation of the subjects' verbal reports of their experiences.

In the present study, a standardized psychological instrument, the Environmental Symptoms Questionnaire (ESQ) (Kobrick and Sampson, 1979; Sampson and Kobrick, 1980), was used to evaluate soldiers' reports of symptoms of heat illness. The ESQ is a 68-item questionnaire that measures a variety of symptoms including headache, dizziness, nausea, thirst, and cramps (Table 14-1). The ESQ is worded in the past tense, and the subject is required to reflect on symptoms experienced during the hours prior to administration. The subject rates each symptom on a 6-point scale ranging from "not at all" to "extreme." The ESQ has been successfully used to assess symptomatology under conditions of high terrestrial altitude (Banderet and Lieberman, 1989; Kobrick and Sampson, 1979; Rock et al., 1987; Sampson and Kobrick, 1980), ambient cold (Johnson et al., 1989), combat field feeding (Hirsch et al., 1984; USACDEC/USARIEM, 1986), and the administration of nerve agent antidote (Kobrick et al., 1990).

METHOD

Subjects

Seventeen healthy male U.S. Army soldiers volunteered to participate in the study. Prior to heat acclimation, all underwent 1 week of dietary stabilization (days 1 to 7) during which consumption of dietary salt was held constant at 8 g per day. On the first (day 8) of 10 days of heat acclimation (days 8 to 17), subjects were randomly, and in a double-blind fashion, assigned to either the 4-g dietary salt group ($n = 8$), or the 8-g dietary salt group ($n = 9$). Examination of selected personal characteristics (age, height, weight, and race) indicated that the two groups were comparable to one another. The subjects assigned to the 4-g salt group averaged 19.8 years old, 71.3 inches tall, and weighed 174.9 pounds; seven were Caucasian and one was Hispanic. The subjects assigned to the 8-g salt group averaged 19.9 years old, 70.9 inches tall, and weighed 169.67 pounds; eight were Caucasian and one was Hispanic.

Procedure

The ESQ was administered to all participants 13 times during the study. To obtain baseline measures during nonheat exposure days when all were consuming a constant 8 g of dietary salt per day, the ESQ was administered during the afternoons of days 1, 4, and 7. On each of the 10 days of heat acclimation (days 8 to 17), the ESQ was administered at the end of the 8 hours of heat exposure.

Subjective reports of heat illness were assessed in two ways: (a) a tabulation of 12 ESQ symptoms selected for their previously established relationship to exercise in the heat (Armstrong et al., 1987), and (b) the formulation and analysis of an overall index of subjective heat illness.

Release 2.1 of the computer-based statistical package Complete Statistical System (CSS) (StatSoft, 1988) was used to perform all statistical analyses.

RESULTS

Tabulation of Selected ESQ Symptoms

The 12 items on the ESQ that are related to the 9 symptoms of heat illness observed by Armstrong et al. (1987) are displayed in Table 14-2 (4-g salt diet) and in Table 14-3 (8-g salt diet) for each subject for each of the 10 heat acclimation days. The 12 symptoms include stomach cramps (item 17), chilly (item 36), dizzy (item 4), warm and sweaty (items 30 and 33), heart beating fast (item 11), irritability and restlessness (items 62 and 63), disturbed coordination (item 7), weakness (item 19), shivering (item 37), and nausea (item 24). Only those symptoms rated at least "1" by the participant (indicating that the symptom was present regardless of how intense it was felt) are listed in the tables. An analysis of variance of the number of symptoms reported as present differed among days, F (9, 135) = 6.10967, $p < .001$, with the mean number of symptoms present being greater, by Duncan post hoc tests ($p < .05$), during the first 2 days of heat acclimation (means = 4.3 and 4.0) than during the remaining 8 heat acclimation days (means = 3.1, 2.9, 3.2, 2.4, 2.5, 2.5, 2.2, and 2.3). Although there was a trend for more symptoms to be reported by subjects in the 4-g diet group (mean = 3.2) than by the 8-g diet group (mean = 2.6), the analysis of variance was not significant with respect to the main effect of diet, F (1,15) = 1.17, $p > .20$; the interaction between diet and heat acclimation day was also not significant, F (9,135) = 1.775, $p > .05$. In Tables 14-4 (4-g salt diet)

TABLE 14-1 U.S. Army Research Institute of Environmental Medicine Environmental Symptoms Questionnaire (ESQ)

Circle the number of each item to correspond to HOW YOU HAVE BEEN FEELING TODAY. PLEASE ANSWER EVERY ITEM. If you did not have the symptom, circle zero (NOT AT ALL).

		Not At All	Slight	Somewhat	Moderate	Quite a Bit	Extreme
1.	I felt lightheaded.	0	1	2	3	4	5
2.	I had a headache.	0	1	2	3	4	5
3.	I felt sinus pressure.	0	1	2	3	4	5
4.	I felt dizzy.	0	1	2	3	4	5
5.	I felt faint.	0	1	2	3	4	5
6.	My vision was dim.	0	1	2	3	4	5
7.	My coordination was off.	0	1	2	3	4	5
8.	I was short of breath.	0	1	2	3	4	5
9.	It was hard to breathe.	0	1	2	3	4	5
10.	It hurt to breathe.	0	1	2	3	4	5
11.	My heart was beating fast.	0	1	2	3	4	5
12.	My heart was pounding.	0	1	2	3	4	5
13.	I had a chest pain.	0	1	2	3	4	5
14.	I had chest pressure.	0	1	2	3	4	5
15.	My hands were shaking or trembling.	0	1	2	3	4	5
16.	I had a muscle cramp.	0	1	2	3	4	5
17.	I had stomach cramps.	0	1	2	3	4	5
18.	My muscles felt tight or stiff.	0	1	2	3	4	5
19.	I felt weak.	0	1	2	3	4	5
20.	My legs or feet ached.	0	1	2	3	4	5
21.	My hands, arms, or shoulders ached.	0	1	2	3	4	5
22.	My back ached.	0	1	2	3	4	5
23.	I had a stomach ache.	0	1	2	3	4	5
24.	I felt sick to my stomach (nauseous).	0	1	2	3	4	5
25.	I had gas pressure.	0	1	2	3	4	5
26.	I had diarrhea.	0	1	2	3	4	5
27.	I felt constipated.	0	1	2	3	4	5
28.	I had to urinate more than usual.	0	1	2	3	4	5
29.	I had to urinate less than usual.	0	1	2	3	4	5
30.	I felt warm.	0	1	2	3	4	5

31.	I felt feverish.	0	1	2	3	4	5
32.	My feet were sweaty.	0	1	2	3	4	5
33.	I was sweating all over.	0	1	2	3	4	5
34.	My hands were cold.	0	1	2	3	4	5
35.	My feet were cold.	0	1	2	3	4	5
36.	I felt chilly.	0	1	2	3	4	5
37.	I was shivering.	0	1	2	3	4	5
38.	Parts of my body felt numb.	0	1	2	3	4	5
39.	My skin was burning or itchy.	0	1	2	3	4	5
40.	My eyes felt irritated.	0	1	2	3	4	5
41.	My vision was blurry.	0	1	2	3	4	5
42.	My ears felt blocked up.	0	1	2	3	4	5
43.	My ears ached.	0	1	2	3	4	5
44.	I couldn't hear well.	0	1	2	3	4	5
45.	My ears were ringing.	0	1	2	3	4	5
46.	My nose felt stuffed up.	0	1	2	3	4	5
47.	I had a runny nose.	0	1	2	3	4	5
48.	I had a nose bleed.	0	1	2	3	4	5
49.	My mouth was dry.	0	1	2	3	4	5
50.	My throat was sore.	0	1	2	3	4	5
51.	I was coughing.	0	1	2	3	4	5
52.	I lost my appetite.	0	1	2	3	4	5
53.	I felt sick.	0	1	2	3	4	5
54.	I felt hungover.	0	1	2	3	4	5
55.	I was thirsty.	0	1	2	3	4	5
56.	I felt tired.	0	1	2	3	4	5
57.	I felt sleepy.	0	1	2	3	4	5
58.	I felt wide awake.	0	1	2	3	4	5
59.	My concentration was off.	0	1	2	3	4	5
60.	I was more forgetful than usual.	0	1	2	3	4	5
61.	I felt worried or nervous.	0	1	2	3	4	5
62.	I felt irritable.	0	1	2	3	4	5
63.	I felt restless.	0	1	2	3	4	5
64.	I was bored.	0	1	2	3	4	5
65.	I felt depressed.	0	1	2	3	4	5
66.	I felt alert.	0	1	2	3	4	5
67.	I felt good.	0	1	2	3	4	5
68.	I was hungry.	0	1	2	3	4	5

SOURCE: Adapted from Kobrick and Sampson (1979) and Sampson and Kobrick (1980).

TABLE 14-2 Subjective Report of Environmental Symptoms Questionnaire Symptoms of Heat Illness: 4-g Salt Diet ($n = 8$)

Subject	Symptoms* on Heat Acclimation Day										Total Symptoms
	1	2	3	4	5	6	7	8	9	10	
1	4 7 11 17 19 30 33	4 11 19 30 33 36	11 19 30 33	19 30 33	19 30 33 62	33 62 63	33 62 63	19 33 62 63	19 33 62 63	19 33 62 63	42
12	7 11 19 30 33 62	4 11 19 30 33 36 62	11 19 30 33 62	11 30 33 62	11 30 33	11 30 33	11 19 33	11 19 30 33	11 30 33	11 30 62	41
13	4 7 11 19 30 33	30 33 62 63	33 62 63	62 63	33 62 63	30 33	11 19 30 33 62 63	30 33	30 33 62 63	19 30 33 62 63	37
11	7 30 33	7 19 30 33 62 63	19 30 33 62 63	30 33 62 63	7 19 30 33 62 63	30 62 63	30 63	30 63	30 63		33

Subject												Total
2	19, 30, 33	19, 30, 33, 62	19, 30, 33, 62	19, 30, 33	19, 24, 30, 33, 62	19, 30, 33, 62	30, 33	30, 33	30, 33	30, 33	31	
22	4, 19, 33, 36	4, 11, 17, 19, 24, 30, 33, 36, 63	17, 19, 36	19, 36	19, 36	19, 36	17, 36	19, 36		36	27	
8	11, 30, 33	11, 30, 33	11, 30, 33	11, 30, 33	30	11, 30	30, 33	11, 30, 33	30, 33	11, 30, 33	25	
6	4, 11, 17, 30, 33	4, 30, 33	30, 33	19, 33	19, 30, 33	33	19, 33	30, 33	33	30, 33	23	
Total	37	42	29	23	27	20	22	21	18	20		259
Mean	4.6	5.3	3.6	2.9	3.4	2.5	2.8	2.6	2.3	2.5		3.2

*Symptoms: 4 = dizzy; 7 = coordination off; 11 = heart beating fast; 17 = stomach cramps; 19 = weakness; 24 = nausea; 30 = warm; 33 = sweaty; 36 = chilly; 37 = shivering; 62 = irritability; 63 = restlessness.

TABLE 14-3 Subjective Report of Environmental Symptoms Questionnaire Symptoms of Heat Illness: 8-g Salt Diet ($n = 9$)

Subject	Symptoms* on Heat Acclimation Day										Total Symptoms
	1	2	3	4	5	6	7	8	9	10	
4	4	7	7	7	7	7	7	7	7	19	53
	7	11	11	11	11	19	19	19	19	30	
	11	19	19	19	19	30	30	30	30	33	
	19	30	30	30	30	33	33	33	33		
	30	33	33	33	33						
	33	63	36	36	36						
	63		37	37							
			63								
25	4	4	30	30	30	30	30	30	30	30	33
	7	30	33	33	33	33	33	33	33	33	
	19	33	62	62	62		62	62	62	62	
	30	62									
	33										
	62										
26	7	30	30	30	30	11	11	30	11	11	32
	11	33	33	33	33	30	30	33	30	30	
	30		63	63	63	33	33	63	33	33	
	33					63			63		
21	4	4	30	30	4	17	30	30	30	30	30
	7	19	33	33	7	30	33	33	33	33	
	19	33			19	33					
	30				24						
	33				30						
					33						
					36						

	1	2	3	4	5	6	7	8	9	10	Total
3	30, 33	30, 33	30, 33	19, 30, 33, 62	19, 30, 33, 62	19, 30, 33	19, 30, 33	30, 33, 62	30, 33	19, 30, 33, 62	29
7	30, 33	11, 30, 33	11, 30, 33	7, 19, 30, 33, 62	30, 33	30, 33	30, 33	30, 33	30, 33	30, 33, 63	26
5	4, 7, 11, 19, 30	30, 33	33		62	62	62, 63	62, 63	62, 63		16
27	4, 19, 30, 33	17	33	33	7, 33	7, 33	33	33	33	33	15
9		30	30	62				62			4
Total	35	24	24	26	28	21	20	21	20	19	238
Mean	3.9	2.7	2.7	2.9	3.1	2.3	2.2	2.3	2.2	2.1	2.6

*Symptoms: 4 = dizzy; 7 = coordination off; 11 = heart beating fast; 17 = stomach cramps; 19 = weakness; 24 = nausea; 30 = warm; 33 = sweaty; 36 = chilly; 37 = shivering; 62 = irritability; 63 = restlessness.

and 14-5 (8-g salt diet), the data from Tables 14-2 and 14-3 are recast to present the 12 symptoms of heat illness and the number of times each symptom was reported each day. Regardless of diet group, the predominant symptoms were warmth, sweatiness, weakness, irritability and restlessness, and rapid heart beat. Both diet groups reported symptoms of dizziness and disturbed coordination to occur most often during the first 2 days of heat acclimation. Chills, shivering, and nausea were rarely reported.

Overall Index of Subjective Heat Illness

To evaluate the subject's overall subjective feelings of heat illness, an index of subjective heat illness was developed. First, all 68 ESQ items were scrutinized for their relationship to clinical descriptions of heat illness (compare with Armstrong et al., 1987; Knochel, 1984; Richards et al., 1979). Twenty-eight were selected for evaluation (items 1, 2, 4, 5, 7, 8, 9, 11, 16, 17, 19, 23, 24, 26, 27, 30, 33, 36, 37, 38, 41, 52, 53, 55, 56, 59, 62, and 63). An initial overall index of subjective illness was calculated for each subject by summing the intensity ratings of the 28 items. This initial index was then used in an item analysis to assess the index's reliability according to Cronbach's alpha statistic (Cronbach, 1951). Initial running of the analysis for all 17 subjects resulted in the deletion of three of the items (items 24, 26, and 37; nausea, diarrhea, and shivering) due to too many missing cases or null variances. An additional three items (items 23, 36, and 59; stomach ache, chilly, and concentration off) were deleted due to negative correlations with the total score. This left 22 ESQ items (Table 14-6) in the final index of subjective heat illness (SHI); Cronbach's alpha statistic for the SHI is 0.86.

To assess the comparability of the two diet groups prior to heat acclimation and when all were still on the 8-g salt diet, a 2×3 (diet group $\times$ diet stabilization day) analysis of variance was conducted on the SHI. This analysis yielded only nonsignificant effects, indicating that both groups were comparable prior to heat acclimation and prior to the implementation of the 4-g salt diet for eight of the subjects. To assess the influence of diet and day of heat acclimation, a 2×10 (diet $\times$ day of heat acclimation) analysis of variance was conducted on the SHI. This analysis yielded a significant main effect for day of heat acclimation, $F(9,135) = 7.179$, $p < .001$, and a significant interaction between diet and day of heat acclimation, $F(9,135) = 2.875$, $p < .01$ (but not a significant main effect for diet, $F(1,15) = 0.397$, $p > .5$).

These data are presented graphically in Figure 14-1 for the ESQ administrations during both the diet stabilization period (days 1 to 7) and the 10 days of heat acclimation (days 8 to 17). Figure 14-1 clearly demonstrates the comparability of the subjects in the two diet groups prior to heat acclimation and the influence on both groups of the heat acclimation. Duncan

TABLE 14-4 Number of Times Each Heat Illness Symptom Was Reported During Heat Acclimation, 4-g Salt Diet ($n = 8$)

	ESQ* Symptom	Heat Acclimation Day										
		1	2	3	4	5	6	7	8	9	10	Total
33	Sweaty	8	8	7	6	6	5	6	6	6	5	63
30	Warm	7	8	6	5	6	5	4	6	5	5	57
19	Weakness	5	5	5	4	5	2	3	3	1	2	35
62	Irritability	1	4	4	3	4	3	2	1	2	3	27
11	Heart beating fast	5	4	3	2	1	2	2	2	1	2	24
63	Restlessness	0	3	2	2	2	2	3	2	3	2	21
36	Chilly	1	3	1	1	1	1	1	1	0	1	11
4	Dizzy	4	4	0	0	0	0	0	0	0	0	8
7	Disturbed coordination	4	1	0	0	1	0	0	0	0	0	6
17	Stomach cramps	2	1	1	0	0	0	1	0	0	0	5
24	Nausea	0	1	0	0	1	0	0	0	0	0	2
37	Shivering	0	0	0	0	0	0	0	0	0	0	0
Total		37	42	29	23	27	20	22	21	18	20	259

*ESQ = Environmental Symptoms Questionnaire.

TABLE 14-5 Number of Times Each Heat Illness Symptom Was Reported During Heat Acclimation, 8-g Salt Diet ($n = 9$)

	ESQ* Symptom	Heat Acclimation Day										
		1	2	3	4	5	6	7	8	9	10	Total
33	Sweaty	7	7	8	7	7	7	7	7	7	7	71
30	Warm	8	7	7	6	6	6	6	6	6	6	64
19	Weakness	5	2	1	3	3	2	2	1	1	2	22
62	Irritability	1	1	1	4	3	1	2	4	2	2	21
7	Disturbed coordination	5	1	1	2	3	2	1	1	1	0	17
11	Heart beating fast	3	2	2	1	1	1	1	0	1	1	13
63	Restlessness	1	1	2	1	1	1	1	2	2	1	13
4	Dizzy	5	2	0	0	1	0	0	0	0	0	8
36	Chilly	0	0	1	1	2	0	0	0	0	0	4
17	Stomach cramps	0	1	0	0	0	1	0	0	0	0	2
37	Shivering	0	0	1	1	0	0	0	0	0	0	2
24	Nausea	0	0	0	0	1	0	0	0	0	0	1
Total		35	24	24	26	28	21	20	21	20	19	238

*ESQ = Environmental Symptoms Questionnaire.

TABLE 14-6 The 22 Environmental Symptoms Questionnaire (ESQ) Items Constituting the Index of Subjective Heat Illness

ESQ Symptom No.	Description
1	Lightheaded
2	Headache
4	Dizzy
5	Faint
7	Coordination off
8	Short of breath
9	Hard to breathe
11	Heart beating fast
16	Muscle cramp
17	Stomach cramps
19	Weak
27	Constipated
30	Warm
33	Sweaty
38	Body parts numb
41	Vision blurry
52	Lost appetite
53	Sick
55	Thirsty
56	Tired
62	Irritable
63	Restless

post hoc tests ($p < .05$) of the means plotted in Figure 14-1 showed that (a) the two diet groups differed from one another only on the first 2 days of heat acclimation, with the 4-g salt group demonstrating significantly more heat illness, and (b) each group acclimated to the heat such that by the fourth day of heat acclimation the SHI had reached a level that did not differ from any of the succeeding days (that is, reduction in the SHI had reached asymptote).

DISCUSSION

Many of the signs and symptoms of heat exhaustion reported by Armstrong et al. (1987) were also prominent in this study. The results of the present study indicate that, regardless of diet group, the predominant symptoms during heat acclimation are warmth, sweatiness, weakness, irritability and restlessness, and rapid heart beat. In addition, dizziness and disturbed coordination occur most often during the first 2 days of heat acclimation.

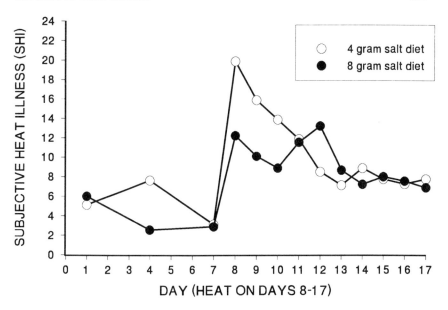

FIGURE 14-1 Mean index of subjective heat illness (SHI) for each test day, where *n* = 17 male soldiers (4-g salt group, *n* = 8; 8-g group, *n* = 9).

On the fifth day of heat acclimation (day 12), there appears to be an increase in subjective heat illness, as measured by the SHI, for the 8-g salt group (see Figure 14-1). Although this "blip" in the curve is statistically nonsignificant, it begs an explanation because it disrupts an otherwise fairly smooth curve to asymptote. To address this issue, an inspection of the daily log notes was conducted. The log notes showed that one of the subjects in the 8-g group (subject 21) reported feeling the "possible onset" of flu-like symptoms on that day. When this subject's entire data set for all days is removed from the analysis, the "blip" on day 12 disappears without changing the rest of the curve. Consequently, this "blip" is likely due to one subject experiencing symptoms unrelated to the treatment procedures on day 12.

CONCLUSIONS

Whether measured by the mean number of heat illness symptoms reported or by an overall index of subjective heat illness (the SHI), subjective reports of heat illness are significantly higher during the first 2 days of heat acclimation than during subsequent days. A diet that includes the daily consumption of 8 g of salt (as compared to 4 g of salt) during heat acclimation results in significantly diminished reports of subjective heat illness during those first 2 days of heat acclimation. After the initial 2 days of heat acclimation, there is no measurable difference in subjective reports of heat illness between the two dietary groups. If subjective heat illness is to be minimized during heat acclimation, and especially if the first 2 days of heat acclimation are significant to military operations, a diet consisting of 8 g of salt per day is preferable to a diet of 4 g of salt per day.

REFERENCES

Armstrong, L.E., R.W. Hubbard, W.J. Kraemer, J.P. DeLuca, and E.L. Christensen
  1987   Signs and symptoms of heat exhaustion during strenuous exercise. Ann. Sports Med. 3:182-189.
Banderet, L.E., and H.R. Lieberman
  1989   Treatment with tyrosine, a neurotransmitter precursor, reduces environmental stress in humans. Brain Res. Bull. 22:759-762.
Cronbach, L.J.
  1951   Coefficient alpha and the internal structure of tests. Psychometrika 16:297-334.
Hirsch, E., H.L. Meiselman, R.D. Popper, G. Smits, B. Jezior, I. Lichton, N. Wenkam, J. Burt, M. Fox, S. McNutt, M.N. Thiele, and O. Dirige
  1984   The effects of prolonged feeding meal, ready-to-eat (MRE) operational rations. Technical Report NATICK/TR-85/035. U.S. Army Natick Research and Development Center, Natick, Mass.
Johnson, R. F., L. G. Branch, and D. J. McMenemy
  1989   Influence of attitude and expectation on moods and symptoms during cold weather military training. Aviat. Space Environ. Med. 60:1157-1162.
Knochel, J.
  1984   Environmental heat illness. Arch. Int. Med. 133:841-864.
Kobrick, J.L., and J.B. Sampson
  1979   New inventory for the assessment of symptom occurrences and severity at high altitude. Aviat. Space Environ. Med. 50:925-929.
Kobrick, J.L., R.F. Johnson, and D.J. McMenemy
  1990   Subjective reactions to atropine/2-PAM chloride and heat while in battle dress uniform and in chemical protective clothing. Milit. Psychol. 2:95-111.
Richards, D., R. Richards, and P.J. Schofield
  1979   Management of heat exhaustion in Sydney's The Sun City-to-Surf fun runners. Med. J. Aust. 2:457-461.
Rock, P.B., T.S. Johnson, A. Cymerman, R.L. Burse, L.J. Falk, and C.S. Fulco
  1987   Effect of dexamethasone on symptoms of acute mountain sickness at Pike's Peak, Colorado (4,300 m). Aviat. Space Environ. Med. 58:668-672.
Sampson, J.B., and J.L. Kobrick
  1980   The Environmental Symptoms Questionnaire: Revisions and new field data. Aviat. Space Environ. Med. 51:872-877.
StatSoft
  1988   CSS (Complete Statistical System) Release 2.1. Tulsa, Okla.: StatSoft.
USACDEC/USARIEM (U.S. Army Combat Developments and Experimentation Center and U.S. Army Research Institute of Environmental Medicine)
  1986   Combat Field Feeding System—Force Development Test and Experimentation (CFFS-FDTE), vol. 1-3. Technical Report Nos. CDEC-TR-85-006A, CDEC-TR-85-006B,

CDEC-TR-85-006C. Fort Ord, Calif.: U.S. Army Combat Developments and Experimentation Center.

USARIEM (U.S. Army Research Institute of Environmental Medicine)
1990   Sustaining Health and Performance in the Desert: A Pocket Guide to Environmental Medicine for Operations in Southwest Asia. Technical Note 91-2. U.S. Army Research Institute of Environmental Medicine, Natick, Mass.

DISCUSSION

PARTICIPANT: I can't remember whether the manipulation of the salt intake preceded the heat exposure or not. Were they instituted at the same time?

DR. JOHNSON: The onset of heat exposure and the manipulation of salt intake occurred on the same date.

PARTICIPANT: So we don't know whether your subjects may have been, say, pre-adapted for 4-gram intakes and what effect that might have had on their initial response to heat exposure. I mean, it is confounded now. Since they are adapting both to the lower salt intake and to the heat at the same time, we are not sure what would have happened if they were first exposed to heat.

PARTICIPANT: Weren't they on 8 grams first?

DR. JOHNSON: Yes, they were all on 8.

PARTICIPANT: It would be interesting to see what would happen if some of them had been on the 4-gram sodium diet during the stabilization period.

DR. JOHNSON: There was a practical reason for conducting the study the way we did. It is unlikely that soldiers would be on a 4-gram sodium diet in garrison prior to going into the field. It is more likely that they would be on at least an 8-gram sodium diet in garrison followed by a decrease in sodium intake per day when deployed to the field.

PARTICIPANT: Was there any evidence at all throughout the study of hyponatremia? I mean, how low did sodium levels ever get in this study?

DR. ARMSTRONG: The sodium levels were normal day to day. However, there was one subject who experienced water intoxication on the very first day.

PARTICIPANT: That is interesting.

DR. ARMSTRONG: He gained 10 pounds in a matter of just a few hours of exercise on the treadmill. He thought that he should drink a lot of water to stay healthy during exercise and heat exposure. Since we were watching for drops in body weight, we did not expect this. He was removed from the study at that point. It was an extremely unusual circumstance, and his data are not included in this presentation. His data are being written up separately as a case study. Other than that, there were no signs of hyponatremia.

PARTICIPANT: With respect to the index of subjective heat illness that you have constructed, can you analyze it using confidence intervals instead and might you get a different interpretation of the results?

DR. JOHNSON: There are many ways that we can analyze the data. We have presented two here: looking for differences between groups based on frequency counts of symptom reports, and conducting traditional analyses of variance on the index of subjective heat illness. Analyses using confidence intervals is a good suggestion but we have not done that here.

PARTICIPANT: One of the things that struck me is the increased reports of heat discomfort under a condition of minimal heat strain. That is, the increase is modest. What might you anticipate with greater heat strain? Since discomfort may be more closely related to changes in skin temperature than to changes in core temperature, might this relationship be the reason for the increase in subjective heat illness?

DR. JOHNSON: There may be such a relationship, but we did not look at relationship to skin temperature changes. We are, however, interested in what these data mean in terms of absolute levels of symptom intensity. That is, reports of subjective heat illness, as measured by the SHI (an intensity index), show that there are significant differences between the groups during the first two days of heat exposure. The data also show that these differences between the groups disappear by the third day of heat exposure, and that the absolute levels have significantly decreased to a much less intense level. We consider these levels as not very intense in an absolute sense because not one person was removed from the heat chamber due to subjective discomfort. In other studies, however, under similar temperature conditions but with the subjects wearing chemical protective clothing, a greater array of symptoms is reported and these symptoms are more intense. Under these condition, subjects do remove themselves because of extreme discomfort.

PARTICIPANT: If I remember correctly, the $V_{O_2 \, max}$ for these subjects was somewhere around 45 to 46 ml per kilogram per minute. Was the incidence of symptoms associated with level of physical fitness?

DR. JOHNSON: All subjects were somewhat uniform in this regard, and we found no relationship between symptoms and fitness levels.

PARTICIPANT: Have you done any studies where you have looked at heat strain and performance?

DR. JOHNSON: We have collected data where we have looked at these variables. We have found that performance of militarily relevant tasks such as marksmanship, is related to heat exposure. Specifically, up to 6 hours exposure to 95°F with 60 percent relative humidity significantly impairs steadiness of the soldier's outstretched arm and hand. Rifle marksmanship for stationary targets, which requires extreme steadiness of the arm and hand, is also impaired during the same heat exposure.

PARTICIPANT: I remember years ago when I was working in the military ergonomics, that subjective ratings depended on who asked the question. For example, if a woman asked male soldiers how they felt, the soldiers tended to report that they felt better than if the questioner was a man.

DR. JOHNSON: That is a good point and it is often overlooked by casual users of subjective report techniques. It is also one of the reasons that we adopted a standardized questionnaire. We wanted to avoid the subtle influences on subjective response due to inadvertent rewording of the questions and due to variability in the characteristics of the questioner. In this study, the questionnaire was always administered by the same person and at a table far removed from the rest of the staff and from other subjects.

PARTICIPANT: Since the administration of the two salt diets was double blind, I am curious as to whether the subjects could guess which diet they had received.

DR. JOHNSON: We did collect the data and found that the subjects were unable to guess at better than a chance level. The double blind procedure was a success.

PARTICIPANT: I missed how the meals were administered.

DR. JOHNSON: The diets were constructed around MREs. For the high salt diet, we used standard off-the-shelf MRE entrees. For the low salt diet, a food engineer altered MREs by removing the sodium glutamate and all the salt-containing preservatives. Ninety percent of the difference in the sodium in the two diets was due to these re-engineered entrees. All other food was obtained from a supermarket. These other foods were mixed so that they looked the same. Taste tests done before the study indicated that independent judges could not tell the difference. Those MRE entrees with the low salt could not be distinguished from those with more salt.

PART IV

Committee Discussion Paper

OVERVIEW

PART IV CONSISTS OF THE PRELIMINARY DISCUSSION PAPER that was written by one committee member, by request of the committee, after the workshop was held. The purpose of this paper was to focus on the area of appetite and summarize some of the critical issues for discussion; to indicate, for the committee, scientific areas where additional information may be needed; and to pose, to the committee, specific questions for pointed discussion during further deliberations. This paper is included to provide further information on the committee deliberation process concerning the nutritional needs for military personnel working in hot environments.

15

Food Intake, Appetite, and Work in Hot Environments

Allison A. Yates[1]

INTRODUCTION

Research to determine the specific internal metabolic mechanisms by which environmental heat affects appetite has focused on measurement of changes in intake induced in animal models in artificial hot environments. External ambient temperature and body temperature, and the regulation thereof, have been looked at in detail in animal models because food intake has been shown to markedly decrease in hot environments in all species of animals studied (Young, 1987), and usually in humans (Mitchell and Edman, 1951).

Internal Mechanisms

The prime theory ascribed to the mechanism by which heat decreases food intake (and therefore appetite) involves thermoregulation and the thermic effect of food. If continued consumption of normal intakes occurs under heat stress conditions, the additional heat required to be dissipated by the normal amounts ingested may result in an inability to dissipate heat adequately. In a series of experiments by Hamilton (1963a), rats, upon exposure to a temperature of 35°C, ate only 2 grams of food during the first 24 hours, compared with a previous intake of more than 20 grams at 24°C; mild (32°C) and severe (35°C) heat stress over 21 days resulted in a contin-

[1] Allison A. Yates, Dean, College of Health and Human Sciences, The University of Southern Mississippi, Southern Station, Box 10075, Hattiesburg, MS 39406-0075

ued lower level of food intake. The marked decrease initially was thought to be due to the initial dehydration; the continued lower level of intake was due to the adaptation to the increased ambient temperature. Body weights in the growing rats dropped initially by as much as 30 grams and then remained constant until the heat stress was removed. These studies have been used as a demonstration of the concept of a body weight set-point lowering effect due to a hot environment (Thompson, 1980).

The "thermostatic" theory of food intake (a decrease in the body weight or fat set-point in response to hot environments) has been proposed as the method by which the body may thermoregulate, in part by decreasing the insulating amount of body fat (Brobeck, 1948). Studies in a number of experimental animals demonstrate a cessation of eating at high temperatures, which indicates that continued eating would probably lead to hyperthermia. The decrease in food intake is thus followed by a decrease in body weight and fat (Jakubczak, 1976).

In investigations of the theory that animals stop eating to prevent hyperthermia, the differences in the resulting thermic effect of food ingested (specific dynamic action) have been implicated. In the series of experiments by Hamilton (1963a), calorie intake of rats fed special diets during mild heat stress was inversely related to the thermogenic effect of the diet selected. It appears that fats may be the preferred energy source in heat stress (Salganik, 1956), and that in severe heat stress, protein is avoided due to the comparatively high amount of heat created (Hamilton, 1963a). With this theory, body temperature should be highly correlated with hunger and satiety. However, there is no consistent observed relationship between the two. Although in 1936 Booth and Strang reported that skin temperature in adults increased 2°C within 10 minutes of eating a high protein meal, a postprandial increase in skin temperature was not found by Stunkard et al. (1962). In dogs, Passmore and Ritchie (1957) found an extremely small rise in skin temperature after a high protein meal while Hamilton (1963a) determined that food consumption and rectal temperature in rats decreased incrementally with temperatures betweens 7° and 32°C, but at 35°C, rectal temperature became elevated, while food intake continued to decrease.

Andersson and Larsson (1961) have shown that heating of the preoptic and anterior hypothalamic regions of the brain (areas that are known to be involved in regulating body temperature) inhibits feeding in animals. Opposite results, however, were obtained by Spector et al. (1968) in rats, when heating of the preoptic medialis region caused increased eating when the temperature of the area was raised to 43°C. Decreased eating occurred in their study when the ambient temperature was raised to 35°C. Local temperature in the anterior hypothalamic area has been reported to drop at the onset of feeding, which is opposite of what would be expected (Hamilton, 1963b). Thus it appears that the effect of brain temperature on feeding may be more a result of external ambient temperature than of localized temperature changes and may be due to the rate of heat flow from the core to the periphery or vice versa, as no single temperature appears to uniquely govern the level of food intake (Spector et al., 1968).

Osmotic factors have also been shown to affect food intake in animals. Ingestion or intubation of hypertonic saline or glucose solutions results in decreased food intake in rats (Ehman et al., 1972; Kozub, 1972). However, intravenous administration of hypertonic infusions resulted in decreased food intake in rats only when the hyperosmolar solution was sodium chloride, but did not affect food intake when the solution was glucose or xylose (Yin and Tsai, 1973). As reviewed by Thompson (1980), this observed decrease in food intake serves as a protective mechanism that is demonstrated under conditions of total water deprivation, which significantly reduces food intake in most species studied, including pigeons (Ziegler et al., 1972). Ad lib food intake dropped to half in rats during a 24-hour period without water (Cizek and Nocenti, 1965), thus demonstrating that food intake and fluid balance are directly related. It appears that observations of decreased food intake in unacclimatized people in tropical climates may, to a large extent, be mediated by hypertonicity associated with initial dehydration, and improve as acclimatization occurs (Bass et al., 1955).

Not only is the stress of a hot environment due to thermoregulation and maintenance hydration, but it may be due to psychic stress as well. Such stress may be initiated by the degree of mental discomfort caused by the heat. Thus the impact of the need to (a) physiologically maintain thermoneutrality, (b) maintain normal hydration in spite of profuse sweating, and (c) feel comfortable in the heat may each affect the individual's appetitie and his/her perceived hunger to a different degree. Researchers cannot distinguish the difference between appetite and hunger in animals due to the lack of methods to communicate feelings; in humans, such information may be important in determining appropriate mechanisms for maintaining body weight and health status in prolonged exposure to heat. If an additional stress due to the situation occurs, such as that resulting from fear of death (as found in war or military conflict), then there may be additive effects on the desire to eat (appetite) or the perceived need to eat (hunger).

OBSERVATIONAL DATA ON INTAKE

A few studies (conducted primarily in foreign countries) do exist in which food intake of adults in hot and/or humid environments has been studied in isolated work environments. Edholm and Goldsmith (1966) reported their study in Bahrain and in the United Kingdom in which two groups of military men were followed in a carefully controlled environment. One group had spent a year in Bahrain prior to the experiment, while the second group was first studied for 12 days in the United Kingdom and then flown to Bahrain where it was joined by the first group. All men then spent the first 4 days in hard work, the next 4 days in mainly sedentary work, and the final 4 days in hard work in tents and outdoors. Both groups then returned to the United Kingdom for a repeat of the 12-day protocol. The daytime temperature in Bahrain rarely fell below 30°C, with a relative humidity of 40 to 90 percent. Energy balance was measured, and similar food was provided to both groups in all settings. The mean food intake in Bahrain was approximately 25 percent less than in the United Kingdom; however, the percentage of calories from fat and carbohydrate was similar, as was the percentage of calories from protein. Both groups lost weight during the 12 days in Bahrain, with the unacclimatized group losing 2.5 kg in 12 days and the acclimatized group losing 1.1 kg. Because weight loss was not quickly recovered upon returning to the United Kingdom, it was thought that the caloric deficit was responsible for the majority of the weight lost in the hot environment. It is apparent, though, that those men previously adapted to the hot environment were less affected by the work schedule, perhaps due to decreased acute dehydration.

Balance studies conducted on an oil tanker in the South Atlantic and the Persian Gulf during the summer season with six male subjects, two of whom were crew members that were involved in heavy work, did not show any directional changes in food intake as a result of heat or acclimatization (Collins et al., 1971; Eddy et al., 1971a,b). However, since the protocol was changed during the study to increase the exercise levels of those who did not initially participate in heavy work, it is difficult to determine whether a decrease in food intake was masked by the increase in energy expenditure in three of the subjects. A number of military studies conducted by the U.S. Department of Defense have looked at garrison and field feeding, food choices and food waste, in addition to tests of the rations developed (Consolazio et al., 1960; Hirsch et al., 1984; Johnson et al., 1947, 1983; Kretsch et al., 1979, 1984, 1986a,b; Richardson et al., 1979). These have all been conducted in only one season, usually fall or spring; thus comparative information regarding summer food choices is not available. A confounding factor in such studies is the presence of air conditioning, which might in itself alter food preferences and intake depending on the length of time the individual is in a conditioned environment where meals are consumed.

A few studies have looked at seasonal body compositional changes and found that there is a decrease in caloric intake and a corresponding decrease in body weight/fat during the summer season as compared to winter. Some studies have also evaluated nutrient intake in adults based on season of the year in hot environments; decreased intake of some vitamins has been reported, such as vitamin A and C (Aldashev et al., 1986), and protein, vitamin C, and total energy (Mommadov and Grafova, 1983), but such studies did not evaluate changes in food preferences or appetite.

Empirical data, based on observations and practices in food service, in both the military and the commercial sectors, indicate a change in food preferences during seasons associated with elevated mean temperature. Few basic studies have attempted specifically to address changing food patterns in self-selected diets due to season. In a study of seasonal variations in self-selected lunches in a large employee cafeteria in Maryland, Zifferblatt et al. (1980) found decreased selection of starches and cooked vegetables, with increased purchases of fruits, salads, yogurt, and cottage cheese, as the noon-time temperature rose (significant at $p < 0.05$). As the temperature increased, average caloric purchases tended to decrease ($p < 0.0529$). It should be noted that the workplace cafeteria, along with the work areas of most of the employees, was kept at 22.2°C (72°F). Therefore, the external temperature may have only moderately influenced appetite.

National surveys have been conducted on food consumption patterns of Americans, but they have not recently gathered data on the same individuals or individuals in similar geographic, and thus environmental, areas at different times of the year to determine if seasonal variation, and consequently changes in temperature, affects appetite (resulting in changes in food intake) or food selection patterns. The 1965-1966 Food Consumption Survey (USDA, 1972) compared household food purchases by season; foods that increased in the summer survey included fresh salad ingredients (tomatoes, lettuce, cucumbers, and so on), salad dressings, cookies, and frozen milk desserts, rice, bread, ground beef, lunch meat, chicken, shellfish, sugar, fresh corn, fresh cantaloupes, other fresh fruits, carbonated beverages, fruit drinks, and alcoholic beverages. Decreased food purchases included fresh milk, table fats, flour, hot cereal, beef roast, sausage, potatoes, fresh dark green leafy vegetables, fresh deep yellow vegetables, oranges, canned vegetables, canned fruit, and soup. Accordingly individuals alter their purchasing behavior during the year, to some extent based on availability and price of food items. Whether appetite (the desire to eat) also changes is unknown from these data.

CONCLUSIONS AND RESEARCH RECOMMENDATIONS

Based on human studies that have documented voluntary decreased food intake in individuals in hot environments and animal studies that have supported the concept of decreased food intake as an adaptive mechanism to ameliorate the increased need for thermoregulation, optimal nutrition is compromised if intake decreases to the extent that inadequate levels of key nutrients are consumed. The following areas of study are recommended in order to determine the exact impact of hot environments on appetite:

• Studies regarding self-selected food patterns of individuals engaged in similar activity in hot versus temperate climates

• Studies that determine the effect of stress on appetite, with temperature as a major variable

When such information is available, then it should be possible to

1. develop basic recommendations for types of foods that should be part of rations in hot environments, and

2. determine if specific supplements with improved palatability should be used when troops are in hot environments where depressed appetite for prolonged periods may prevent adequate nutrient intake.

REFERENCES

Aldashev, A.A., B.I. Kim, O.A. Kolesova, V.L. Reznik, and V.V. Subach
    1986   Indices of the nutritional status of workers in the oil and gas production industry adapting to the extreme conditions of an arid zone. (in Russian) Vopr. Pitan. May-June (3):25-28.
Andersson, B., and B. Larsson
    1961   Influence of local temperature changes in the preoptic area and rostral hypothalamus on the regulation of food and water intake. Acta Physiol. Scand. 52:75-89.
Bass, D.E., C.R. Kleeman, M. Quinn, A. Henschel, and A.H. Hegnauer
    1955   Mechanisms of acclimatization to heat in man. Med. Anal. Rev. 34:323-380.
Booth, G., and J.M. Strang
    1936   Changes in temperature of the skin following ingestion of food. Arch. Intern. Med. 57:533-543.
Brobeck, J.R.
    1948   Food intake as a mechanism of temperature regulation. Yale J. Biol. and Med. 20:545-552.
Cizek, L.J., and M.R. Nocenti
    1965   Relationship between water and food ingestion in the rat. Am. J. Physiol. 208:615-620.
Collins, K.J., T.P. Eddy, A. Hibbs, A.L. Stock, and E.F. Wheeler
    1971   Nutritional and environmental studies on an ocean-going oil tanker. 2. Heat acclimatization and nutrient balances. Brit. J. Industr. Med. 28:246-258.
Consolazio, C.F., R. Shapiro, J.E. Masterson, and P.S.L. McKinzie
    1960   Report of caloric requirements of men working in an extremely hot desert environment, Yuma, Arizona July-August, 1959, U.S. Army Medical Research and Nutrition Laboratory, Fitzsimons General Hosptial, Report No. 246, July, 1960.
Eddy, T.P., A.L. Stock, and E.F. Wheeler
    1971a   Nutritional and environmental studies on an ocean-going oil tanker. 3. Energy balances and physique. Brit. J. Industr. Med. 28:330-341.
Eddy, T.P., E.F. Wheeler, and A.L. Stock
    1971b   Nutritional and environmental studies on an ocean-going oil tanker. 4. The diet of seamen. Brit. J. Industr. Med. 28:342-352.
Edholm, O.G, and R. Goldsmith
    1966   Food intakes and weight changes in climatic extremes. Proc. Nutr. Soc. 25:113-119.

Ehman, G.K., D.J. Albert, and J.L. Jamieson
1972   Injections into the duodenum and the induction of satiety in the rat. Can. J. Psychol.
        25:147-166.
Hamilton, C.L.
1963a   Interactions of food intake and temperature regulation in the rat. J. Comp. Physiol.
        Psychol. 56:476-488.
1963b   Hypothalamic temperature records of a monkey. Proc. Soc. Exptl. Biol. Med.
        112:55-57.
Hirsch, E., H.L. Meiselman, R.D. Popper, G. Smits, B. Jezior, I. Lichton, M.
        Wenkam, J. Brut, M. Fox, S. McNutt, M.N, Thiele, and O. Dirige
1984   The effects of prolonged feeding meal, ready-to-eat (MRE) operational rations,
        Technical Report NATICK/TR-85/035, U.S. Army Natick Research and Develop-
        ment Center, Natick, MA, October, 1984.
Jakubczak, L.F.
1976   Food and water intakes of rats as a function of strain, age, temperature, and body
        weight. Physiol. Behav. 17:251-258.
Johnson, R.E., and R.M. Kark
1947   Feeding Problems in Man as Related to Environment. An Analysis of United
        States and Canadian Army Ration Trials and Surveys, 1941-1946, Quartermaster
        Food and Container Institute for the Armed Forces, Research and Development
        Branch, U.S. Army Medical Nutrition Laboratory, Chicago, April, 1947.
Johnson, H.L., R.A. Nelson, J.E. Canham, J.H. Skala, C.F. Consolazio, and H.E. Sauberlich
1983   Comparisons of utilizations and nutrient contents of A rations and short order
        meals at the Air Force Dining Facility, Lowry Air Force Base, Denver, Colo-
        rado—July, 1971. Letterman Army Institute of Research Report No. 140, San
        Francisco, March, 1983.
Kozub, F.J.
1972   Male-female differences in response to stomach loads of hypertonic NaCl in rats.
        Psychon. Sci. 28:149-151.
Kretsch, M.J., D.D. Schnakenberg, R.D. Fults, R.A. Nelson, Y.C. LeTellier, and J.E. Canham
1979   Nutrient intakes and some socioeconomic characteristics of Twentynine Palms
        Marine Corps personnel before food service system modifications—March, 1977,
        Letterman Army Institute of Research Report No. 65, San Francisco, June, 1979.
Kretsch, M.J., H.E. Sauberlich, and J.H. Skala
1984   Nutritional status assessment of marines before and after the installation of the
        "multi-restaurant" food service system at the Twentynine Palms Marine Corps
        Base, California, Letterman Army Institute of Research Report No. 192, San Fran-
        cisco, December, 1984.
Kretsch, M.J., P.M. Conforti, and H.E. Sauberlich
1986a   Nutrient intake evaluation of male and female cadets at the United States Military
        Academy, West Point, New York, Letterman Army Institute of Research Report
        No. 218, San Francisco, April, 1986.
Kretsch, M.J., P.M. Conforti, H.L. Johnson, and H.E. Sauberlich
1986b   Effects of energy intake and expenditure on weight gain and percent body fat of
        male and female cadets at the United States Military Academy, West Point, New
        York. Letterman Army Institute of Research Report No. 225, San Francisco, Sep-
        tember, 1986.
Mitchell, H.H., and M. Edman
1951   Nutrition in Climatic Stress. Pp. 50-51. Springfield, Ill.: Charles C. Thomas.
Mommadov, I.M., and V.A. Grafova
1983   Daily diet and ascorbic acid intake in man during work in the Arid zone. Hum.
        Physiol. 9(4):224-228.

Passmore, R., and F.J. Ritchie
   1957   The specific dynamic action of food and the satiety mechanism. Brit J. Nutr. 11:79-85.
Richardson, R.P., D.P. Leitch, B.M. Hill, P.M. Short, G. Turk, H.L. Meiselman, L.E. Symington, R. Porter, and D, Schnakenberg
   1979   A New Foodservice System Concept for Aircraft Carriers, Technical Report Natick/ TR/80/007, U.S. Army Natick Research and Development Command, Natick, December, 1979.
Salganik, R.I.
   1956   Nutrition in high environmental temperatures. Vopr. Pitan. (Russian) 33:3-11.
Spector, N.H., J.R. Brobeck, and C.L. Hamilton
   1968   Feeding and core temperature in albino rats: Changes induced by preoptic heating and cooling. Science 161:286-288.
Stunkard, A.J., W.L. Clovis, and S.M. Free
   1962   Skin temperature after eating, evidence bearing upon a thermostatic control of food intake. Am. J. Med. Sci. 244:126-130.
Thompson, C.I.
   1980   Controls of Eating. New York, N.Y.: Spectrum Publications.
USDA (U.S. Department of Agriculture)
   1972   Food Consumption of Households in the U.S., Seasons and Year 1965-66. March 1972 Report 12, MC 7473(72). Agricultural Research Service, Washington, D.C.: U.S. Government Printing Office.
Yin, T.H., and C.T. Tsai
   1973   Effects of glucose on feeding in relation to routes of entry in rats. J. Comp. Physiol. Psychol. 85:258-264.
Young, B.A.
   1987   The effect of climate upon intake. Pp. 163-190 in the Nutrition of Herbivores, J.B. Hacker and J.H. Ternourth eds. New York, N.Y.: Academic Press.
Ziegler, H.P., H.L. Green, and J. Siegel
   1972   Food and water intake and weight regulation in the pigeon. Physiol. Behav. 8:127-134.
Zifferblatt, S.M., C.S. Wilbur, and J.L. Pinsky
   1980   Influence of ecologic events on cafeteria food selections: Understanding food habits. J. Am. Diet. Assoc. 76:9-14.

APPENDIXES

A

Military Recommended Dietary Allowances, AR 25-40 (1985)

The most recent revision of the Military Recommended Dietary Allowances (MRDAs) are included in Army Regulation 25-40 (U.S. Army, 1985). The entire regulation has been included on the following pages for reference and comparison with existing RDAs and issues related to nutritional needs in hot environments. No changes other than page formatting were made to the text. Note that this regulation is a joint regulation and presents the nutrition responsibilities for the Army, Navy, and Air Force. As described in Chapter 1, this regulation is currently under revision. Further information concerning this regulation can be obtained by writing to: Headquarters, Department of the Army (SGPS-CO-B), 5109 Leesburg Pike, Falls Church, VA 22041-2358. Copies of the original AR 25-40 can be obtained by writing to the address listed at the end of the regulation.

Headquarters   ***Army Regulation 40-25/Naval**
Departments of the Army,   **Command Medical Instruction**
the Navy, and the Air Force   **10110.1/Air Force Regulation**
Washington, DC   **160-95**
15 May 1985

Medical Services

Nutrition Allowances, Standards, and Education

Summary. This joint regulation on nutrition allowances, standards, and education has been revised. It defines the nutrition responsibilities of The Surgeons General of the Army, the Navy, and the Air Force. This regulation—

a. Provides a current statement of the military recommended dietary allowances.

b. Sets nutrient standards for packaged rations.

c. Provides a standardized nutrient density index for normal and re- duced calorie menu planning.

d. Provides nutrition education guidance to assist the military in pro- moting a healthful diet.

Applicability. This regulation applies to all active elements of the Army, Navy, and Air Force. It also applies to the Reserve Components of these Services.

Impact on New Manning System. This regulation does not contain infor- mation that affects the New Manning System.

Supplementation. Supplementation of and exceptions to this regulation are prohibited without prior approval from HQDA (DASG-PSP), WASH DC 20310-2300; Department of the Navy, Naval Medical Command, WASH DC 20732; or HQ USAF/SGB, Bolling AFB, WASH DC 20332-6188, for each respective Service. Nutrient standards prescribed in table 2-3 for opera- tional and restricted rations are not subject to exception.

Interim changes. Interim changes to this regulation are not official unless they are authenticated by The Adjutant General, Headquarters, Department of the Army (HQDA). Users will destroy interim changes on their expira- tion dates unless sooner superseded or rescinded.

Suggested improvements. The Army office of primary interest in this regulation is the Office of The Surgeon General, HQDA. Army users are invited to send comments and suggested improvements on DA Form 2028 (Recommended Changes to Publications and Blank Forms) directly to HQDA (DASG-PSP), WASH DC 20310-2300. Other users may send comments and recommendations through normal channels to their respective Surgeons General: Naval Medical Command, ATTN: MEDCOM-312, Navy Department, WASH DC 20372, for the NAVY; and HQ USAF/SGB, WASH DC 20332-6188, for the Air Force.

Contents

Chapter 1
Introduction

1-1. Purpose
This regulation defines the nutrition responsibilities of The Surgeons General of the Army, Navy, and Air Force by—
  a. Establishing dietary allowances for military feeding.
  b. Prescribing nutrient standards for packaged rations.
  c. Providing, basic guidelines for nutrition education as prescribed in DOD 1338.10-M.

1-2. References
  a. Required Publications.
    (1) DOD Manual 1338.10-M, Manual for the Department of Defense Food Service Program. (Cited in para 1-1.)
    (2) TB MED 507/NAVMED P-5052-5/AFP 160-1, Occupational and Environmental Health: Prevention, Treatment, and Control of Heat Injury. (Cited in para 2-5*i*.)
  b. Related publications. (A related publication is merely a source of additional information. The user does not have to read it to understand this regulation.)
    (1) *Recommended Dietary Allowances*, ninth revised edition, 1980. (Copies may be obtained from the Office of Publications, National Academy of Sciences, 2101 Constitution Avenue, WASH DC 20418.)
    (2) United States Department of Agriculture Handbook 8 Series, *Composition of Foods, Raw, Processed, and Prepared*. (Copies may be obtained from the Superintendent of Documents, US Government Printing Office, WASH DC 20402.)

1-3. Explanation of abbreviations and terms
Abbreviations and special terms used in this regulation are explained in the glossary.

1-4. Responsibilities
  a. The Surgeon General, Department of the Army (TSG, DA). TSG, DA, will act as the Department of Defense (DOD) Executive Agent for Nutrition and will—
    (1) Establish dietary allowances for military personnel subsisting under normal operating conditions.
    (2) Establish nutrient standards for packaged rations.
    (3) Adjust dietary allowances and nutrient standards to meet variations in age, sex, body size, physical activity, climate, or other conditions that may influence nutritional requirements.

(4) Evaluate current and proposed operational rations. Recommend adjustments and other actions to ensure that the nutrient composition of the rations as offered for consumption meets the nutritional requirements of personnel in all operational environments.

(5) Coordinate the development of nutrition education programs for all Services.

(6) Provide qualified representatives to advise committees which support the DOD Food Service Program in matters that affect the nutritional quality of the military diet.

b. The Surgeons General of the Army, Navy, and Air Force. TSGs will—

(1) Review requests and make appropriate recommendations for deviations from established nutritional standards.

(2) Evaluate adjustments to planned diets (menus). Make recommendations to ensure that the nutrient composition of the diet as offered will promote and maintain health.

(3) Evaluate the nutritional status of personnel and report nutritional deficiencies or excesses.

(4) Recommend standard methods to assess body composition.

(5) Provide nutritional guidance to the Services' weight control and physical fitness programs.

(6) Develop and implement a Service-wide nutrition education program for military personnel and their dependents. Provide information to motivate the consumption of a nutritionally adequate diet that contains all of the macronutrients and micronutrients needed to promote health and to maintain desirable body weight.

(7) Assist in providing food service personnel with knowledge and skills of proper food preparation that will maintain the nutritional value of foods.

(8) Provide qualified representatives to—

(a) Advise local food service organizations, such as menu boards, on matters that affect the nutritional quality of meals prepared and consumed.

(b) Serve as consultants to installation commanders on the development and evaluation of nutritional aspects of the Services' weight control and physical fitness programs.

Chapter 2
Nutritional Allowances and Standards

2-1. Military recommended dietary allowances

a. Table 2-1 prescribes military recommended dietary allowances (MRDA) for military personnel. These allowances are adapted from the National Academy of Sciences/National Research Council publication *Recommended Dietary Allowances* (RDA), ninth revised edition, 1980. MRDA are the daily essential nutrient intake levels presently considered to meet the known nutritional needs of practically all 17- to 50-year old, moderately active military personnel.

b. MRDA are intended for use by professional personnel involved in menu planning, dietary evaluation on a population basis, nutrition education, nutrition research, and food research and development. MRDA are based on estimated nutritional requirements. They provide broad dietary guidelines for healthy military personnel.

c. MRDA represent recommended daily nutrient intake levels, which should meet the physiological requirements of nearly all healthy military personnel. The energy allowances shown in table 2-1 represent ranges of caloric intake reflecting wide variations in energy requirements among individuals at similar levels of activity. These energy allowances are designed to maintain desirable body weight for healthy service members under conditions of moderate physical activity in an environment compatible with thermal comfort. The allowances are not to be interpreted as individual requirements. Also, they may not apply to personnel requiring special dietary treatment for conditions such as infection, chronic disease, trauma, unusual stress, pregnancy, lactation, or weight reduction. The allowances are subject to adjustments as outlined in paragraphs 2-3 and 2-4.

d. MRDA refer to the nutrient concentrations of edible portions of food offered for consumption. Nutrient losses may occur during food processing and preparation. These nutrient losses must be considered when nutrient composition tables are used to compare menus or food products with these allowances. The most recent edition of the United States Department of Agriculture Handbook 8 series, *Composition of Foods, Raw, Processed, and Prepared,* will be used as the standard reference nutrient composition data base.

2-2. Estimated safe and adequate daily dietary intakes

Table 2-2 is based on the RDA and provides estimated safe and adequate adult dietary intake ranges for selected nutrients, which are known to be essential in the diet, but for which recommended levels of intake have not been established.

2-3. Nutrient standards for operational and restricted rations

Table 2-3 prescribes nutrient standards, which are the criteria for evaluating the nutritional adequacy of operational and restricted rations. Operational rations include the individual combat ration such as the meal, combat, individual (MCI); the meal, ready-to-eat (MRE); and other rations (A, B, or T) used to support operations in the field. A level of 3600 kilocalories (kcal) is required for operational rations to meet energy demands associated with extended field operations. (See para 2-4.) Total fat calories should not exceed 40 percent of the energy value of the operational ration or 160 grams (gm). It is essential that ration planners compensate for losses of nutrients, such as ascorbic acid, thiamin, riboflavin, niacin, and pyridoxine (vitamin B6), which may occur during storage of operational and restricted rations.

a. Nutritionally complete, individual operational rations such as the MCI and MRE must be formulated so that the nutrient content of each day's ration satisfies these nutrient standards. It is desirable that each combat meal provides one-third of the nutrient standard.

b. Under certain operational scenarios such as long-range patrol, assault and reconnaissance, and other situations where resupply is unavailable, it may be necessary for troops to subsist for periods (up to 10 days) on a restricted ration. To minimize loss of performance, the restricted ration should provide 1100 to 1500 kilocalories, 50 to 70 grams of protein, and a minimum of 100 grams of carbohydrate on a daily basis. Vitamins and minerals should be provided at the levels prescribed in table 2-3. This restricted ration is not appropriate for use under extreme, cold climates.

c. The survival food packet is a packaged food bar of approximately 400 kilocalories derived from carbohydrates. The low protein content spares body water by reducing the obligatory water demand caused by consuming high protein foods. The nutrient standards for operational and restricted rations do not apply to the survival food packet. This packet is designed to be consumed for periods of less than 4 consecutive days.

2-4. Energy requirements

The following factors affect individual energy requirements:

a. Age. MRDA are intended for men and women 17 to 50 years of age. Upon completion of growth, energy requirements for adults gradually decline with age due to a reduced resting metabolic rate and curtailment in physical activity. Within the 17 to 50 year military age range, age-related differences in caloric allowances appear to be minimal under conditions of similar physical activity.

b. Body size. The energy allowances are established for average sized personnel, which represent approximately 70 percent of the military personnel between the ages of 17 and 50 years. (See table 2-1.) To maintain desirable body weight, caloric intake must be adjusted for variable energy requirements due to individual differences in lean body mass reflected by body size. Large individuals (such as those with greater height and appropriately higher weight) have slightly higher resting, basal metabolic rates. They, therefore, require more total energy per unit of time for activities that involve moving body mass over distance. Smaller sized individuals require fewer calories.

  c. Physical activity. Differences in energy needs are largely due to differences in the amount of time an individual performs moderate and heavy work tasks in contrast to light or sedentary activities. MRDA for energy in table 2-1 are for military personnel who are moderately active and living in a temperate climate or in a thermally neutral environment. Total energy requirements are influenced by the intensity and duration of physical activity. For example, a day of moderate physical activity may include 8 hours of sleeping, 12 hours of light activity, and 4 hours of moderate to heavy activity. For military personnel doing heavy work or involved in prolonged, vigorous physical training, the recommended caloric allowance should be increased by at least 25 percent (approximately 500 to 900 kilocalories).

  d. Climate. MRDA for energy intake are established for personnel in a temperate climate. (See table 2-1.) When there is prolonged exposure to cold or heat, energy allowances may need adjustment.

  (1) *Cold environment.* In a cold environment (mean temperature less than 14 °C (57.2 °F), the energy cost of work for garrison troops is approximately 5 percent greater than in a warmer environment. There is an additional 2 to 5 percent increase in energy expenditure associated with carrying the extra weight of heavy, cold weather clothing and footgear (the "hobbling" effect). Garrison personnel may require an extra 150 to 350 kilocalories per day under these conditions. Energy allowances of 4500 calories for men and 3500 calories for women are required to support adequately clothed troops maneuvering for prolonged periods (several hours) with heavy gear on foot, snowshoes, and skis over snow- or ice-covered terrain. This increased energy allowance does not apply to troops stationed in cold climates who are engaged in moderate activity within a garrison setting.

  (2) *Hot environment.* In a hot climate, loss of appetite may cause a voluntary but undesirable reduction in caloric intake below the level of need. This loss of appetite may be most noticeable after troops have arrived in a hot environment and before the process of acclimatization is completed. When personnel are required to perform the same amount of work in a hot environment as in a temperate environment, the caloric expenditure will be increased. Little adjustment appears to be necessary for a change in environmental temperature between 20 °C (68 °F) and 30 °C (86 °F). It is desirable under conditions of moderate physical activity to increase the caloric allowance by at least 0.7 percent for every degree centigrade rise in

average ambient temperature above 30 °C (86 °F). Daily energy requirements under extremely hot conditions (greater than 40 °C (104 °F), may reach 56 kcal/kilogram (kg) of body weight.

(3) *Nuclear, biochemical, and chemical environment.* Certain conditions will require special guidance and nutrient formulation not described in this regulation. One such condition is when troops are operating in contaminated environments for more than 6 hours while wearing protective clothing.

2-5. Nutrient discussion

a. Protein. MRDA for protein are based, in part, on an estimated nutritional requirement of 0.8 gm/day/kg of body weight. (See table 2-1.) For military personnel within the reference weight range, protein recommendations are set between 48 to 63 gm/ day, for males and 37 to 50 gm/day for females. These computed protein levels have been further increased to 100 gm/day for male and 80 gm/day for female personnel. This increase reflects usual intake patterns and helps to maintain a high level of palatability and food acceptance among military personnel. These allowances are based on the consumption of a diet containing mixed proteins of animal and vegetable origin. A total day's protein intake of more than 100 gm/day has not been shown to improve heavy physical performance.

b. Fat. Fats are important in the diet to furnish energy, provide essential fatty acids, transport fat soluble vitamins and aid in their absorption, increase palatability, and give meal satisfaction. It is becoming increasingly clear that excessive amounts to total fat may lead to an increased risk of coronary heart and vascular disease. For this reason, it is recommended that the calories derived from total dietary fat should not exceed 35 percent under garrison feeding conditions. Higher proportions of fat calories are acceptable in combat, arctic, or other operational rations to increase caloric density. Emphasis should be placed on planning the military menu with lower fat concentrations while maintaining acceptability. A reduction of fat calories in the diet can be achieved by lowering added fats during food preparation and replacing foods high in fat with lean meats, fish, poultry, low fat milk, and other low fat dairy products in the military menu. As fat calories are reduced in the diet, it is recommended that the current level of about 7 percent of caloric intake as polyunsaturated fat be maintained to ensure an adequate intake of essential fatty acids.

c. Carbohydrate. Carbohydrates should contribute approximately 50 to 55 percent of the total dietary energy. It is recommended that simple, refined, and other processed sugars provide only about 10 percent of total dietary energy. The remaining carbohydrate calories should come from complex carbohydrates such as starches and naturally occurring sugars found in fruits, vegetables, and milk.

d. Calcium and phosphorus. MRDA are the same for both calcium (Ca) and phosphorus (P), although a wide variation in the Ca:P ratio is tolerated. In the presence of adequate vitamin D nutriture, a ratio of between 1:1 to 1.5:1 is nutritionally desirable.

e. Iron, ascorbic acid, and animal protein. The absorption of iron, a nutrient involved in maintaining optimal aerobic fitness, can be significantly affected by the composition of foods in a particular meal. Heme iron from animal protein sources is better absorbed (approximately 23 percent) than nonheme iron (approximately 3 to 8 percent) which is found in both animal and in many plant food sources. Certain cereal and legume proteins are known to reduce the bioavailability of nonheme iron. The nonheme iron absorption rate can be more than doubled when nonheme iron is consumed with a modest serving of meat, fish, poultry, or a source of ascorbic acid (vitamin C) at the same meal. The dietary iron allowance for females and 17- to 18-year old males is 18 milligrams (mg)/day, or 7.5 and 5.6 mg/1000 calories respectively. Moderately active female personnel consuming an average of 2400 calories per day may require supplemental iron to meet the recommended 18 mg/day. Issuing supplemental iron should be done on an individualized basis after a medical evaluation.

f. Iodine. Wide variation occurs in the amount of iodine present in food and water. All table and cooking salt used should be iodized to ensure an adequate intake of 150 micrograms (mcg) of iodine per day.

g. Fluoride. Fluoride is an essential nutrient which is found in the enamel of teeth and bone. This nutrient is an important factor in preventing tooth decay. Fluoride may confer some protection against certain degenerative bone diseases. Fluoride is found in varying amounts in most foods and water supplies. Maintaining a fluoride concentration of about 1 mg/liter (1 part per million) in water supplies has proven to be safe, economical, and efficient in reducing the incidence of dental caries.

h. Sodium. Sodium is the principal cation involved in maintaining osmotic equilibrium and extracellular fluid volume in the body.

(1) Under conditions of normal ambient temperature and humidity, the healthy adult can maintain sodium balance with an intake of as little as 150 mg/day (381 milligrams of salt). While daily intake below 2000 milligrams of sodium are generally considered upalatable, 3300 milligrams of sodium/day represents a lower acceptable limit to which the American population can adapt. The average young civilian male consumes approximately 5500 milligrams of sodium/day in food plus an additional 20 percent (1000 milligrams) as added salt. Although dietary levels of sodium for the military population are unknown, the average intake may well exceed the civilian level. The goal for the sodium content in foods as served within military dining facilities is 1700 milligrams of sodium/1000 kcal. (See table 3-1.)

(2) Hard physical work in a high ambient temperature greatly increases the amount of sodium lost in sweat. Sodium losses may reach levels as high as 8000 mg/day (20 grams of salt). Whenever more than 3 liters of water per day are required to replace sweat losses, extra salt intake may be required. The need for extra salt depends on the severity of sweat losses and the degree of acclimatization. Sodium should be replaced through food in both nondiscretionary form and as added salt.

i. Water. As caloric requirements are increased, water needs are also increased. During periods of light to moderate activity in a temperate climate, 1 milliliter of water per calorie expended is a reasonable intake goal. Water requirements may increase from 50 to 100 percent for personnel living in a hot climate expending similar energy levels. Water requirements may increase threefold above normal under conditions of heavy work in a hot environment. Even in cold climates sweat rates and, consequently, water needs may be quite high due to the hot microclimate that can develop under insulated clothing during heavy physical activity. Inadequate water intakes can be accompanied by a disturbance in electrolyte balance with a resultant performance decrement. (See TB MED 507/NAVMED P-5052-5/AFP 160-1.) Under conditions of normal dietary intake, the preferred fluid to replace losses is cool water. Electrolyte- and sugar-containing solutions are not necessary since glucose and electrolytes are adequately replenished in the normal diet. Under certain conditions, electrolyte and sugar solutions may actually impair rather than enhance performance.

TABLE 2-1 MRDA for selected nutrients[1]

Nutrient	Unit	Male	Female
Energy[2,3]	Kcal MJ	3200(2800-3600) 13.4(11.7-15.1)	2400(2000-2800 10.0(8.4-11.7)
Protein[4]	gm	100	80
Vitamin A[5]	mcg RE	1000	800
Vitamin D[6,7]	mcg	5-10	5-10
Vitamin E[8]	mg TE	10	8
Ascorbic Acid	mg	60	60
Thiamin (B_1)	mg	1.6	1.2
Riboflavin (B_2)	mg	1.9	1.4
Niacin[9]	mg NE	21	16
Vitamin B_6	mg	2.2	2.0
Folacin	mcg	400	400
Vitamin B_{12}	mcg	3.0	3.0
Calcium[7]	mg	800-1200	800-1200
Phosphorus[7]	mg	800-1200	800-1200
Magnesium[7]	mg	350-400	300
Iron[7]	mg	10-18	18
Zinc	mg	15	15
Iodine	mcg	150	150
Sodium	mg	See note[10]	See note[10]

[1]MRDA for moderately active military personnel, ages 17 to 50 years, are based on the *Recommended Dietary Allowances*, ninth revised edition, 1980.

[2]Energy allowance ranges are estimated to reflect the requirements of 70 percent of the moderately active military population. One megajoule (MJ) equals 239 kcals.

[3]Dietary fat calories should not contribute more than 35 percent of total energy intake.

[4]Protein allowance is vased on an estimated protein requirement of 0.8 gm/kilograms (kg) desirable body weight. Using the reference body weight ranges for males of 60 to 79 kilograms and for females of 46 to 63 kilograms, the protein requirement is approximately 48 to 64 grams for males and 37 to 51 grams for females. These amounts have been approximately doubled to reflect the usual protein consumption levels of Americans and to enhance diet acceptability.

[5]One microgram of retinol equivalent (mcg RE) equals 1 microgram of retinol, or 6 micrograms betacarotene, or 5 international units (IU)

TABLE 2-1 *Continued*

[6]As cholecalcifero, 10 micrograms of cholecalcifero equals 400 IU of vitamin D.

[7]High values reflect greater vitamin D, calcium, phosphorus, magnesium, and iron requirements for 17- to 18-year olds than for older ages.

[8]One milligram of alpha-tocopherol equivalent (mg TE) equals 1 milligram d-alpha-tocopherol.

[9]One milligram of niacin equivalent (mg NE) equals 1 milligram niacin or 60 milligrams dietary tryptophan.

[10]The safe and adequate levels for daily sodium intake of 1100 to 3300 mg published in the RDA are currently impractical and unattainable within military food service systems. However, an average of 1700 milligrams of sodium per 100 kilocalories of food served is the target for military food service systems. This level equates to a daily sodium intake of approximately 5500 milligrams for males and 4100 milligrams for females.

TABLE 2-2 Estimated safe and adequate daily dietary intake ranges of selected vitamins and minerals[1]

Nutrition	Unit	Amount
Vitamins		
Vitamins K	mcg	70-140
Biotin	mcg	100-200
Pantothenic Acid	mg	4-7
Trace Elements[2]		
Fluoride	mg	1.5-4.0
Selenium	mcg	50-200
Molybdenum	mg	0.15-0.50
Copper	mg	2-3
Manganese	mg	2.5-5.0
Chromium	mcg	50-200
Electrolytes		
Potassium	mg	1875-5625
Chloride	mg	1700-5100

[1]This table is based on the Recommended Dietary Allowances, ninth edition, 1980, table 10, "Estimated Safe and Adequate Daily Dietary Intakes of Selected Vitamins and Minerals." Estimated ranges are provided for these nutrients because sufficient information upon which to set a recommended allowance is not available. Values reflect a range of recommended intake over an extended period of time.

[2]Since toxic levels for many trace elements may only be several times the usual intakes, the upper levels for the trace elements given in this table should not be habitually exceeded.

TABLE 2-3 Nutritional standards for operational and restricted rations

Nutrient	Unit[1]	Operational rations	Restricted rations[2,4]
Energy	Kcal	3600	1100-1500
Protein	gm	100	50-70
Carbohydrate	gm	440	100-200
Fat	gm	160 (maximum)	50-70
Vitamin A	mcg RE	1000	500
Vitamin D	mcg	10	5
Vitamin E	mg TE	10	5
Ascorbic Acid	mg	60	30
Thiamin	mg	1.8	1.0
Riboflavin	mg	2.2	1.2
Niacin	mg NE	24	13
Vitamin B_6	mg	2.2	1.2
Folacin	mcg	400	200
Vitamin B_{12}	mcg	3	1.5
Calcium	mg	800	400
Phosphorus	mg	800	400
Magnesium	mg	800	400
Iron	mg	18	9
Zinc	mg	15	7.5
Sodium	mg	5000-7000[5]	2500-3500[5]
Potassium	mg	1875-5625	950-2800

[1]See notes in table 2-1 for explanation of units.

[2]Values are minimum standards at the time of consumption unless shown as a range or a maximum level.

[3]The operational ration includes the MCI, MRE, A, B, and T rations.

[4]Restricted rations are for use under certain operational scenarios such as long-range patrol, assault, and reconnaissance when troops are required to subsist for short periods (up to 10 days) on an energy restricted ration.

[5]These values do not include salt packets.

Chapter 3
Military Menu Guidance

3-1. Nutrient density index

a. Table 3-1 lists selected nutrients from the MRDA (table 2-1) for which adequate food composition data are presently available on a nutrient density basis. A nutrient density index (NDI) is provided for both the general military diet and for the reduced calorie menu. (See para 3-2.) The NDI is a technique for evaluating the nutritional adequacy of individual foods, recipes, meals, and cycle menus.

b. The nutrient concentrations per 1000 calories in table 3-1 are based on the recommended calorie intake for healthy male and female personnel at moderate levels of activity. A single nutrient value is recommended for both sexes to simplify use. Because of lower caloric requirements for women, the NDI is generally higher for the female than for the male. Female nutrient values have been adopted for most nutrient densities except for iron and sodium.

c. The computed iron density represents an interpolation between the male and female MRDA for iron. Six milligrams of iron per 1000 calories is considered reasonable and consistent with the amounts of iron found in the usual food supply. This iron density may be inadequate for women. (See para 2-5*e.*)

d. The NDI for sodium is a target to be achieved in foods as served in military dining facilities.

e. The lower female MRDA for calcium and phosphorus were used to compute the NDI for calcium and phosphorus.

f. Personnel subsisting on a 1500-calorie meal plan require a diet that is nutritionally more dense. Guidance for this type of diet is in the column headed "Reduced calorie menu amount" in table 3-1.

g. It is emphasized that the purpose of representing the MRDA in terms of nutrient densities is for menu evaluation, not for calculating nutrient requirements.

h. The NDI may serve as an important basic tool for nutrition education within the military.

3-2. Reduced calorie menu (1500 kcal)

In support of the military physical fitness and weight control programs, each military dining facility will offer a nutritionally adequate reduced menu (1500 to 1600 kcal/day). Each meal should contain approximately 500 kilocalories except when serving line constraints or unique mission requirements make this impractical. The specified NDI for the reduced calorie menu in table 3-1 provides guidance for reviewing the nutritional quality of the menu. The calories derived from total dietary fat should not exceed 35 percent in the reduced calorie menu. Implementation procedures and exceptions to policy for a reduced calorie menu will be prescribed by each military service.

TABLE 3-1 Nutrient density index per 1000 calories for menu planning

Nutrient	Unit	Military diet amount	Reduced calorie menu amount
Protein	gm	33	53
Vitamin A	mcg RE	333	533
Ascorbic Acid	mg	25	40
Thiamin (B_1)	mg	0.5	0.7[1]
Riboflavin (B_2)	mg	0.6	0.8[2]
Niacin	mg	6.7	8.7[3]
Calcium	mg	333	533
Phosphorus	mg	333	533
Magnesium	mg	125	200
Iron	mg	6.0[4]	6.0[4]
Sodium	mg	1700	1700

[1]NDI for thiamin is based on a minimum recommended allowance of 1.0 mg/day.

[2]NDI for riboflavin is based on a minimum recommended allowance of 1.2 mg/day.

[3]NDI for niacin is based on a minimum recommended allowance of 13.0 mg/day.

[4]Iron supplementation is recommended for female personnel subsisting on a 1500 kilocalories diet. Levels higher than 6 mg/1000 calories are difficult to attain in a conventional US diet.

Chapter 4
Nutrition Education

4-1. Introduction
The following statements about a healthful diet are suggested guidelines to promote optimal fitness in the general military population. Each of the military services should incorporate these guidelines in their nutritional education programs. These statements should guide modification in food procurement policy, food preparation, recipe formulation, and menu development.

4-2. General guidelines for a healthful diet
a. Eat a wide variety of nutritious foods. A well-balanced diet must provide about 50 nutrients, including essential amino acids, carbohydrates, essential fatty acids, vitamins, minerals, water, and dietary fiber. No single food item supplies all the essential nutrients in the amounts required by the body. The greater the variety of foods consumed, the less likely is the chance of developing either a deficiency or an excess of any nutrient. Selection of a diet from a variety of food groups ensures a well-balanced intake of the numerous macronutrients and micronutrients. These groups include—
    (1) Whole grains, enriched cereals, and breads.
    (2) Fruits and vegetables.
    (3) Dry peas and beans.
    (4) Meats, poultry, fish, and eggs.
    (5) Dairy products.
    b. Maintain ideal body weight. Personnel should strive to maintain ideal body weight by consuming only as much energy as is expended. To lose weight, calorie intake should be reduced by decreasing total food intake, especially fats, oils, sugars, and alcohol. Also, physical activity should be increased.
    c. Avoid excessive dietary fat. Consumption of fats and oils should be limited during weight reduction and weight maintenance because fats and oils have a high energy density. Military personnel who are identified as being "at risk" of heart disease should reduce saturated fats and cholesterol in their diet and proportionately increase their intake of polyunsaturated fats.
    d. Eat foods with adequate starch and fiber. Complex carbohydrates should be increased to make up any calorie deficit due to reduction of fat and refined sugar calories. Emphasis should be placed on fiber-rich foods such as whole grain products, vegetables, and mature legumes.
    e. Avoid too much sugar. The major health hazard from eating too much sugar is dental caries. Also, excessive intake of refined sugars may displace other foods that are important sources of essential nutrients.

f. Avoid too much salt. Under normal conditions, an adequate but safe daily intake ranges from 3 to 8 grams (.105 to .28 ounce) of salt (1100 to 3300 milligrams of sodium). Regular consumption of highly salted foods may result in excessive sodium intake. Personnel who are "at risk" of high blood pressure should avoid highly salted foods.

g. Avoid excessive alcohol consumption. Alcoholic beverages have a low nutrient density (that is, they are high in calories and low in other nutrients). Alcoholic beverages can displace valuable nutrient-rich foods in the diet. Impulsive alcohol consumption may lead to acute ethanol toxicity. Sustained, excessive alcohol consumption alters the way nutrients are utilized in the body and may contribute to liver disease and neurological disorders.

GLOSSARY

Section I
Abbreviations

Ca	calcium
DA	Department of the Army
DOD	Department of Defense
gm	gram (1 gm = .035 ounce)
IU	international unit
HQDA	Headquarters, Department of the Army
kcal	kilocalorie
kg	kilogram (2.2 pounds)
lb	pound
mcg	microgram (.000000035 ounce)
mg	milligram (.000035 ounce)
MCI	meal, combat, individual
MJ	megajoule (239 kilocalories)
MRDA	military recommended dietary allowances
MRE	meal, ready-to-eat
NDI	nutrient density index
NE	niacin equivalent
oz	ounce (28.571428 grams)
P	phosphorus
RDA	recommended dietary allowance
RE	retinol equivalent
TSG	The Surgeon General
TE	alpha-tocopherol equivalent

Section II
Terms

Kilocalorie

Energy provided to the body in the form of kilocalories—commonly called calories. One kcal is defined as the amount of heat necessary to raise 1 kg (liter) of water from 15 °C to 16 °C (59 °F to 60.8 °F). The joule is the accepted international unit of energy. To convert kcal to joules multiply by the factor of 4.2. (Example: 9 kcals = 37.8 joules.)

Macronutrients

Nutrients essential for human nutrition in relatively large amounts; examples are carbohydrates, protein, calcium, phosphorus, and sodium.

Micronutrients
Nutrients essential for human nutrition in relatively small amounts; examples are the vitamins, iron, zinc, and copper.

Operational ration
A specialty designed ration normally composed of nonperishable items for use under actual or simulated combat conditions. This ration is used in peacetime for emergencies or contingencies, travel, and training.

Ration
The allowance of food for the subsistence of one person for 1 day.

Reference body weight range
A body weight range that covers the average weight for male (60 to 79 kg (132 to 173 lb)) and female (46 to 63 kg (101.2 to 138.6 lb)) military personnel based on average height data. This range is used in this regulation to estimate protein requirements which are computed on a per kilogram body weight basis.

Restricted ration
A light weight, operational ration requiring no further preparation, providing suboptimal levels of energy and nutrients, and intended for short-range patrols.

By Order of the Secretaries of the Army, the Navy, and the Air Force:

JOHN A. WICKHAM, JR
General, United States Army
Chief of Staff

Official:
DONALD J. DELANDRO
Brigadier General, United States Army
The Adjutant General

W. M. McDERMOTT, JR.
Rear Admiral, MC, United States Navy
Commander, Naval Medical Command

CHARLES A. GABRIEL
General, United States Air Force
Chief of Staff

Official:
JAMES H. DELANEY
Colonel, United States Air Force
Director of Administration

Distribution:

Army:
Active Army, ARNG, USAR: To be distributed in accordance with DA Form 12-9A, requirements for AR, Medical Services: Applicable to all Army elements—B.

Navy/Marine Corps:
Ships and stations having Medical Personnel; NAVSUP—CO, NAVFSSO (20); MARCORPS CODE IV plus 7000163 (10). Stocked: CO, NAVPUBFORMCEN, 5801 Tabor Ave., Philadelphia, PA 19120.

Air Force: F.

---

*U.S. GOVERNMENT PRINTING OFFICE: 1985-461-029:10199

B

Nutritional Needs in Hot Environments— A Selected Bibliography

On the following pages is a selection of references dealing with nutritional requirements in hot environments. This bibliography was compiled from the joint reference lists of the 15 chapters in this report, selected references from a computer-based literature search conducted in 1991, and references recommended by the invited speakers as background reading for the workshop participants. As a result, references that are historical in nature are included in this listing with the most current studies of nutrition in the heat.

Adlerkreutz, H., K. Kosunen, K. Kuoppasalmi, A. Pakarinen, and S. Karonen
   1977   Plasma hormones during exposure to intense heat. Proc. Cong. Int. Med. 13:346-355.
Adolph, E.F., and associates
   1947   Physiology of Man in the Desert. New York: Interscience Publishers.
Agricultural Research Service (ARS)
   1972   Food Consumption of Households in the U.S., Seasons and Year 1965-66. Report no. 12, MC 7473(72). Washington, D.C.: U.S. Government Printing Office. March.
Aldashev, A.A., B.I. Kim, O.A. Kolesova, V.L. Reznik, and V.V. Subach
   1986   Indices of the nutritional status of workers in the oil and gas production industry adapting to the extreme conditions of an arid zone. (in Russian) Vopr. Pitan. May-June (3):25-28.

Allan, J.R., and C.G. Wilson
1971   Influence of acclimatization on sweat sodium concentration. J. Appl. Physiol. 30:708-712.
Anderson, R.A., M.M. Polansky, and N.A. Bryden
1984   Strenuous running: Acute effects on chromium, copper, zinc and selected variables in urine and serum of male runners. Biol. Trace Elem. Res. 6:327-336.
Anderson, R.A., N.A. Bryden, M.M. Polansky, and P.A. Deuster
1988   Exercise effects on chromium excretion of trained and untrained men consuming a constant diet. J. Appl. Physiol. 64:249-252.
Andersson, B., and B. Larsson
1961   Influence of local temperature changes in the preoptic area and rostral hypothalamus on the regulation of food and water intake. Acta Physiol. Scand. 52:75-89.
Andron, R.I.
1991   Gastrointestinal bleeding in runners. Ann. Intern. Med. 114(5):429.
Anonymous
1953   Background of symposium on nutrition under climatic stress. (Reprinted from Activities Report, 5(2):1-12. Published by The Research and Development Associates, Food and Container Institute, Inc.)
Armstrong, L.E., and K.B. Pandolf
1988   Physical training, cardiorespiratory physical fitness and exercise-heat tolerance. Pp. 199-226 in Human Performance Physiology and Environmental Medicine at Terrestrial Extremes, K.B. Pandolf, M.N. Sawka, and R.R. Gonzalez, eds. Indianapolis, Ind.: Benchmark Press.
Armstrong, L.E., D.L. Costill, W.J. Fink, M. Hargreaves, I. Nishibata, D. Bassett, and D.S. King
1985a   Effects of dietary sodium on body and muscle potassium content during heat acclimation. Eur. J. Appl. Physiol. 54:391-397.
Armstrong, L.E., R.W. Hubbard, P.C. Szlyk, W.T. Matthew, and I.V. Sils
1985b   Voluntary dehydration and electrolyte losses during prolonged exercise in the heat. Aviat. Space Environ. Med. 56:765-70
Armstrong, L.E., D.L. Costill, and W.J. Fink
1985c   Influence of dehydration on competitive running performance. Med. Sci. Sports Exerc. 17:456-461.
Armstrong, L.E., R.W. Hubbard, B.H. Jones, and J.T. Daniels
1986   Preparing Alberto Salazar for the heat of the 1984 Olympic Marathon. Physician Sportsmed. 14(3):73-81.
Armstrong, L.E., D.L. Costill, and W.J. Fink
1987   Changes in body water and electrolytes during heat acclimation: Effects of dietary sodium. Aviat. Space Environ. Med. 58:143-148.
Armstrong, L.E., R.W. Hubbard, W.J. Kraemer, J.P. DeLuca, and E.L. Christensen
1987   Signs and symptoms of heat exhaustion during strenuous exercise. Ann. Sports Med. 3:182-189.
Armstrong, L.E., J.P. De Luca, E.L. Christensen, and R.W. Hubbard
1990   Mass-to-surface area index in a large cohort. Am. J. Phys. Anthropol. 83:321-329.

Aruoma, O.I., T. Reilly, D. MacLaren, and B. Halliwell
 1988   Iron, copper and zinc concentrations in human sweat and plasma; the effect of exercise. Clin. Chim. Acta 177:81-88.
Ashworth, A., and A.D.B. Harrower
 1967   Protein requirements in tropical countries: Nitrogen losses in sweat and their relation to nitrogen balance. Br. J. Nutr. 21(4):833-843.
Avellini, B.A., E. Kamon, and J.T. Krajewski
 1980   Physiological responses of physically fit men and women to acclimation to humid heat. J. Appl. Physiol. Respirat. Environ. Exercise Physiol. 49(2):254-261.
Balaban, E.P., J.V. Cox, P. Snell, R.H. Vaugh, and E.P. Frenkel
 1989   The frequency of anemia and iron deficiency in the runner. Med. Sci. Sports Exerc. 21:643-648.
Banderet, L.E., and H.R. Lieberman
 1989   Treatment with tyrosine, a neurotransmitter precursor, reduces environmental stress in humans. Brain Res. Bull. 22:759-762.
Barclay, G.R., and L.A. Turnberg
 1988   Effect of moderate exercise on salt and water transport in the human jejunum. Gut 29:816-820.
Bartoshuk, L.M., K. Rennert, H. Rodin, and J.C. Stevens
 1982   Effects of temperature on the perceived sweetness of sucrose. Physiol. Behav. 28:905-910.
Baska, R.S., F.M. Moses, and P.A. Deuste
 1990   Cimetidine reduces running-associated gastrointestinal bleeding. Dig. Dis. Sci. 35(8):956-960.
Bass, D.E., C.R. Kleeman, M. Quinn, A. Henschel, and A.H. Hegnauer
 1955   Mechanisms of acclimatization to heat in man. Med. Anal. Rev. 34:323-380.
Bean, W.B., and L.W. Eichna
 1943   Performance in relation to environmental temperature. Reactions of normal young men to a simulated desert environment. Fed. Proc. 2:144-158.
Beighton, P.
 1971   Fluid balance in the Sahara. Nature 223(317):275-277.
Beisel, W.R., R.F. Goldman, and R.J.T. Joy
 1968   Metabolic balance studies during induced hyperthermia in man. J. Appl. Physiol. 24(1):1-10.
Beller, G.A., J.T. Maher, L.H. Hartley, D.E. Bass, and W.E.C. Wacker
 1975   Changes in serum and sweat magnesium levels during work in the heat. Aviat. Space Environ. Med. 46:709-712.
Bonner, R.M., M.H. Harrison, C.J. Hall, and R.J. Edwards
 1976   Effect of heat acclimatization on intravascular responses to acute heat stress in man. J. Appl. Physiol. 41:708-713.
Booth, G., and J.M. Strang
 1936   Changes in temperature of the skin following the ingestion of food. Arch. Int. Med. 57:533-543.

Brandenberger, G., V. Candas, M. Follenius, J. Libert, and J. Kahn
   1986   Vascular fluid shifts and endocrine responses to exercise in the heat:
          Effects of rehydration. Eur. J. Appl. Physiol. 55:123-129.
Brebner, D.F., and D.M. Kerslake
   1964   The time course of the decline in sweating produced by wetting the skin.
          J. Physiol. (Lond.) 175:295-302.
Brobeck, J.R.
   1948   Food intake as a mechanism of temperature regulation. Yale J. Biol.
          Med. 20:545-552.
Brouha, L., P.E. Smith, Jr., R. De Lanne, and M.E. Maxfield
   1960   Physiological reactions of men and women during muscular activity and
          recovery in various environments. J. Appl. Physiol. 16:133-140.
Brouns, F., W.H.M. Saris, and N.J. Rehrer
   1987   Abdominal complaints and gastrointestinal function during long-lasting
          exercise. Int. J. Sports Med. 8:175-189.
Brown, N.E., M.M. McKinley, L.E. Baltzer, and C.F. Opurum
   1985   Temperature preferences for a single entree. J. Am. Diet. Assoc. 85:1339-
          1341.
Brune, M., B. Magnusson, H. Persson, and L. Hallberg
   1986   Iron losses in sweat. Am. J. Clin. Nutr. 43:438-443.
Burch, G.E., and N.P. DePasquale
   1962   Hot Climates, Man and His Heart. Springfield, Ill.: Charles C. Thomas.
Burse, R.L.
   1979   Sex differences in human thermoregulatory response to heat and cold
          stress. Hum. Factors 21:687-699.
Buskirk, E.R.
   1951   The Effect of Heat on Nutrient Requirements: Animal Experiments. Ex-
          cerpt from: H.H. Mitchell and M. Edman Chapter III Diet in a Hot Envi-
          ronment. Pp. 42-95 in Nutrition and Climatic Stress. Springfield, Ill.:
          Charles C. Thomas.
   1981   Some nutritional considerations in the conditioning of athletes. Ann. Rev.
          Nutr. 1:319-350.
Buskirk, E.R., and D.E. Bass
   1957   Climate and Exercise. Technical Report EP-61, U.S. Army Quartermaster
          Research and Development Center, Natick, Mass.
Buskirk, E.R., P.F. Iampietro, and B.E. Welch
   1957   Variations in resting metabolism with changes in food, exercise and cli-
          mate. Metabolism 6:144-153.
Calvino, A.M.
   1986   Perception of sweetness: The effects of concentration and temperature.
          Physiol. Behav. 36:1021-1028.
Chen, J.D., Z.Y. Yang, S.H. Ma, and Y.C. Zhen
   1990   The effects of *Actinidia sinensis* Planch (kiwi) drink supplementation on
          athletes training in hot environments. J. Sports Med. Phys. Fitness 30:181-
          184.

Clarkson, P.M.
    1991   Vitamins and trace minerals. Pp. 123-175 in Ergogenics: Enhancement of
            Performance in Exercise and Sport. Vol. 4 of Perspectives in Exercise
            Science and Sports Medicine. Indianapolis, Ind.: Benchmark Press.
Cleland, T.S., S.M. Horvath, and M. Phillips
    1969   Acclimatization of women to heat after training. Int. Z. Angew. Physiol.
            27:15-24.
Collier, G.
    1989   The economics of hunger, thirst, satiety and regulation. Pp. 136-154 in
            The Psychology of Human Eating Disorders: Preclinical and Clinical Per-
            spectives. New York: Vol. 575 of the Annals of the New York Academy
            of Sciences.
Collins, K.J., and J.S. Weiner
    1962   Observations on arm-bag suppression of sweating and its relationship to
            thermal sweat-gland fatigue. J. Physiol. (Lond.) 161:538-556.
    1968   Endocrinological aspects of exposure to high environmental temperature.
            Physiol. Rev. 48:785-839.
Collins, K.J., T.P Eddy, A. Hibbs, A.L. Stock, and E.F. Wheeler
    1971   Nutritional and environmental studies on an ocean-going oil tanker. 2.
            Heat acclimatization and nutrient balances. Br. J. Indu. Med. 28(3):246-
            258.
Conn, J.W.
    1949   Acclimatization to heat. Adv. Int. Med. 3:337.
    1963   Aldosteronism in man: Some clinical and climatological aspects. Part 1.
            J. Am. Med. Assoc. 183:775-781.
Consolazio, C.F.
    1963   The energy requirements of men living under extreme environmental con-
            ditions. 3. Extremely hot environments. Pp. 65-77 in World Review of
            Nutrition and Dietetics. vol. 27, G.H. Bourne, ed. New York: Hafner
            Publishing.
    1966   Nutrient requirements of troops in extreme environments. Army Research
            and Development Newsmagazine 11:24-27.
Consolazio, C.F., and R. Shapiro
    1964   Energy requirements of men in extreme heat. Pp. 121-124 in Environ-
            mental Physiology and Psychology in Arid Conditions: Proceedings of
            the Lucknow Symposium. Liège, Belgium: United Nations.
Consolazio, C.F., F. Konishi, R.V. Ciccolini, J.M. Jamison, E.J. Sheehan, and
            W.F. Steffen
    1960   Food consumption of military personnel performing light activities in a
            hot desert environment. Metabol. 9(5):435-442.
Consolazio, C.F., R. Shapiro, J.E. Masterson, and P.S.L. McKinzie
    1960   Caloric Requirements of Men Working in an Extremely Hot Desert Envi-
            ronment. Report No. 246. Denver, Colo.: United States Army Medical
            Research and Nutrition Laboratory.
    1961   Energy requirements of men in extreme heat. J. Nutri. 73:126-134.

Consolazio, C.F., Le Roy O. Matoush, R.A. Nelson, R.S. Harding, and J.E. Canham
  1963   Excretion of sodium, potassium, magnesium and iron in human sweat and the relation of each to balance and requirements. J. Nutr. 79:407-415.
Consolazio, C.F., Le Roy O. Matoush, R.A. Nelson, and G.A. Leveille
  1963   The Excretion of Lipid and Lipid Substances in Human Sweat. Report No. 280. United States Army Medical Research and Nutrition Laboratory. Denver, Colo.
Consolazio, C.F., Le Roy O. Matoush, R.A. Nelson, J.A. Torres, and C.J. Isaac
  1963   Environmental temperature and energy expenditures. J. Appl. Physiol. 18:65-68.
Consolazio, C.F., R.A. Nelson, Le Roy O. Matoush, R.C. Hughes, and P. Urone
  1964   Trace mineral losses in sweat. Pp. 1-12 in report no. 284 of U.S. Army no. 3A12501A283 (Military Internal Medicine), Subtask no. 03 (Biochemistry), U.S. Army Medical Research and Nutrition Laboratory, Fitzimmons General Hospital, Denver, Colo.
Consolazio, C.F., Le Roy O. Matoush, R.A. Nelson, G.J. Isaac, and J.E. Canham
  1966   Comparisons of nitrogen, calcium and iodine excretion in arm and total body sweat. Am. J. Clin. Nutri. 18:443-448.
Consolazio, C.F., H.L. Johnson, and H.J. Krzywicki
  1970   Energy metabolism during exposure to extreme environments. Unnumbered report. U.S. Army Medical Research and Nutrition Laboratory, Fitzsimmons General Hospital. Denver, Colo.
Costill, D.L., R. Cote, E. Miller, T. Miller, and S. Wynder
  1975   Water and electrolyte replacement during repeated days of work in the heat. Aviat. Space Environ. Med. 46:795-800.
Costill, D.L., R. Cote, and W. Fink
  1976   Muscle water and electrolytes following varied levels of dehydration in man. J. Appl. Physiol. 40:6-11.
Couzy, F., P. Lafargue, and C.Y. Guezennec
  1990   Zinc metabolism in the athletes: Influence of training, nutrition and other factors. Int. J. Sports Med. 11:263-266.
Crowdy, J.P., M.F. Haisman, and H. McGavock
  1971   The effects of a restricted diet on the performance of hard and prolonged physical work. Report 2/71. Army Personnel Research Establishment.
Crowdy, J.P., C.F. Consolazio, A.L. Forbes, M.F. Haisman, and D.W. Worsley
  1982   The metabolic effects of a restricted food intake on men working in a tropical environment. Hum. Nutri.: Appl. Nutri. 36:325-344.
Davies, J., M. Harrison, L. Cochrane, R. Edwards, and T. Gibson
  1981   Effect of saline loading during heat acclimatization on adrenocortical hormones. J. Appl. Physiol. 50:605-612.
de Castro, J.M.
  1988   Physiological, environmental, and subjective determinants of food intake in humans: A meal pattern analysis. Physiol. Behav. 44:651-659.
de Castro, J.M., and E.S. de Castro
  1989   Spontaneous meal patterns of humans: Influence of the presence of other people. Am. J. of Clin. Nutr. 50:237-247.

de Castro, J.M., J. McCormick, M. Pederson, and S.N. Kreitzman

1986   Spontaneous human meal patterns are related to preprandial factors regardless of natural environmental constraints. Physiol. Behav. 38:25-29.

Deuster, P.A., S.B. Kyle, P.B. Moser, R.A. Vigersky, A. Singh, and E.B. Schoomaker.

1986   Nutritional survey of highly trained women runners. Am. J. Clin. Nutr.
45:954-962.

Deuster, P.A., B.A. Day, A. Singh, L. Douglass, and P.B. Moser-Veillon

1989   Zinc status of highly trained women runners and untrained women. Am.
J. Clin. Nutr. 49:1295-1301.

Dill, D.B.

1938   Life, Heat and Altitude. Cambridge, Mass.: Harvard University Press.

1985   The Hot Life of Man and Beast. P. 185. Springfield, Ill.: Charles C.
Thomas.

Dill, D.B., H.T. Edwards, P.S. Bauer, and E.J. Levenson

1930/   Physical performance in relation to external temperature. Arbeitsphysiologie
1931   3:508-518.

Dill, E.B., L.F. Soholt, D.C. McLean, T.F. Drost, Jr., and M.T. Loughran

1977   Capacity of young males and females for running in desert heat. Med.
Sci. Sports. 9(3)137-142.

Dimri, G.P., M.S. Malhotra, J. Sen Gupta, T.S. Kumar, and B.S. Aora

1980   Alterations in aerobic-anaerobic proportions of metabolism during work
in heat. Eur. J. Appl. Physiol. 45:43-50.

Donhoffer, S., and J. Vonotzky

1947   The effect of environmental temperature on food selection. Am. J. Physiol.
150:329-333.

Dreon, D.M., and G.E. Butterfield

1986   Vitamin B_6 utilization in active and inactive young men. Am. J. Clin.
Nutr. 43:816-824.

Drinkwater, B.L., ed.

1986   Female Endurance Athletes. Champaign, Ill.: Human Kinetics Publishers.

Early, R.G., and B.R. Carlson

1969   Water-soluble vitamin therapy in the delay of fatigue from physical activity in hot climatic conditions. Int. Z. Angew. Physiol. 27:43-50.

Eddy, T.P., A.L. Stock, and E.F. Wheeler

1971a   Nutritional and environmental studies on an ocean-going oil tanker. 3.
Energy balances and physique. Brit. J. Indu. Med. 28:330-341.

Eddy, T.P., E.F. Wheeler, and A.L. Stock

1971b   Nutritional and environmental studies on an ocean-going oil tanker. 4.
The diet of seamen. Brit. J. Indu. Med. 28:342-352.

Edelman, B., D. Engell, P. Bronstein, and E. Hirsch

1986   Environmental effects on the intake of overweight and normal-weight
men. Appetite 7:71-83.

Edholm, O.G., and R. Goldsmith

1966   Food intakes and weight changes in climatic extremes. Proc. Nutri. Soc.
25(2):113-119.

Edholm, O.G., R.H. Fox, R. Goldsmith, I.F.G. Hampton, C.R. Underwood, E.J. Ward, H.S. Wolf, J.M. Adam, and J.R. Allan
1964   Report to the Medical Research Council, London: Army Personnel Research Committee, No. APRC64/65. [cited in Edholm, O.G., and R. Goldsmith (1966). Food intakes and weight changes in climatic extremes. Proceedings of the Royal Nutritional Society 25:113-119].

Edison, A.O., R.H. Silber, and D.M. Tennent
1945   The effects of varied thiamine intake on the growth of rats in tropical environment. Am. J. Physiol. 144:643-651.

Eichna, L.W., C.R. Park, N. Nelson, S.M. Horvath, and E.D. Palmes
1950   Thermal regulation during acclimatization in a hot, dry (desert type) environment. Am. J. Physiol. 163:585-597.

Engell, D., and E. Hirsch
1991   Environmental and sensory modulation of fluid intake in humans. Pp. 382-390 in Thirst: Psychological and Physiological Aspects, D.J. Ramsey and D. Booth, eds., London: Springer-Verlag.

Finberg, J.P.M., and G.M. Berlyne
1977   Modification of renin and aldosterone response to heat by acclimatization in man. J. Appl. Physiol. 42:554-558.

Finberg, J.P.M., M. Katz, H. Gazit, and G.M. Berlyne
1974   Plasma renin activity after acute heat exposure in nonacclimatized and naturally acclimatized man. J. Appl. Physiol. 36:519-523.

Fink, W.J., D.L. Costill, and W.J. Van Handel
1975   Leg muscle metabolism during exercise in the heat and cold. Eur. J. Appl. Physiol. 34:183-190.

Follenius, M., G. Brandenberger, B. Reinhardt, and M. Simeoni
1979   Plasma aldosterone, renin activity, and cortisol responses to heat exposure in sodium depleted and repleted subjects. Eur. J. Appl. Physiol. 41:41-50.

Fordtran, J.S., and B. Saltin
1967   Gastric emptying and intestinal absorption during prolonged severe exercise. J. Appl. Physiol. 23(3):331-335.

Francesconi, R., J.T. Maher, G. Bynum, and J. Mason
1977   Recurrent heat exposure: Effects on plasma and urinary sodium and potassium in resting and exercising men. Aviat. Space Environ. Med. 48:399-404.

Francesconi, R.P., M.N. Sawka, and K.B. Pandolf
1983   Hypohydration and heat acclimation: Plasma renin and aldosterone during exercise. J. Appl. Physiol.: Respirat. Environ. Exercise Physiol. 55(6):1790-1794.

1984   Hypohydration and acclimation: Effects on hormone responses to exercise/heat stress. Aviat. Space Environ. Med. 55:365-369.

Francesconi, R.P., M.N. Sawka, K.B. Pandolf, R.W. Hubbard, A.J. Young, and S. Muza
1985   Plasma hormonal responses at graded hypohydration levels during exercise/heat stress. J. Appl. Physiol. 59(6):1855-1860.

Francesconi, R.P., P. C. Szlyk, I.V. Sils, N. Leva, and R.W. Hubbard
  1989   Plasma renin activity and aldosterone: Correlations with moderate hypohydration. Aviat. Space Environ. Med. 60:1172-1177.

Galvao, E.G.
  1950   Human heat production in relation to body weight and body surface. J. Appl. Physiol. 3:21.

Gathiram, P., M.T. Wells, J.G. Brock-Utne, B.C. Wessels, and S.L. Gaffin
  1987   Prevention of endotoxaemia by non-absorbable antibiotics in heat stress. J. Clin. Pathol. 40:1364-1368.

Gengler, W.R., F.A. Martz, H.D. Johnson, G.F. Krause, and L. Hahn
  1970   Effect of temperature on food and water intake and rumen fermentation. J. Dairy Sci. 53:434-437.

Gisolfi, C.V.
  1973   Work-heat tolerance derived from interval training. J. Appl. Physiol. 35:349-354.

Gisolfi, C.V., N.C. Wilson, and B. Claxton
  1977   Work-heat tolerance of distance runners. Ann. N.Y. Acad. Sci. 301:139-150.

Gleeson, M., J.D. Robertson, and R.J. Maughan
  1987   Influence of exercise on ascorbic acid status in man. Clin. Sci. 73:501-505.

Glenn, J.F., R.E. Burr, R.W. Hubbard, M.Z. Mays, R.J. Moore, B.H. Jones, and G.P. Krueger, eds.
  1990   Sustaining Health and Performance in the Desert: A Pocket Guide to Environmental Medicine for Operations in Southwest Asia. Technical Note 91-2. United States Army Research Institute of Environmental Medicine. Natick, Mass.

Gonzalez, R.R., L.G. Berglund, and A.P. Gagge
  1978   Indices of thermoregulatory strain for moderate exercise in the heat. J. Appl. Physiol. 44:889-899.

Graber, C.D., R.B. Reinhold, and J.G. Breman
  1971   Fatal heatstroke. J. Am. Med. Assoc. 216:1195-1196.

Green, B.G.
  1986   Sensory interactions between capsaicin and temperature in the oral cavity. Chem. Sens. 11:371-382.
  1990   Effects of thermal, mechanical, and chemical stimulation on the perception of oral irritation. Pp. 171-192 in Chemical Senses. Vol. 2, Irritation, B.G. Green, J.R. Mason, and M.R. Kare, eds. New York: Marcel Dekker.
  1991   Oral chemesthesis: The importance of time and temperature for the perception of chemical irritants. Pp. 107-123 in Sensory Science Theory and Applications in Foods, H.T. Lawless, and B.P. Klein, eds. New York: Marcel Dekker.

Green, B.G., and S.P. Frankmann
  1987   The effect of cooling the tongue on the perceived intensity of taste. Chemical Senses 12(4):609-619.
  1988   The effect of cooling on the perception of carbohydrate and intensive sweeteners. Physiol. Behav. 43:515-519.

Green, B.G., S.J. Lederman, and J.C. Stevens
1979   The effect of skin temperature on the perception of roughness. Sens. Proc. 3:327-333.

Greenleaf, J.E., B.L. Castle, and W.K. Ruff
1972   Maximal oxygen uptake, sweating and tolerance to exercise in the heat. Int. J. Biometeor. 16(4):375-387.

Greenleaf, J.E., P.J. Brock, L.C. Keil, and J.T. Morse
1983   Drinking and water balance during exercise and heat acclimation. J. Appl. Physiol. 54:414-419.

Grucza, R., J.-L. Lecroart, G. Carette, J.-J. Hauser, and Y. Houdas
1987   Effect of voluntary dehydration on thermoregulatory responses to heat in men and women. Eur. J. Appl. Physiol. 56:317-322.

Guilland, J., T. Penaranda, C. Gallet, V. Boggio, F. Fuchs, and J. Klepping
1989   Vitamin status of young athletes including the effects of supplementation. Med. Sci. Sports Exerc. 21:441-449.

Gutteridge, J.M.C., D.A. Rowley, B. Halliwell, D.F. Cooper, and D.M. Heeley
1985   Copper and iron complexes catalytic for oxygen radical reaction in sweat from human athletes. Clin. Chim. Acta 145:267-273.

Hamilton, C.L.
1963   Hypothalamic temperature records of a monkey. Proc. Soc. Exptl. Biol. Med. 112:55-57.
1963   Interactions of food intake and temperature regulation in the rat. J. Comp. Physiol. Psychol. 56:476-488.
1967   Food and temperature. Pp. 303-317 in Handbook of Physiology: Section 6, vol. 1, C.F. Code, ed. Washington, D.C.: American Physiological Society.

Hamilton, C.L., and J.R. Brobeck
1964   Food intake and temperature regulation in rats with rostral hypothalamic lesions. Am. J. Physiol. 207:291-297.

Harrison, M.H.
1985   Effects of thermal stress and exercise on blood volume in humans. Physiol. Rev. 65(1)149-209.

Havenith, G., and H. van Middendorp
1990   The relative influence of physical fitness, acclimatization state, anthropometric measures and gender on individual reactions to heat stress. Eur. J. Appl. Physiol 61:419-427.

Helgheim, I., O. Hetland, S. Nilsson, F. Ingjer, and S.B. Stromme
1979   The effects of vitamin E on serum enzyme levels following heavy exercise. Eur. J. Appl. Physiol. 40:283-289.

Henane, R.
1980   Acclimatization to heat in man: Giant or windmill, a critical reappraisal. Pp. 275-284 in Pecs: Proceedings of the 28th International Congress of Physiological Science, F. Obal and G. Benedek, eds. New York: Pergamon.

Henschel, A., H.L. Taylor, J.M. Brôzek, O. Mickelsen, and A. Keys
1944   Vitamin C and ability to work in hot environments. Am. J. Trop. Med. Hyg. 24:259-264.

Henschel, A., H.L. Taylor, O. Mickelsen, J.M. Brôzek, and A. Keys
1944 The effect of high vitamin C and B intake on the ability of man to work in hot environments. Fed. Proc. 3:18.

Herbert, W.E., and P.M. Ribisl
1972 Effects of dehydration upon physical working capacity of wrestlers under competitive conditions. Res. Q. Am. Assoc. Health Phys. Educ. 43:416-421.

Hindson, T.C.
1970 Ascorbic acid status of Europeans resident in the tropics. Br. J. Nutr. 24:801-802.

Hirsch, E., H.L. Meiselman, R.D. Popper, G. Smits, B. Jezior, I. Lichton, M. Wenkam, J. Brut, M. Fox, S. McNutt, M.N, Thiele, and O. Dirige
1984 The effects of prolonged feeding meal, ready-to-eat (MRE) operational rations. Technical Report NATICK/TR-85/035. Natick, Mass.: U.S. Army Natick Research and Development Center.

Hubbard, R.W., and L.E. Armstrong
1988 The heat illnesses: Biochemical, ultrastructural, and fluid-electrolyte considerations. Pp. 305-360 in Human Performance Physiology and Environmental Medicine at Terrestrial Extremes, K.B. Pandolf, M.N. Sawka, and R.R. Gonzalez, eds. Indianapolis, Ind.: Benchmark Press.

Hubbard, R.W., L.E. Armstrong, P.K. Evans, and J.P. DeLuca
1986 Long-Term Water and Salt Deficits—A Military Perspective. Pp. 29-48 in Predicting Decrements in Military Performance Due to Inadequate Nutrition: Proceedings of a Workshop. Washington, D.C.: National Academy Press.

Iampietro, P.F., J.A. Vaughn, A. MacLead, B.E. Welch, J.G. Marcinek, J.B. Mann, M.P. Grotheer, and T.E. Friedemann
1956 Caloric intake and energy expenditure of eleven men in a desert environment. Report No. EP-40. U.S. Army Quartermaster Research and Development Center, Natick, Mass.

Jakubczak, L.F.
1976 Food and water intakes of rats as a function of strain, age, temperature, and body weight. Physiol. Behav. 17:251-258.

Johnson, R.E.
1943 Nutritional standards for men in tropical climates. Gastroenterology 1:832-900.

Johnson, R.E., and R.M. Kark
1946 Feeding Problems in Man as Related to Environment. An Analysis of United States and Canadian Army Ration Trials and Surveys. Chicago, Ill.: Quartermaster Food and Container Institute for the Armed Forces.
1947 Environment and food intake in man. Science. 105:378-379.
1947 Feeding Problems in Man as Related to Environment. An Analysis of United States and Canadian Army Ration Trials and Surveys, 1941-1946. Chicago, Ill.: Quartermaster Food and Container for the Armed Forces, Research and Development Branch, Office of the Quartermaster General.

Johnson, H.L., R.A. Nelson, J.E. Canham, J.H. Skala, C.F. Consolazio, and H.E. Sauberlich
  1983   Comparisons of utilizations and nutrient contents of A rations and short order meals at the Air Force Dining Facility, Lowry Air Force Base, Denver, Colorado—July, 1971. Report No. 140. San Francisco, Calif.: Letterman Army Institute of Research.

Johnson, H.L., R.A. Nelson, and C.F. Consolazio
  1988   Effects of electrolyte and nutrient solutions on performance and metabolic balance. Med. Sci. Sports Exerc. 20:26-33.

Johnson, R.F., L.G. Branch, and D.J. McMenemy
  1989   Influence of attitude and expectation on moods and symptoms during cold weather military training. Aviat. Space Environ. Med. 60:1157-1162.

Jooste, P.L., and N.B. Strydom
  1979   Improved mechanical efficiency derived from heat acclimation. S. Afr. J. Res. Sport Phys. Ed. Rec. 2:45-53.

Kark, R.M.
  1954   Studies on troops in the field. Pp. 193-195 in Nutrition under Climatic Stress, H. Spector and M.S. Peterson, eds. Washington, D.C.: National Academy of Sciences/National Research Council.

Kark, R.M., H.F. Alton, E.D. Pease, W.B. Bean, C.R. Henderson, R.E. Johnson, and L.M. Richardson
  1947   Tropical deterioration and nutrition. Clinical and biochemical observations on troops. Medicine 26:1-40.

Keen, C.L., and R.M. Hackman
  1986   Trace elements in athletic performance. Pp. 51-65 in Sport, Health and Nutrition: 1984 Olympic Scientific Congress Proceedings, vol. 2, F.I. Katch, ed. Champaign, Ill.: Human Kinetics.

Kelso, T.B., W.G. Herbert, F.C. Gwazdauskas, F.L. Goss and J.L. Hess
  1984   Exercise-thermoregulatory stress and increased plasma b-endorphin/b-lipotropin in humans. J. Appl. Physiol. 57:444-449.

Kendall, A.C.
  1972   Rickets in the tropics and sub-tropics. Cent. Afr. J. Med. 18:47-49.

Kenney, M.J., and C.V. Gisolfi
  1986   Thermal regulation: Effects of exercise and age. Pp. 133-143 in Sports Medicine for the Mature Athlete. Indianapolis, Ind.: Benchmark Press.

Kerslake, D.M., ed.
  1972   The Stress of Hot Environments. Cambridge, England: Cambridge University Press.

Keys, A., and A. Henschel
  1941   High vitamin supplementation (B_1, nicotinic acid and C) and the response to intensive exercise in U.S. Army infantrymen. Am. J. Physiol. 133:350-351.

  1942   Vitamin supplementation of U.S. Army rations in relation to fatigue and the ability to do muscular work. J. Nutr. 23:259-269.

Keys, A., A.F. Henschel, O. Mickelsen, and J.M. Brôzek
  1943   The performance of normal young men on controlled thiamine intakes. J. Nutr. 26:399-415.

Keys, A., A.F. Henschel, O. Mickelsen, J.M. Brôzek, and J.H. Crawford
1944   Physiological and biochemical functions in normal young men on a diet
        restricted in riboflavin. J. Nutr. 27:165-178.
Keys, A., J. Brôzek, A. Henschel, O. Mickelsen, and L.L. Taylor
1950   The Biology of Human Starvation. Minneapolis, Minn.: University of
        Minnesota Press.
King, D.S., D.L. Costill, W.J. Fink, M. Hargreaves, and R.A. Fielding
1985   Muscle metabolism during exercise in the heat in unacclimatized and
        acclimatized humans. J. Appl. Physiol. 59:1350-1354.
Kirby, C.R., and V.A. Convertino
1986   Plasma aldosterone and sweat sodium concentrations after exercise and
        heat acclimation. J. Appl. Physiol. 61:967-970.
Kirwan, J.P., D.L. Costill, H. Kuipers, M.J. Burrell, W.J. Fink, J.E. Kovaleski, and
        R.A. Fielding
1987   Substrate utilization in leg muscle of men after heat acclimation. J.
        Appl. Physiol. 63:31-35.
Klausen, K., D.B. Dill, E.E. Phillips, and D. McGregor
1967   Metabolic reactions to work in the desert. J. Appl. Physiol. 22:292-296.
Klesges, R.C., D. Bartsch, J.D. Norwood, D. Kautzman, and S. Haugrud
1984   The effects of selected social and environmental variables on the eating
        behavior of adults in the natural environment. Int. J. Eating Disord. 3:35-
        41.
Knochel, J.P.
1984   Environmental heat illness. Arch. Int. Med. 133:841-864.
Knochel, J.P., and R.M. Vertel
1967   Salt loading as a possible factor in the production of potassium depletion,
        phabdomyolysis, and heat injury. Lancet 1(491)659-661.
Kobrick, J.L., R.F. Johnson, and D.J. McMenemy
1990   Subjective reactions to atropine/2-PAM chloride and heat while in battle
        dress uniform and in chemical protective clothing. Milit. Psychol. 2(2):95111.
Korhonen, H., and M. Harri
1986   Seasonal changes in energy economy of farmed polecat as evaluated by
        body weight, food intake and behavioral strategy. Physiol. Behav. 37:777-
        783.
Koslowski, S., and B. Saltin
1964   Effect of sweat loss on body fluids. J. Appl. Physiol. 19:1119-1124.
Kosunen, K.J., A.J. Pakarinen, K. Kuoppasalmi, and H. Adlerkreutz
1976   Plasma renin activity, angiotensin II, and aldosterone during intense heat
        stress. J. Appl. Physiol. 41:323-327.
Kotze, H.F., W.H. Van der Walt, G.G. Rogers, and N.B. Strydom
1977   Effects of plasma ascorbic acid levels on heat acclimatization in man. J.
        Appl. Physiol. 42:711-716.
Kraly, F.S., and E.M. Blass
1976   Increased feeding in rats in a low ambient temperature. Pp. 77-89 in
        Hunger: Basic Mechanisms and Clinical Implications, D. Novin, ed. New
        York: Raven Press.

Kretsch, M.J., D.D. Schnakenberg, R.D. Fults, R.A. Nelson, Y.C. LeTellier, and
J.E. Canham
1979   Nutrient intakes and some socioeconomic characteristics of Twentynine
Palms Marine Corps personnel before food service system modifications—
March, 1977. Report No. 65. June. San Francisco, Calif.: Letterman Army
Institute of Research.
Kretsch, M.J., Sauberlich, H.E., and J.H. Skala
1984   Nutritional status assessment of marines before and after the installation
of the "multi-restaurant" food service system at the Twentynine Palms
Marine Corps Base, California. Report No. 192. December. San Francisco, Calif.: Letterman Army Institute of Research.
Kretsch, M.D., P.M. Conforti, H.L. Johnson, and H.E. Sauberlich
1986   Effects of energy intake and expenditure on weight gain and percent
body fat of male and female cadets at the United States Military Academy, West Point, New York. Report No. 225. September. San Francisco,
Calif.: Letterman Army Institute of Research.
Ladell, W.S.S.
1945   Thermal sweating. Br. Med. Bull. 3:175-179.
1957   Disorders due to heat. Trans. R. Soc. Trop. Med. Hyg. 51:189-216.
Ladell, W.S.S., J.C. Waterlow, and M.F. Hudson
1954   Desert climate: Physiological and clinical observations. Lancet 2:491-
497.
Lamanca, J.J., E.M. Haymes, J.A. Daly, R.J. Moffatt, and M.F. Waller
1988   Sweat iron loss of male and female runners during exercise. Int. J. Sports
Med. 9:52-55.
Lane, H.W.
1989   Some trace elements related to physical activity: Zinc, copper, selenium,
chromium, and iodine. Pp. 301-307 in Nutrition in Exercise and Sports,
J.E. Hickson and I. Wolinsky, eds. Boca Raton, Fla.: CRC Press.
Lang, J.K., K. Gohil, L. Packer, and R.F. Burk
1987   Selenium deficiency, endurance exercise capacity, and antioxidant status
in rats. J. Appl. Physiol. 63:2532-2535.
Lawless, H.T.
1984   Oral chemical irritation: Psychophysical properties. Chem. Sens. 9:143-
157.
Leklem, J.E., and T.D. Shultz
1983   Increased plasma pyridoxal 5'-phosphate and vitamin B_6 in male adolescents after a 4500-meter run. Am. J. Clin. Nutr. 38:541-548.
Lester, L.S., and F.M. Kramer
in   The effects of heating on food acceptability and consumption. J. Foodserv.
press   Systems.
Lester L.S., F.M. Kramer, J. Edinberg, S. Mutter, and D.B. Engell
1990   Evaluation of the canteen cup stand and ration heater pad: Effects on
acceptability and consumption of the meal, ready-to-eat in a cold weather
environment. Technical Report Natick TR-90/008L. U.S. Army Natick
Research, Development and Engineering Center, Natick, Mass.

Levitz, L.
1975   The susceptibility of feeding to external control. Pp. 53-60 in Obesity in Perspective, G.A. Bray, ed. Department of Health, Education, and Welfare Publication No. NIH 75-708. Washington, D.C.: U.S. Government Printing Office.

Lichton, I.J., J.B. Miyamura, and S.W. McNutt
1988   Nutritional evaluation of soldiers subsisting on meal, ready-to-eat operational rations for an extended period: Body measurements, hydration, and blood nutrients. Am. J. Clin. Nutr. 48:30-37.

Lijnen, P., P. Hespel, R. Fagard, R. Lysens, E. Vanden Eynde, and A. Amery
1988   Erythrocyte, plasma and urinary magnesium in men before and after a marathon. Eur. J. Appl. Physiol. 58:252-256.

Logue, A.W.
1986   The Psychology of Eating and Drinking. New York: W.H. Freeman.

Macari, M., S.M.F. Zuim, E.R. Secato, and J.R. Guerreiro
1986   Effects of ambient temperature and thyroid hormones on food intake by pigs. Physiol. Behav. 36:1035-1039.

MacGregor, R.G.S., and G.L. Loh
1941   The influence of a tropical environment upon the basal metabolism, pulse rate and blood pressure in Europeans. J. Physiol. (London) 99:496-509.

Marriott, B.M., and C. Rosemont
1991   Fluid Replacement and Heat Stress: Proceedings of a Workshop. 2nd printing. Washington, D.C.: National Academy Press.

Mason, E.D.
1934   The basal metabolism of European women in South India and the effect of change in climate on European and South Indian women. J. Nutr. 8:695.

McBurney, D.H., V.B. Collings, and L.M. Glanz
1973   Temperature dependence of human taste response. Physiol. Behav. 11:89-94.

McDonald, R., and C.L. Keen
1988   Iron, zinc, and magnesium nutrition and athletic performance. Sports Med. 5:171-184.

Meyers, A.W., A.J. Stunkard, and M. Coll
1980   Food accessibility and food choice. Arch. Gen. Psychiatry 37:1133-1135.

Miescher, E., and Suzanne M. Fortner
1989   Responses to dehydration and rehydration during heat exposure in young and older men. Am. J. Physiol. 257(26):1050-1056.

Mills, C.A.
1941   Environmental temperatures and thiamine requirements. Am. J. Physiol. 133:525-532.

Mitchell, H.H., and M. Edman
1949   Research Reports—Nutrition and Resistance to Climatic Stress with Particular Reference to Man. Chicago, Ill.: Quartermaster Food and Container Institute for the Armed Forces.
1951   Nutrition and Climatic Stress. Springfield, Ill.: Charles C. Thomas.

1951   Nutrition and Resistance to Climatic Stress with Particular Reference to Man. Springfield, Ill.: Charles C. Thomas.

Miyamura, J.B., S.W. McNutt, I.J. Lichton, and N.S. Wenkam
1987   Altered zinc status of soldiers under field conditions. J. Am. Diet. Assoc. 87:595-597.

Mommadov, I.M., and V.A. Grafova
1983   Daily diet and ascorbic acid intake in man during work in the Arid zone. Human Physiol. 9(4):224-228.

Morimoto, T., Z. Slabochova, R.K. Naman, and F. Sargent II.
1967   Sex differences in physiological reactions to thermal stress. J. Appl. Physiol. 22:526-532.

Muza, S.R., N.A. Pimental, H.M. Cosimini, and M.N. Sawka
1988   Portable ambient air microclimate cooling simulated desert and tropic conditions. Aviat. Space Environ. Med. 59:553-558.

Nadel, E.R.
1983   Effects of temperature on muscle metabolism. Pp. 134-143 in Biochemistry of Exercise, H.G. Knuttgen, J.A. Vogel, and J. Poortmans, eds. Champaign, Ill.: Human Kinetics Publishers.

Nadel, E.R., E. Cafarelli, M.F. Roberts, and C.B. Wenger
1979   Circulatory regulation during exercise in different ambient temperatures. J. Appl. Physiol. 46:430-437.

Nadel, E.R., S.M. Fortney, and C.B. Wenger
1980   Effect of hydration state on circulatory and thermal regulations. J. Appl. Physiol. 49:715-721.

National Research Council
1989   Diet and Health: Implications for Reducing Chronic Disease Risk. Report of the Committee on Diet and Health, Food and Nutrition Board. Washington, D.C.: National Academy Press.
1989   Recommended Dietary Allowances, 10th ed. Washington, D.C.: National Academy Press.

Nielsen, B.
1969   Thermoregulation in rest and exercise. Acta Physiol. Scand. Suppl. 323.

Nielsen, B., G. Savard, E.A. Richter, M. Hargreaves, and B. Saltin
1990   Muscle blood flow and muscle metabolism during exercise and heat stress. J. Appl. Physiol. 69:1040-1046.

Nielsen, M.
1970   Heat production and body temperature during rest and work. Pp. 205-214 in Physiological and Behavioral Temperature Regulation, J.D. Hardy, A.P. Gagge, and J.A.J. Stolwijk, eds. Springfield, Ill.: Charles C. Thomas.

Neufer, P.D., A.J. Young, and M.N. Sawka
1989   Gastric emptying during exercise: Effects of heat stress and hypohydration. Eur. J. Appl. Physiol. 58:433-439.

Norman, E.J., and R.M. Gaither
1991   Review of Army Food Related Operations in Hot Desert Environments. Technical Report Natick/TR-91/008. United States Army Natick Research, Development and Engineering Center. Natick, Mass.

Olha, A.E., V. Klissouras, J.D. Sullivan, and S.C. Skoryna
   1982   Effect of exercise on concentration of elements in the serum. J. Sports
           Med. Phys. Fitness 22:414-425.
Orr, J.B., and J.L. Gilks
   1931   Studies of nutrition: The physique and health of two African tribes. Med.
           Res. Coun. London, Spec. Rep., Series 155:82.
Owen, M.D., K.C. Kregel, P.T. Wall, and C.V. Gisolfi
   1986   Effects of ingesting carbohydrate beverages during exercise in the heat.
           Med. Sci. Sports Exerc. 18(5):568-575.
Pandolf, K.B., B.S. Cadarette, M.N. Sawka, J.J. Young, R.P. Francesconi, and
   R.G. Gonzales
   1988   Thermoregulatory responses of middle-aged and young men during dry-
           heat acclimation. J. Appl. Physiol. 65(1)65-71.
Pangborn, R.M., R.B. Chrisp, and L.L. Bertolero
   1970   Gustatory, salivary, and oral thermal responses to solutions of sodium
           chloride at four temperatures. Percept. Psychophy. 8:69-75.
Paolone, A.M., C.L. Wells, and G.T. Kelly
   1978   Sexual variations in thermoregulation during heat stress. Aviat. Space
           Environ. Med. 49(5):715-719.
Paulus, K., and A.M. Reisch
   1980   The influence of temperature on the threshold values of primary tastes.
           Chem. Sens. 5:11-21.
Penicaud, L., D.A. Thompson, and J. Le Magnen
   1986   Effects of 2-deoxy-d-glucose on food and water intake and body tem-
           perature in rats. Physiol. Behav. 36:431-435.
Petersen, E.S., and H. Vejby-Christensen
   1973   Effect of body temperature on steady-state ventilation and metabolism in
           exercise. Acta Physiol. Scand. 89:342-351.
Pimental, N.A., H.M. Cosimini, M.N. Sawka, and C.B. Wenger
   1987   Effectiveness of an air-cooled vest using selected air temperature and
           humidity combinations. Aviat. Space Environ. Med. 58:119-124.
Pitts, G.C., R.E. Johnson, and C.F. Consolazio
   1944   Work in the heat as affected by intake of water, salt, and glucose. Am. J.
           Physiol. 142:253-259.
Piwonka, R.W., and S. Robinson
   1967   Acclimation of highly trained men to work in severe heat. J. Appl. Physiol.
           22:9-12.
Poda, G.A.
   1979   Vitamin C for heat symptoms? Ann. Intern. Med. 91(4):657.
Popper, R., G. Smits, H.L. Meiselman, and E. Hirsch
   1989   Eating in combat: A survey of U.S. Marines. Milit. Med. 154:619-623.
Refinetti, R.
   1988   Effects of food temperature and ambient temperature during a meal on
           food intake in the rat. Physiol. Behav. 43:245-247.
Richards, D., R. Richards, and P.J. Schofield
   1979   Management of heat exhaustion in Sydney's The Sun City-to-Surf fun
           runners. Med. J. Aust. 2:457-461.

Richardson, R.P., D.P. Leitch, B.M. Hill, P.M. Short, G. Turk, H.L. Meiselman, L.E. Symington, R. Porter, and D. Schnakenberg
1979   A New Foodservice System Concept for Aircraft Carriers, Technical Report Natick/TR/80/007. December. Natick, Mass.: U.S. Army Natick Research and Development Command.

Roberts, M.F., C.B. Wenger, J.A.J. Stolwijk, and E.R. Nadel
1977   Skin blood flow and sweating changes following exercise and heat acclimation. J. Appl. Physiol. 43:133-137.

Robinson, S., and S.D. Gerking
1947   Thermal balance of men working in severe heat. Am. J. Physiol. 149:476-488.

Robinson, S., and A.H. Robinson
1954   Chemical composition of sweat. Physiol. Rev. 34:202-220.

Robinson, S., D.B. Dill, J.W. Wilson, and M. Nielsen
1941   Adaptations of white men and Negroes to prolonged work in humid heat. Am. J. Trop. Med. 21:261-287.

Robinson, S., E.S. Turrell, H.S. Belding, and S.M. Horvath
1945   Rapid acclimatization to work in hot climates. Am. J. Physiol. 140:168-176.

Robinson, S., H.S. Belding, C.F. Consolazio, S.M. Horvath, and E.S. Turrell
1986   Acclimatization of older men to work in heat. J. Appl. Physiol. 20(4):583-586.

Rolls, B.J., I.C. Fedoroff, J.F. Guthrie, and L.J. Laster
1990   Effects of temperature and mode of presentation of juice on hunger, thirst and food intake in humans. Appetite 15:199-208.

Rose, L.I., D.R. Carroll, S.L. Lowe, E.W. Peterson, and K.H. Cooper
1970   Serum electrolyte changes after marathon running. J. Appl. Physiol. 29:449-451.

Rose, M.S., R.P. Francesconi, L. Levine, B. Shukitt, A.V. Cardello, P.H. Warren, I. Munro, L. Banderet, P.M. Poole, P. Frykman, and M.N. Sawka
1987   Effects of a NBC Nutrient Solution on Physiological and Psychological Status During Sustained Activity in the Heat. Report No. T25-87. United States Army Research Institute of Environmental Medicine. Natick, Mass.

Rose, M.S., P.C. Szlyk, R.P. Francesconi, L.S. Lester, L. Armstrong, W. Matthew, A.V. Cardello, R.D. Popper, I. Sils, G. Thomas, D. Schilling, and R. Whang
1988   Effectiveness and Acceptability of Nutrient Solutions in Enhancing Fluid Intake in the Heat. Report No. T10-89. United States Army Research Institute of Environmental Medicine. Natick, Mass.

Rothwell, N.J., and M.J. Stock
1986   Influence of environmental temperature on energy balance, diet-induced thermogenesis and brown fat activity in "cafeteria"-fed rats. Br. J. Nutr. 56:123-129.

Rowell, L.B., J.R. Blackmon, R.H. Martin, J.A. Mazzarella, and R.A. Bruce
1965   Hepatic clearance of indocyanine green in man under thermal and exercise stresses. J. Appl. Physiol. 20:384-394.

Rowell, L. B., H.J. Marx, R.A. Bruce, R.D. Conn, and F. Kusumi
1966   Reductions in cardiac output, central blood volume and stroke volume with thermal stress in normal men during exercise. J. Clin. Invest. 45:1801-1816.

Rowell, L.B., K.K. Kraning II, J.W. Kennedy, and T.O. Evans
1967   Central circulatory responses to work before and after acclimatization. J. Appl. Physiol. 22:509-518.

Rowell, L.B., G.L. Brengelmann, J.B. Blackmon, R.D. Twiss, and F. Kusumi
1968   Splanchnic blood flow and metabolism in heat-stressed man. J. Appl. Physiol. 24:475-484.

Rowell, L.B., G.L. Brengelmann, J.A. Murray, K.K. Kraning II, and F. Kusumi
1969   Human metabolic responses to hyperthermia during mild to maximal exercise. J. Appl. Physiol. 26:395-402.

Rozin, P., L. Ebert, and J. Schull
1982   Some like it hot: A temporal analysis of hedonic responses to chili pepper. Appetite 3:13-22.

Salganik, R.I.
1956   Nutrition in high environmental temperatures. (in Russian) Vopr. Pitan. 33:3-11.

Saltin, B.
1964   Aerobic and anaerobic work capacity after dehydration. J. Appl. Physiol. 19:1114-1118.

Saltin, B., A.P. Gagge, U. Bergh, and J.A.J. Stolwijk
1972   Body temperatures and sweating during exhaustive exercise. J. Appl. Physiol. 32:635-643.

Sargent, F., and R.E. Johnson
1957   The Physiological Basis for Various Constituents in Survival Rations. Part 4. An Integrative Study of the All-Purpose Survival Ration for Temperate, Cold and Hot Weather. Wright Air Development Center Technical Report 53-484. Wright-Patterson Air Force Base, Ohio: Wright Air Development Center.

Sawka, M.N., and K.B. Pandolph
1990   Effects of body water loss on exercise performance and physiological functions. Pp. 1-8 in Perspectives in Exercise Science and Sports Medicine, Vol. 3, Fluid Homeostasis During Exercise, C.V. Gisolfi and D.R. Lamb, eds. Indianapolis, Ind.: Benchmark Press

Sawka, M.N., and C.B. Wenger
1988   Physiological responses to acute exercise-heat stress. Pp. 1-38 in Human Performance Physiology and Environmental Medicine at Terrestrial Extremes, K.B. Pandolf, M.N. Sawka, and R.R. Gonzalez, eds. Indianapolis, Ind.: Benchmark Press.
1988   Physiological responses to acute exercise-heat stress. Pp. 97-151 in Human Performance Physiology and Environmental Medicine at Terrestrial Extremes, K.B. Pandolf, M.N. Sawka, and R.R. Gonzalez, eds. Indianapolis, Ind: Benchmark Press.

Sawka, M.N., K.B. Pandolf, B.A. Avellini, and Y. Shapiro
  1983   Does heat acclimation lower the rate of metabolism elicited by muscular
          exercise? Aviat. Space Environ. Med. 54:27-31.
Sawka, M.N., A.J. Young, B.S. Cadarette, L. Levine, and K.B. Pandolf
  1985   Influence of heat stress and acclimation on maximal aerobic power. Eur.
          J. Appl. Physiol. 53:294-298.
Schacter, S., and L.N. Friedman
  1974   The effects of work and cue prominence on eating behavior. Pp. 11-14 in
          Obese Humans and Rats, S. Schachter and J. Rodin, eds. Potomac, Md.:
          Earlbaum Associates.
Scott, M.L.
  1975   Environmental influences on ascorbic acid requirements in animals. Ann.
          N.Y. Acad. Sci. 258:151-155.
Sen Gupta, J., P. Dimri, and M.S. Malhotra
  1977   Metabolic responses of Indians during sub-maximal and maximal work in
          dry and humid heat. Ergonomics 20:33-40.
Senay, L.C., and R. Kok
  1977   Effects of training and heat acclimatization on blood plasma contents of
          exercising men. J. Appl. Physiol. Respir. Environ. Exerc. Physiol. 43:591-
          599.
Shapiro, R., and C.F. Consolazio
  1959   Energy Requirements of Men Exposed to Solar Radiation and Heat. Re-
          port No. 240. United States Army Medical Research and Nutrition Labo-
          ratory. Denver, Colo.
Shapiro, Y., K.B. Pandolf, and R.F. Goldman
  1982   Predicting sweat loss response to exercise, environment and clothing.
          Eur. J. Appl. Physiol. 48:83-96.
Shvartz, E., Y. Shapiro, A. Magazanik, A. Meroz, H. Birnfeld, A. Mechtinger, and
          S. Shibolet
  1977   Heat acclimation, physical fitness and responses to exercise in temperate
          and hot environments. J. Appl. Physiol. 43:678-683.
Siegel, A.J.
  1988   Medical conditions arising during sports. Pp. 221-223 in Women and
          Sports: Physiology and Sports Medicine, M.M. Shangold and G. Mirkin,
          eds. Philadelphia: F.A. Davis Company.
Singh, A., B.L. Smoak, K.Y. Patterson, L.G. LeMay, C. Veillon, and P. A. Deuster
  1991   Biochemical indices of selected trace minerals in men: Effect of stress.
          Am. J. Clin. Nutr. 53:126-131.
Smiles, K.A., and S. Robinson
  1971   Sodium ion conservation during acclimatization of men to work in the
          heat. J. Appl. Physiol. 31:63-69.
Smith, R.E., Editor-in-Chief
  1965   Proceedings of the International Symposium on Temperature and Alti-
          tude. Kyoto, Japan. Bethesda, Md.: Federation of American Societies for
          Experimental Biology.

Smoland, J., O. Korhonen, and R. Ilmarinen
  1990   Responses of young and older men during prolonged exercise in dry and humid heat. Eur. J. Appl. Physiol. 61:413-418.
Snyder, A.C., L.L. Dvorak, and J.B. Roepke
  1989   Influence of dietary iron source on measures of iron status among female runners. Med. Sci. Sports Exerc. 21:7-10.
Spector, H., and M.S. Peterson, eds.
  1954   Nutrition Under Climatic Stress. 1952. Advisory Board on Quartermaster Research and Development—A Symposium. Committee on Foods, National Academy of Sciences, Washington, D.C.: National Research Council.
Spector, N.H., J.R. Brobeck, and C.L. Hamilton
  1968   Feeding and core temperature in albino rats: Changes induced by preoptic heating and cooling. Science 161:286-288.
Stevens, J.C., and B.G. Green
  1978   Temperature-touch interaction: Weber's phenomenon revisited. Sens. Proc. 2:206-219.
Stolwijk, J.A.J., B. Saltin, and A.P. Gagge
  1968   Physiological factors associated with sweating during exercise. Aerospace Med. 39:1101-1105.
Strydom, N.B., C.H. Wyndham, C.G. Williams, J.F. Morrison, G.A.G. Bredell, A.J.S. Benade, and M. Von Rahden
  1966   Acclimatization to humid heat and the role of physical conditioning. J. Appl. Physiol. 21:636-642.
Strydom, N.B., H.F. Kotze, W.H. Van der Walt, and G.G. Rogers
  1976   Effect of ascorbic acid on rate of heat acclimatization. J. Appl. Physiol. 41:202-205.
Stunkard, A.J., W.L. Clovis, and S.M. Free
  1962   Skin temperature after eating, evidence bearing upon a thermostatic control of food intake. Am. J. Med. Sci. 244:126-130.
Sutton, J.R., and R.M. Brock
  1986   Sports Medicine for the Mature Athlete. Indianapolis: Benchmark Press, Inc.
Swiergiel, A.H., and D.L. Ingram
  1986   Effect of diet and temperature acclimation on thermoregulatory behavior in piglets. Physiol. Behav. 36:637-642.
Szlyk, P., I.V. Sils, R.P. Francesconi, R.W. Hubbard, and L.E. Armstrong
  1989   Effects of water temperature and flavoring on voluntary dehydration in man. Physiol. Behav. 45:639-647.
Taylor, H.L., A. Henschel, O. Mickelsen, and A. Keys
  1944   The effect of sodium chloride intake on the work performance of man during exposure to dry heat and experimental heat exhaustion. Am. J. Physiol. 140:439-451.
Taylor, N.A.S.
  1986   Eccrine sweat glands. Adaptations to physical training and heat acclimation. Sports Med. 3:387-397.

Thompson, C.I.
1980   Controls of Eating. New York, N.Y.: Spectrum Publications.
Tin-May-Than, Ma-Win-May, Khin-Sann-Aung, and M. Mya-Tu
1978   The effect of vitamin B_{12} on physical performance capacity. Br. J. Nutr. 40:269-273.
Tsuchiya, K., and M. Iriki
1980   Effects of spinal cord cooling and heating on gastrointestinal motility in spinal-intact and acutely spinalized dogs. Ital. J. Gastroenterol. 12:255-259.
Tucker, R.G., O. Mickelsen, and A. Keys
1960   The influence of sleep, work, diuresis, heat, acute starvation, thiamine intake and bed rest on human riboflavin excretion. J. Nutr. 72:251-261.
Uhari, M., A. Pakarinen, J. Hietala, T. Nurmi, and K. Kouvalainen
1983   Serum iron, copper, zinc, ferritin, and ceruloplasmin after intense heat exposure. Eur. J. Appl. Physiol. 51:331-335.
USARIEM (U.S. Army Research Institute of Environmental Medicine)
1990   Sustaining Health and Performance in the Desert: A Pocket Guide to Environmental Medicine for Operations in Southwest Asia. Technical Note 91-2. U.S. Army Research Institute of Environmental Medicine, Natick, Mass.
Van Rij, A.M., M.T. Hall, G.L. Dohm, J. Bray, and W.J. Pories
1986   Changes in zinc metabolism following exercise in human subjects. Biol. Trace Element Res. 10:99-106.
Weiner, J.S., J.O.C. Willson, H. El-Neil, and E.F. Wheeler
1972   The effect of work level and dietary intake on sweat nitrogen losses in a hot climate. Br. J. Nutri. 27(3):543-52.
Weinman, K.P., Z. Slabochova, E.M. Bernauer, T. Morimoto, and F. Sargent II
1967   Reactions of men and women to repeated exposure to humid heat. J. Appl. Physiol. 22:533-538.
Welch, B.E., E.R. Buskirk, and P.F. Iampietro
1958   Relation of climate and temperature to food and water intake in man. Metabol. 7(2):141-148.
Wenger, C.B.
1988   Human heat acclimatization. Pp. 153-197 in Human Performance Physiology and Environmental Medicine at Terrestrial Extremes, K.B. Pandolf, M.N. Sawka, and R.R. Gonzalez, eds. Indianapolis, Ind.: Benchmark Press.
Wheeler, E.F., H. El-Neil, J.O. Willson, and J.S. Weiner
1973   The effect of work level and dietary intake on water balance and the excretion of sodium, potassium and iron in a hot climate. Br. J. Nutri. 30(1):127-137.
Williams, C.G., G.A.G. Bredell, C.H. Wyndham, N.B. Strydom, J.F. Morrison, J. Peter, P.W. Fleming, and J.S. Ward
1962   Circulatory and metabolic reactions to work in heat. J. Appl. Physiol. 17:625-638.
Williams, M.H.
1989   Vitamin supplementation and athletic performance, an overview. Int. J. Vitam. Nutr. Res. 30:161-191.

Wyndham, C.H.
1977   Heatstroke and hyperthermia in marathon runners. Pp. 129-138 in The Marathon: Physiological, Medical, Epidemiological and Psychological Studies, P. Milvy, ed. New York, N.Y.: New York Academy of Science.

Wyndham, C.H., J.F. Morrison, and C.G. Williams
1965   Heat reactions of male and female Caucasians. J. Appl. Physiol. 20:357-364.

Wyndham, C.H., A.J.A. Benade, C.G. Williams, N.B. Strydom, A. Golden, and A.J.A. Heynes
1968   Changes in central circulation and body fluid spaces during acclimatization to heat. J. Appl. Physiol. 25:586-593.

Wyndham, C.H., G.G. Rogers, L.C. Senay, and D. Mitchell
1976   Acclimatization in a hot, humid environment: Cardiovascular adjustments. J. Appl. Physiol. 40:779-785.

Yoshimura, H.
1970   Anemia during physical training (sports anemia). Nutr. Rev. 28:251-253.

Young, A.J.
1990   Energy substrate utilization during exercise in extreme environments. Pp. 65-117 in Exercise and Sport Sciences Reviews, vol. 18, K.B. Pandolf and J.O. Holloszy, eds. Baltimore, Md: Williams & Wilkins.

Young, A.J., M.N. Sawka, L. Levine, B.S. Cadarette, and K.B. Pandolf
1985   Skeletal muscle metabolism during exercise is influenced by heat acclimation. J. Appl. Physiol. 59:1929-1935.

Zellner, D.A., W.F. Stewart, P. Rozin, and J.M. Brown
1988   Effect of temperature and expectations on liking for beverages. Physiol. Behav. 44:61-68.

Ziegler, H.P., H.L. Green, and J. Siegel
1972   Food and water intake and weight regulation in the pigeon. Physiol. Behav. 8:127-134.

Zifferblatt, S.M., C.S. Wilbur, and J.L. Pinsky
1980   Influence of ecologic events on cafeteria food selections: Understanding food habits. J. Am. Diet. Assoc. 76:9-14.

C

Biographical Sketches

COMMITTEE ON MILITARY NUTRITION RESEARCH

RICHARD L. ATKINSON Since 1986, he has been Professor of Internal Medicine at Eastern Virginia Medical School and Associate Chief of Staff for Research and Development at the Department of Veterans Affairs Medical Center in Hampton, Virginia. He received an M.D. degree from the Medical College of Virginia. His research interests are in nutrition, particularly in obesity and the regulation of body weight and energy balance.

WILLIAM R. BEISEL In 1985, he joined the Department of Immunology and Infectious Diseases at The Johns Hopkins School of Hygiene and Public Health, teaching courses as a part-time Adjunct Professor. This followed retirement after 43 years as an Army Physician (Internist) and Senior Executive civilian. While with the Army, he did comprehensive basic and clinical research studies to define the complex of metabolic, endocrine, physiologic, and nutritional responses to infection, and their interrelationships with the immune system.

VALERIE McC. BREEN *(FNB Staff, Project Assistant)* is currently Project Assistant for the Committee on Military Nutrition Research, Food and Nutrition Board, Institute of Medicine, Washington, D.C. She has a bachelor of science degree in biological and physical sciences from Indiana University. Before coming to the Institute of Medicine she was on a three year diplomatic assignment in Paris, France.

JOHANNA T. DWYER (*Food and Nutrition Board, Liaison*) is Professor of Medicine and Community Health at Tufts University School of Medicine and also at the Tufts School of Nutrition. She is also Senior Scientist at the U. S. Department of Agriculture (USDA) Human Nutrition Research Center on Aging at Tufts. She holds the D.Sc. from the Harvard School of Public Health. Research interests include energy balance, dietary aspects of disease, and special physiological stresses and diet.

JOEL GRINKER is currently a Professor in the Human Nutrition Program, School of Public Health, a Professor in Pediatrics at the Medical School, and a member of the Center for Human Growth and Development at the University of Michigan. She received a Ph.D. in experimental social psychology from New York University and was the recipient of a Russell Sage Foundation Fellowship at the Rockefeller University in biochemistry, biology, and behavior. After 15 years at Rockefeller University in the laboratory of Human Behavior and Metabolism, she moved to the University of Michigan to become Chair of the Program in Human Nutrition. Major areas of interest are in obesity, specifically the development and maintenance of obesity through the life span.

EDWARD S. HORTON is Professor and Chairman of the Department of Medicine at the University of Vermont College of Medicine, Burlington, Vermont. He is a graduate of Harvard Medical School and received his training in internal medicine, and endocrinology and metabolism, at Duke University. Since 1967, he has been at the University of Vermont where his major research has involved studies of the regulation of energy expenditure in humans, the interrelationships between obesity and diabetes mellitus, and the mechanisms of insulin resistance in skeletal muscle and adipose tissue. He is particularly interested in the effects of exercise and physical conditioning on insulin sensitivity, and the regulation of glucose transport and metabolism in skeletal muscle. He is immediate Past President of the American Diabetes Association and a Past President of the American Society for Clinical Nutrition.

G. RICHARD JANSEN is Emeritus Professor of Nutritional Science and formerly Head of the Department of Food Science and Human Nutrition at Colorado State University. His Ph.D. in biochemistry was from Cornell University. His research interests deal primarily with protein nutrition, and he has co-authored a book on diet and health issues. Prior to his appointment at Colorado State, he was a research fellow at the Merck Institute. He served in the United States Air Force from 1950 to 1953.

GILBERT A. LEVEILLE is Vice President of Research and Technical Services for Nabisco Brands, Inc. Prior to joining Nabisco in 1986 he was Director of Nutrition and Health for General Foods, and from 1971 to 1980 was Professor and Chairman of the Department of Food Science and Human Nutrition at Michigan State University. He holds a Ph.D. in nutrition and biochemistry from Rutgers University. His areas of research interest include carbohydrate and lipid metabolism, obesity and metabolic adaptations to diet.

BERNADETTE M. MARRIOTT (*FNB Staff, Program Director*) is Program Director for the Committee on Military Nutrition Research, Food and Nutrition Board, Institute of Medicine. She has a Ph.D. degree in psychology from the University of Aberdeen, Scotland, and a B.Sc. degree in biochemistry/immunology and postdoctoral laboratory experience in trace mineral nutrition. Prior to joining the Institute of Medicine staff, she held university and medical school faculty positions at Johns Hopkins University, the University of Puerto Rico, and Goucher College. Her areas of research interest include bioenergetic modeling and social influences of food selection in human and nonhuman primates.

JOHN A. MILNER Since 1989 he has been Professor and Head of the Nutrition Department at The Pennsylvania State University. He has a Ph.D. degree in nutrition from Cornell University. He has a broad background in both fundamental and applied nutrition. His own research deals with the role of the diet as a modifier of cancer risk.

ROBERT O. NESHEIM (*Committee Chairman*) He retired as Vice President, Science and Technology, for the Quaker Oats Company, Chicago, Illinois, in 1983, and in 1991, as President of Advanced Healthcare, Inc., Monterey, California. He earned a Ph.D. degree in nutrition from the University of Illinois and has had extensive experience in research management. He has been involved in food and nutrition issues for many years, serving on many national committees, including the Food and Nutrition Board and the Food Advisory Committee, Office of Technology Assessment, U.S. Congress. He is a Fellow of the American Institute of Nutrition.

JAMES G. PENLAND is a Research Psychologist at the USDA Agriculture Research Service, Grand Forks Human Nutrition Research Center and Adjunct Professor of Psychology at the University of North Dakota, where he received a Ph.D. in experimental cognitive psychology in 1984. For the past six years, his research has focused on the effects of trace element nutrition on neurophysiologic, cognitive, and emotional function relevant to performance demands placed on adults in our society. Recent research has addressed dietary involvement in brain electrophysiology during sleep and waking, attention and memory performance, mood states, sensory function, and menstrual and menopausal distress. His research program includes both human and animal studies.

JOHN E. VANDERVEEN Since 1975, he has been the Director, Division of Nutrition at the Food and Drug Administration. He is responsible for planning, developing, and implementing programs that provide scientific knowledge required to carry out the Food, Drug, and Cosmetic Act with respect to the field of nutrition. His duties also include providing scientific counsel in the formation of regulations and regulatory programs in the broad field of nutrition and food labeling, as well as providing nutritional review of petitions submitted for regulatory actions, exemptions and/or food additive approvals. He earned a Ph.D. degree in chemistry from the University of New Hampshire.

ALLISON A. YATES is Dean of the College of Health and Human Sciences at the University of Southern Mississippi and associate professor of foods and nutrition. She has a Ph.D. degree in nutrition from the University of California at Berkeley, and an M.S. in public health from UCLA, and is a registered dietitian. She currently serves as Project Director for the Division of Applied Research of the National Food Service Management Institute. Her areas of expertise are in food habits, diet composition, and protein and energy interrelationships.

AUTHORS

LAWRENCE E. ARMSTRONG is Assistant Professor of Exercise Sciences at the Human Performance Laboratory of The University of Connecticut, with a joint appointment in the Department of Physiology and Neurobiology. From 1983 to 1990 he conducted human research at the U.S. Army Research Institute of Environmental Medicine, Heat Research Division, Natick, Massachusetts. He is a Fellow of the American College of Sports Medicine and a member of the American Physiological Society and the Aerospace Medical Association. He serves as an Editorial Board member and/or reviewer for five scientific journals, including the *International Journal of Sport Nutrition* and *Aviation, Space, and Environmental Medicine*. He is the Past President of the New England Chapter of the American College of Sports Medicine.

ELDON W. ASKEW is Chief of the Military Nutrition Division at the U.S. Army Research Institute of Environmental Medicine in Natick, Massachusetts. Colonel Askew received his doctoral degree in nutrition sciences and biochemistry from the Michigan State University, and has served in many key positions in the U.S. Army Medical Research and Development Command. His areas of specialization include biochemical adaptation to exercise training, the role of nutrition in exercise, and nutrition in environmental extremes.

ELSWORTH R. BUSKIRK is Professor of Applied Physiology Emeritus at the Pennsylvania State University. He received his Ph.D. in physiological hygiene from the University of Minnesota in 1954 and spent the next three years at the Environmental Research Laboratories, Natick, Massachusetts. He subsequently moved to the National Institute of Arthritis and Metabolic Diseases at the National Institutes of Health where he worked on metabolic problems, primarily obesity. In 1963 he organized the Laboratory for Human Performance Research at Penn State, became its first director, and was instrumental in establishing a graduate program in physiology that continues. In 1988 he was granted an endowed professorship at Penn State as the Mrs. Robert A. Noll Professor of Human Performance. He is a past president of the American College of Sports Medicine and has served two terms as editor of its professional journal. He has also been active in the affairs of the American Physiological Society having served on several of its committees and as an associate editor for the *Journal of Applied Physiology*. He remains active with the American Heart Association as a member of its Research Committee.

PRISCILLA M. CLARKSON is a Professor of Exercise Science at the University of Massachusetts at Amherst. She is a member of the Exercise Countermeasures Group at Johnson Space Center, National Aeronautics and Space Administration, a member of the Gatorade Sports Science Institute, and an inducted member of the American Academy of Physical Education. Her research interests include muscle soreness and exercise-induced muscle damage, sports nutrition, especially with regard to vitamin and mineral requirements, and dance medicine.

WILLIAM C. CURTIS, JR. is a Research Medical Officer in the Thermal Physiology and Medicine Division of the U.S. Army Research Institute of Environmental Medicine. With an M.D. degree from Howard University, he completed both residency training and served as physician-in-charge of the Hypertension Clinic at Cook County Hospital. His areas of specialty include anti-hypertension drugs, heat tolerance of former heat injured patients, and test volunteer safety and performance.

RALPH P. FRANCESCONI is a Supervisory Research Chemist and Chief of the Comparative Physiology Division at the U.S. Army Research Institute of Environmental Medicine in Natick, Massachusetts. In this capacity much of his research effort has been focused on endocrinological responses of humans during and subsequent to acute or recurrent exercise in hot environments, and he has written extensively on this subject.

CARL V. GISOLFI is Professor of Exercise Science and Physiology and Biophysics at the University of Iowa. He earned his Ph.D. degree in anatomy and physiology at Indiana University. He is a past president of the American

College of Sports Medicine. His research interests include (a) the role of gastrointestinal function in fluid and electrolyte homeostasis during rest and exercise, (b) mechanisms of circulatory insufficiency during heat stroke, and (c) molecular mechanisms of thermotolerance and heat-acclimatization.

BARRY G. GREEN is a Member of the Monell Chemical Senses Center where he heads the program in Sensory Irritation. An experimental psychologist with an expertise in physchophysical measurement, he has researched a wide variety of topics in the areas of human somatosensation and the chemical senses since 1975. His current work focuses on the chemical sensitivity of the skin and its relationship to the senses of taste, olfaction, temperature, and pain.

C. PETER HERMAN is Professor of Psychology at the University of Toronto, Canada. He received his Ph.D. in psychology from Columbia University, taught at Northwestern University, and has been at the University of Toronto since 1976. His research specialty is behavioral aspects of eating and dieting in humans.

EDWARD S. HIRSCH is Research Psychologist at the U.S. Army Natick Research, Development and Engineering Center. He received a Ph.D. in physiological and comparative psychology from Rutgers University. His interest in environmental influences on human feeding behavior stems from his earlier work on ecological influences on energy intake and patterns of ingestion in non-human animals.

ROGER W. HUBBARD is a Supervisory Biological Scientist and Director of the Environmental Pathophysiology Directorate at the U.S. Army Research Institute of Environmental Medicine in Natick, Massachusetts. He has pioneered the use of the laboratory rat as an appropriate model for human heatstroke and has also proposed the energy depletion model of heat injury. He has authored or co-authored multiple signal works on the mechanisms and etiology of heat injury.

RICHARD F. JOHNSON is Research Psychologist in the Military Performance and Neuroscience Division at the U.S. Army Research Institute of Environmental Medicine (USARIEM), Natick, Massachusetts. He received his Ph.D. in psychology (1970) from Brandeis University, where he was both a National Aeronautics and Space Administration Trainee and a Woodrow Wilson Dissertation Fellow. Prior to joining USARIEM in 1984, he served as a captain in the U.S. Army Medical Service Corps (1970-1972), was a National Institute of Mental Health grantee (1972-1976), and was a research psychologist with the U.S. Army Natick Research and Development Laboratories (1976-1983). He is senior lecturer in psychology at Northeastern University and is the author of numerous publications in areas of psychophysiology, experimental research methodology, hypnosis, and stress. He is a fellow of both the American Psychological Association and the American Psychological Society, and is Past President of the Natick Chapter of Sigma Xi, The Scientific Research Society. He is currently studying the effects of environmental extremes (cold, heat, humidity) and protective systems (protective clothing, treatment drugs, training) on vigilance and psychomotor behavior.

CARL L. KEEN is a Professor of Nutrition and Internal Medicine at the University of California at Davis. He earned his doctoral degree in Nutrition with a specialty in physiological biochemistry at the University of California at Davis. His research interests include the study of the influence of maternal diet on embryonic and fetal development, and the functional consequences of stress and disease-induced changes in mineral metabolism.

F. MATTHEW KRAMER is currently a Research Psychologist at the U.S. Army Natick Research, Development, and Engineering Center. He received a Ph.D. in counseling psychology from the Pennsylvania State University, and completed postdoctoral work at the University of Minnesota and the University of Pennsylvania. Dr. Kramer's interests focus on understanding human food habits, that is, the factors underlying food selection, intake, and acceptability.

NATALIE M. LEVA is a Biochemistry Technician in the Comparative Physiology Division of the U.S. Army Research Institute of Environmental Medicine in Natick, Massachusetts. She has a bachelor's degree in science from the University of Massachusetts, and specializes in the areas of radioimmunoassay and biological statistics.

WILLIAM T. MATTHEW has served as a Research Biologist with the U.S. Army Research Institute of Environmental Medicine since 1968 and is currently a member of the Biophysics and Biomedical Modeling Division. His primary area of interest is environmental stress assessment methodologies and their application to military training and operational settings.

DONNA J. MERULLO, nee McMenemy, is currently a Research Psychologist with GEO-CENTER, INC. assigned to the U.S. Army Research Institute of Environmental Medicine (USARIEM). She received a B.S. degree from Tufts University in 1983 and began working as a research assistant for the Boston University Center for Technology and Policy. In 1985, she joined the USARIEM Health and Performance Division as a research psychologist. She has been a representative to the Office for Military Performance Assessment Technology and is a member of Sigma Xi, The Scientific Research Society. She has participated in numerous research studies investigating the effects of extreme environments, nutrition, and medications on human performance.

ROBERT J. MOORE is currently a Research Biochemist with the U.S. Army Institute of Surgical Research at Ft. Sam Houston, Texas. Captain Moore received the Ph.D. from the Virginia Polytechnic Institute, and was commissioned in the Medical Service Corps in 1988. His areas of specialization include carbohydrate nutrition and its role in load-bearing and endurance, nutrient requirements while working in the heat, and energy expenditure.

KENT B. PANDOLF is the Director of the Environmental Physiology and Medicine Directorate at the U.S. Army Research Institute of Environmental Medicine, and holds the rank of Adjunct Professor of Health Sciences at Boston University and Adjunct Clinical Professor of Sports Biology at Springfield College. He received his Ph.D. and M.P.H. from the University of Pittsburgh in environmental/exercise physiology. His current research interests involve the physiological evaluation of human performance during environmental and/or exercise stress.

MICHAEL N. SAWKA currently holds the positions of Chief, Thermal Physiology and Medicine Division at the U.S. Army Research Institute of Environmental Medicine, and Associate Professor at Massachusetts General Hospital. He received B.S. (1973) and M.S. (1974) degrees from East Stroudsburg University and his Ph.D. (1977) degree from Southern Illinois University. Dr. Sawka's research interests are in the areas of environmental and exercise physiology as well as rehabilitation medicine.

PATRICIA C. SZLYK is a Research Physiologist in the Comparative Physiology Division at the U.S. Army Research Institute of Environmental Medicine in Natick, Massachusetts. With a doctoral degree in cardiovascular/respiratory physiology from the State University of New York, Buffalo, she has published extensively in multidisciplinary journals on the effects of environmental stress on performance/thermal physiology.

C. BRUCE WENGER has been a Research Pharmacologist at the U.S. Army Research Institute of Environmental Medicine in Natick, Massachusetts since 1984. He received his M.D. and Ph.D. degrees from Yale University. His research interests include human circulatory responses to thermal stress, and the epidemiology and pathophysiology of heat illness.

ANDREW J. YOUNG is a Research Physiologist and Leader of the Cold Physiology Working Group in the Thermal Physiology and Medicine Division of the U.S. Army Research Institute of Environmental Medicine, Natick, Massachusetts. He attended the Virginia Military Institute where he received a B.S. in biology in 1974, and the North Carolina State University where he received a Ph.D. in physiology in 1977. Dr. Young's major research interest concerns the physiological basis of adaptations in human performance during acclimatization to environmental extremes of high altitude, heat, and cold. He is a Fellow of the American College of Sports Medicine, and a member of the Scientific Research Society of North American and the American Physiological Society. In addition to serving as a reviewer for such journals as *Arctic, Aviation, Space and Environmental Medicine*, and *The Journal of Applied Physiology*, Dr. Young is on the Editorial Board of *Medicine and Science in Sports and Exercise*.

Index

A

Acclimatization/acclimation
    age and, 14, 15
    air-conditioning and, 196, 199–200
    and aldosterone levels, 268, 274
    and appetite, 19–20, 107, 109, 200–201
    B complex vitamin supplementation and, 148–149
    body weight and, 107–108, 195
    defined, 7, 108
    dietary requirements following, 107–108
    and energy requirements, 19, 29–30, 45, 109
    and exercise, 62–63, 262
    and food intake, 28, 29–30, 48, 185
    and gastrointestinal functioning, 81
    and gender differences in response to heat stress, 13–14
    glycogen sparing effect, 65
    heat illness symptoms during, 288–290
    and lactate levels, 65, 66
    and metabolic rate, 11, 59, 61, 63, 104–105, 108

NaCl balance during, 247–255, 259–260, 268–269
    and nitrogen loss from sweating, 206
    and oxygen uptake, 59, 62, 105, 108
    physique and, 194–195
    and plasma renin activity, 268, 269, 274
    and plasma volume, 274
    and sodium/NaCl intakes, 17–18, 248, 262, 270, 277
    and sweat rates, 16, 90, 91, 92, 93, 95, 96
    and thermoregulation, 7, 16, 55, 70, 92
    vitamin C and, 48–49, 148–149, 152, 159, 160, 169
    see also Temperature (environmental)
Acute-phase response, 122, 123, 125, 126–127
Adiposity, and sweating response, 96
Adrenocorticotropic hormone synthesis, 150
Aero Medical Laboratory, 97
Aerobic fitness
    age and, 14
    nitrogen losses and, 111

363